Lethal but Legal

Lethal but Legal

CORPORATIONS, CONSUMPTION,
AND PROTECTING
PUBLIC HEALTH

NICHOLAS FREUDENBERG

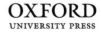
OXFORD
UNIVERSITY PRESS

OXFORD
UNIVERSITY PRESS

Oxford University Press is a department of the University of Oxford.
It furthers the University's objective of excellence in research, scholarship,
and education by publishing worldwide.

Oxford   New York
Auckland   Cape Town   Dar es Salaam   Hong Kong   Karachi
Kuala Lumpur   Madrid   Melbourne   Mexico City   Nairobi
New Delhi   Shanghai   Taipei   Toronto

With offices in
Argentina   Austria   Brazil   Chile   Czech Republic   France   Greece
Guatemala   Hungary   Italy   Japan   Poland   Portugal   Singapore
South Korea   Switzerland   Thailand   Turkey   Ukraine   Vietnam

Oxford is a registered trademark of Oxford University Press
in the UK and certain other countries.

Published in the United States of America by
Oxford University Press
198 Madison Avenue, New York, NY 10016

Library of Congress Cataloging-in-Publication Data
Freudenberg, Nicholas, author.
Lethal but legal : corporations, consumption, and protecting public health / Nicholas Freudenberg.
    p. ; cm.
Includes bibliographical references and index.
ISBN 978–0–19–993719–6 (hardback); 978–0–19–049537–4 (pbk.)
I. Title.
[DNLM: 1. Public Health.   2. World Health.   3. Chronic Disease—epidemiology.
4. Industry.   5. Internationality.   6. Socioeconomic Factors. WA 530.1]
RA441
362.1—dc23
2013023752

9 8 7 6 5 4 3 2 1
Printed in the United States of America
on acid-free paper

Contents

Preface

Never before in human history has the gap between the scientific and economic potential for better health for all and the reality of avoidable premature death been greater. In the past, babies died in infancy, women in childbirth, workers from injuries or occupational diseases, and people of all ages from epidemics of infectious disease exacerbated by inadequate nutrition, contaminated water, and poor sanitation. For the most part, the world lacked the resources and the understanding to eliminate these problems. As societies developed; as science, technology, and medicine advanced; and as people organized to improve their standards of living, more and more of the world's population attained the living conditions that support better health and longer lives.

Today, the world still confronts the global health challenges of the last century. Epidemics of malaria, HIV infection, tuberculosis, and other communicable diseases still threaten well-being and economic development in many poor countries. More than a billion people live in urban slums where the average lifespan can be 35 years, half of that in better-off places where residents have certain access to adequate nutrition, clean water, and sanitation.

Now new threats have emerged. Deaths from chronic conditions like heart disease, cancer, diabetes, and stroke have surged, today accounting for more than 60 percent of the world's deaths. Injuries have become the leading cause of death for young people around the world. Everywhere, from the wealthiest nations like the United States to the poorest countries in Africa, Asia, and Latin America, the proportion of deaths from these causes of death are growing. These premature deaths and preventable illnesses and injuries impose new suffering on individuals, families, and communities. They burden economies and taxpayers and jeopardize the improvements in health brought about by the public health advances of the previous two centuries.

Alarmingly, these new epidemics are not the result of the poverty and squalid living conditions that caused illness and death in the past, even though chronic disease and injuries afflict the poor much more than the rich. Nor are they the result of ignorance and inadequate science. For the most part, we understand the causes of these illnesses and injuries enough to prevent them. What we lack is the political will to implement the needed preventive measures. Even worse, in some cases the growing health burden is the *result* of new science and technology, which have been used to promote profit rather than prevent illness. These new epidemics of chronic diseases and injuries are instead the *consequence* of what most people thought were the remedies for poverty-related ill health: economic growth, better standards of living, and more comfortable lifestyles.

While many factors contributed to this global health transformation, *Lethal but Legal* focuses on what I consider to be most important and most easily modifiable cause: the triumph of a political and economic system that promotes consumption at the expense of human health. In this book, I describe how this system has enabled industries like alcohol, automobiles, firearms, food and beverages, pharmaceuticals, and tobacco—pillars of the global consumer economy—to develop products and practices that have become the dominant cause of premature death and preventable illness and injuries. This system was born in the United States and has now spread around the world.

In a global economy that focuses relentlessly on profit, enhancing the bottom line of a few hundred corporations and the income of their investors has become more important than realizing the potential for good health that the world's growing wealth and the advances in science, technology, and medicine have enabled. This tension between private accumulation and public well-being is not new. But in the twenty-first century, it has come to shape our economy and politics in ways that profoundly threaten democracy, human well-being, and the environment that supports life. Paradoxically, the increasing concentration of power in the small number of the world's multinational corporations also presents new opportunities to create another healthier and more just future.

In *Lethal but Legal*, I argue that, for the United Sates and the world to achieve their articulated goals of better health for all and a more equal distribution of advances in health, we will need to redesign the system that has evolved to promote consumption at the expense of well-being. Succeeding in this task will require taking on the world's most powerful corporations and their allies. Only the naïve or foolish would underestimate the enormity of this challenge. But neither nature, human evolution, nor fate created the new burdens of chronic diseases and injuries. Rather, it was human decisions, made in corporate boardrooms, advertising and lobbying firms, and legislative and judicial chambers.

In the last few decades, the directors of a few hundred corporations have changed the world to suit their needs, and as a result set the stage for the twenty-first–century epidemics. Surely the world's people, supported by social movements, honest governments, health professionals, and scientists can take back our health, as we have done so many times before when special interests challenged human well-being.

Three paths led me to write this book. First, as a public health practitioner, I have worked for three decades with community and advocacy organizations, churches, government agencies, and other researchers to develop, implement, and evaluate programs and policies to improve the health of low-income populations. In these efforts, this work has frequently come into conflict with special interests. Paint companies and landlords opposed efforts to eliminate childhood lead poisoning because it jeopardized profits. Pharmaceutical companies charged so much for the drugs that could have kept HIV infection or diabetes under control that the people who needed these medicines could not afford them. Fast food and soda companies promoted their high fat, sugar, and calorie products to children who were becoming obese and overweight and therefore at high risk of diabetes and other diet-related diseases. When the groups I worked with suggested policies or programs to limit these harmful practices, corporations used their political clout to thwart these proposed remedies.

In this work, the corporate role in promoting disease was not our main focus, but repeatedly we were stymied when we tried to make prevention the priority. I wanted to understand how one small sector of society had accumulated the power to block health progress. I wanted to devise useful strategies that my frustrated students and colleagues could use to overcome this resistance they encountered.

The second path to this book was my work as a public health researcher and teacher. My research has focused on understanding how social forces influence health and inequalities in health. My teaching seeks to prepare public health professionals and researchers to take action to reduce the forces that damage health. Like many other researchers, I have come to appreciate the profound influence of what have been called the *social determinants* of health: the day-to-day conditions in which ordinary people live, the political processes that govern society, and the stratifications of wealth and power that characterize today's world.

But I have also been frustrated by the lack of impact of this new research on social determinants of health. Too often, researchers *describe* the causes of ill health without illuminating solutions. Too often the solutions they propose—ending the stratification systems—seem pie-in-the-sky, however worthy this goal may be. For me, analyzing the specific pathways by which the business and political decisions that corporations make improve or harm health promises new insights on a key social determinant of health. These insights can then guide policies to improve health and find a better balance between private profit and public well-being.

The third path is my experiences as an activist. I came of age politically in the antiwar and student movements of the 1960s. Over the years, I have had the privilege of participating in or writing about these and other movements: the environmental justice, labor, and women's movements of the 1970s and 1980s; the HIV and health care reform movements of the 1980s and 1990s; and most recently, the food justice movement. In these encounters, I have been fascinated to observe how communities mobilize to confront the threats they perceive and how movements learn from each other—or fail to do so. Too often the health campaigns against the tobacco, food, and alcohol corporations that market unhealthy products or the "Big Pharma" efforts to promote diseases only they can cure seem isolated, missing the opportunity to find new allies and win bigger victories. In the book, I hope to discover common ground across the disparate arenas where people are organizing to change harmful corporate practices.

The aftermath of the 2008 financial crisis further stimulated my activist juices. The evidence suggests that banks and other financial institutions engaged in risky practices that led our economy to the brink of meltdown. But when the public demanded stronger oversight of the financial sector and prosecution of those who had thrown so many people out of their homes, jobs, and communities, "Big Business" blamed the problems on the government and on the foolish consumers these lenders had targeted. If one sector of Big Business could evade any responsibility for the most serious financial crisis since the Great Depression, surely the consumer sector would try the same strategy to avoid taking action to reduce the slow-motion crisis of chronic diseases and injuries that their products and practices are causing. This book is my effort to prevent such a future.

Some public health researchers are uncomfortable traveling on both the research and advocacy roads. To me they are two paths to the same destination: more just and healthy societies. My friend Dr. Jeremiah Stamler, a founder of modern cardiovascular epidemiology and a veteran of many battles with the food and pharmaceutical industries, once told me, "If a researcher isn't willing to follow his data into the policy arena, who will?" In looking to combine the roles of researcher and activist, I am inspired by the founders of public health— people such as Rudolf Virchow, Louis Villerme, Edwin Chadwick, and Alice Hamilton—who demonstrated that it is possible to both study and act in the political arena to change the conditions that make people sick.

When I speak in public about the impact of corporations on health, people sometimes ask if I am against corporations. This seems like asking if one is against families, religion, or government. People created these institutions over the course of human history to solve particular problems. Of course corporations have made important contributions to creating a better world, and of course they are here to stay in one form or another for the foreseeable future.

But the question today is whether our political and economic arrangements maximize the benefits that corporations bring to humanity and minimize the harms. It does seem to me that many of society's most serious problems— income inequality, compromised democracy, environmental deterioration, and accelerating climate change—are related to the current dominance of corporations. My goal in *Lethal but Legal* is to explore how corporations contribute to our society's most important health problems and what we can do to reduce this burden of premature death and preventable illness. If our efforts to reduce corporate-induced health problems also contribute to reducing other harms that corporations cause, so much the better.

Another question I am asked is why I have chosen to focus on only (!) six industries. I have chosen to limit *Lethal but Legal* to the alcohol, automobile, firearms, food and beverage, pharmaceutical, and tobacco industries for a few reasons. These six are central to the global consumer economy, the largest portion of the world's economy today and in the future. They have a profound influence on health behavior, lifestyle, and the physical environment. As a result, their products and practices are associated with a significant proportion of the global burden of disease, as I explain in Chapter 2. Finally, researchers have extensively documented their impact on health, and health authorities and social movements have taken action to reduce the threats these industries pose, providing a body of evidence to inform action. Friends and colleagues often urge me to add more industries to my portfolio of interest: energy, entertainment, tourism, gaming, health care, and petrochemicals, to name a few. I encourage other researchers to investigate these other important influences on health but believe my already broad focus gives me more than enough to cover in this book.

For readers who want a roadmap, let me briefly summarize the journey this book covers. In Chapter 1, I describe the practices of three industries that have since World War II had a profound impact on heath in the United States. The fast food, soda, and snacks sectors of the food industry produce the products most associated with the rise in obesity and diet-related health problems like diabetes. As a result of successes in controlling its practices in the United States, the tobacco industry has moved its lethal marketing campaigns to countries like Russia, Mexico, and Indonesia. The alcohol industry has developed and marketed products to win over new populations: teens and young adults, women, and blacks and Latinos. As a result, these groups are now seeing some of the alcohol-related health problems previously concentrated among white men. I use these three stories to illustrate the rise of what I call the *corporate consumption complex,* a network of corporations, financial institutions, banks, trade associations, advertising, lobbying and legal firms, and others that promote what I call "hyperconsumption," a pattern of consuming that is directly linked to premature mortality and preventable illness or injury. Like the military-industrial complex that jeopardized American values during the Cold War, today the corporate consumption complex threatens public health, democracy, and sustainable economic development.

Chapter 2 examines the state of global health today and charts the rise of chronic condition diseases (called non-communicable diseases in most parts of the world) and injuries here in the United States and in emerging nations like Brazil, India, and China. I analyze the theories that have been proposed to explain these increases, including population aging, the conquest of infectious diseases, and changes in lifestyles related to health. I describe three more industries that contribute to injuries and chronic conditions: the, automobile, firearms and pharmaceutical industries, and summarize the growing evidence that the business and political practices of these and the three industries described in Chapter 1 have become the major modifiable causes of today's top killers. I also compare changing harmful corporate practices as a solution to two other intervention strategies often proposed by policymakers and researchers: applying biomedical advances to the prevention and treatment of chronic diseases and modifying the unhealthy lifestyles of individuals who smoke, eat, or drink too much or act in other ways that hurt their health.

How did this political and economic system that promotes consumption arise? How is it different from earlier stages of free market economies? In Chapter 3, I seek to answer these questions by telling the story of changes in corporate power and practices since 1970. While the consumer economy started much earlier, I make the case that domestic and global threats to the power of U.S. corporations in that period were the precipitating cause of the transformation that has led to today's health problems. I also examine how the 2008 global economic crisis both threatened and strengthened the corporate consumption complex.

In Chapter 4, I dissect the corporate consumption complex today, profiling a few key players and describing its anatomy and the particular ways it uses its power to achieve its goals. I examine two prototypical members of the complex, the McDonald's Corporation and the Pharmaceutical Research and Manufacturers Association, showing the webs that bind the corporate consumption complex together. Today, even if its members do not always agree on everything, the complex has become the dominant voice on public policy and public health in the world.

The corporate consumption complex uses its political clout when it needs to, but much of its impact is due to its success in promulgating and broadcasting an ideology that supports its values and justifies its actions, even when they have been shown to cause millions of preventable deaths. In Chapter 5, I describe key elements of that ideology and the mechanisms that corporations and their allies use to advance that ideology. Using public opinion polling data, I also examine to what extent people here in the United States and elsewhere accept or challenge the tenets of this ideology.

The corporate consumption complex hatched in the United States but is now a global force. In Chapter 6, I describe how corporations have set the rules for international trade and how they use organizations like the World Trade Organization, the North American Free Trade Agreement and other trade groups to advance their business goals, often at the expense of public health. By examining some key current conflicts—on global tobacco control, setting public health standards for food advertising to children, and deciding when health considerations can trump corporate patent protections, I illuminate the global issues that divide public health advocates and corporate leaders.

In the last two chapters of *Lethal but Legal,* I ask how we can reverse the accelerating epidemics of chronic conditions and injuries. What have we learned from the myriad of efforts to change harmful corporate practices? What are the elements of a political, policy, and scientific agenda that will enable the world to realize its vast potential for reducing human suffering and inequalities in health?

Chapter 7 provides an overview and analysis of several strategies that have been used to reduce corporate practices that harm health. I describe six efforts—one from each of the six industries—to change harmful corporate practices, describing the strategies the organizations and movements used, their accomplishments and limitations, and the lessons they learned. While these disparate strands of activity have different goals and operate in different settings, they share a commitment to protecting public health by taking on special interests that profit at the expense of health, and using flexible and creative strategies to realize their health objectives. I analyze the barriers to a unified movement to modify health-damaging corporate practices and suggest the pathways by which we can weave these strands into a transformative force for improving health in the United States and around the world.

Finally, in Chapter 8, I describe how we can restore the balance between corporations and government; between profit and public health. I suggest actions that can challenge the current dominance of the corporate consumption complex and examine alternative paths to prosperity and well-being. I propose several specific policy goals designed to bring together the diverse strands of the emerging challengers to the corporate consumption complex and to speed the process of changing harmful corporate practices.

In the current political climate, these proposals may seem idealistic, even naïve. But in a society committed to public health and democracy, they would be common sense. Public opinion polls show that the majority of Americans support these propositions and would choose policies that achieve these objectives. Recently, some researchers estimated that if current trends in obesity and diabetes continued, our children and grandchildren can expect to have shorter life spans than we do.[1] To escape the possibility of bequeathing our children a world where the public health gains of recent centuries have been reversed, we will need new ideas, new policies, new political will, and new action. Converting these ideas into the practical steps that can restore the balance between government and business constitutes the public health priority of our time.

Acknowledgments

Like raising a child, writing a book takes a village, and I am grateful to my many fellow villagers who generously gave their time, intelligence, and support. In late 2012, several colleagues working in related fields met to critique the book at Roosevelt House, Hunter College's public policy institute, in the history-infused former home of Franklin and Eleanor Roosevelt. The advice I received from Sue Atkinson, Cheryl Healton, Gerald Markowitz, John McDonough, Jennifer Pomeranz, Nancy Romer, David Rosner, and Richard Wilkinson helped make *Lethal but Legal* a much better book.

I have been fortunate to have Hunter College of the City University of New York as my academic home for more than 30 years. Its mission, its students, and its support for my work have made every day I have spent there a pleasure. I especially thank President Jennifer Raab, Provost Vita Rabinowitz, and Deans Ken Olden and Neal Cohen for their ongoing support and encouragement. My faculty colleagues at the City University of New York School of Public Health, and especially Susan Klitzman and Marilyn Auerbach, have created an academic environment where we can together strive to create the twenty-first–century public health practice and research that will over time contribute to the goal of achieving health for all.

Over the past several years, many students have worked with me to gather and organize the evidence presented in this book, some as research assistants, and others as part of course work. I thank Marissa Anto, Sarah Bradley, Bill Cabin, Monica Gagnon, Alexandra Lewin, Kim Libman, Zoe Meleo-Erwin, Salwa Nassar, Estelle Raboni, Monica Serrano, and Erica Sullivan. Emily Franzosa played an especially important role in getting the book ready for production.

Other colleagues have inspired, challenged, and supported my work on corporations and health, some by reading and critiquing sections of the book, others as sources and sounding boards. For this, I thank Sandro Galea, Rene Jahiel, David Jernigan, Michele Simon, Jerry Stamler, David Vlahov, and Bill Wiist.

None of these individuals nor any institution with which I am affiliated bears responsibility for the opinions expressed in the book or for any errors of fact or judgement—those are mine alone.

Another neighborhood in my village of support has helped turn my ideas into an actual book. I am appreciative of the guidance from my book agent, Alice Martell, and my always enthusiastic and helpful editor at Oxford University Press, Chad Zimmerman.

On the home front, my partner Wendy Chavkin and our son Sasha read and commented on chapters, listened to my rants, and in general put up with my many years fixation on this project. Their indispensable support made my village whole.

Nicholas Freudenberg
New York
August 2013

Part One

DEFINING THE PROBLEM

1

Manufacturing Disease

Unhealthy Products Become Ubiquitous

Every day, corporate managers make decisions about what products to make and how and where to market them. These seemingly ordinary choices, the lifeblood of our market economy, shape our environment and lifestyles so pervasively that their influence is all but invisible. But, increasingly, what corporations decide also shapes our patterns of health and disease. Today, the decisions made by executives and managers in the food, tobacco, alcohol, pharmaceutical, firearms, automobile, and other industries have a far greater impact on public health than the decisions of health officials, hospital directors, and doctors. Moreover, evidence suggests that the impact of corporations on our health, lifestyle, economy, international trade, and political systems is growing.

Meanwhile, governments around the world have abdicated their responsibility for protecting public health by reducing their oversight of business, privatizing key services, weakening regulations, and making individuals more responsible for their health. In this chapter, I will explore how and why this happened by focusing on three industries whose products have each contributed to millions of premature deaths and preventable illnesses in the United States and around the world. These profiles show how the food and beverage, tobacco, and alcohol industries have used sophisticated marketing, lobbying and public relations, and product design to magnify the harm that their products cause.

The industry profiles also reveal an unexpected silver lining. According to the World Health Organization and independent scientists, the products of the food, tobacco, and alcohol industries have become primary causes of the rising global burden of chronic diseases, now the world's leading killers.[1,2,3] If recent changes in the business and political practices of a few dozen of the world's largest food, tobacco, and alcohol corporations have accelerated these epidemics, then changing these practices has the potential to reverse these increases.

Food and Beverage Corporations: Appropriating Science and Technology to Market Overconsumption

Food companies introduce more than 20,000 new products into the global marketplace each year, a twenty-fold increase from 1970.[4] U.S. supermarkets today stock an average 38,000 products, five times more than 20 years ago.[5,6] McDonald's has more than 800 products on its menu, from the signature Big Mac to Cinnamon Melts, a breakfast treat composed of 50 distinct ingredients.[7] The decisions that companies make about the products they develop and market create the cornucopia from which consumers choose what to eat.

To make these decisions, food companies have come to rely on new input from such disciplines as evolutionary biology, biochemistry, neuroscience, food technology, and engineering. In the past few decades, the food industry has used insights from the frontiers of today's science and technology to design, produce, and sell more kinds of food to more consumers. Concentration of the supermarket, fast food, and beverage sectors enabled fewer but bigger food companies to generate the profits needed to afford the best science and technology money could buy. In appropriating modern science to enhance profitability, the industry has directly contributed to the world's most serious health problems.

The use of science and technology in the development, marketing, and retailing of fast food, children's cereals, and sweetened beverages shows how food companies use new knowledge to increase consumption of products that are most closely linked to growing global epidemics of obesity, diabetes, and other diet-related diseases.

PRODUCT DESIGN: HYPERPALATABLE FOODS BRING PROFIT . . . AND OBESITY

"Hyperpalatable foods" have been defined as foods that provide eaters with greater physiological and psychological rewards than traditional foods.[8] They blend or layer fat, salt, and sugar, and include several flavorings and additives. A comparison of a few traditional and hyperpalatable foods in the table below (Table 1.1) shows that hyperpalatable foods are higher in the fats, sugars, and sodium (salt) associated with today's chronic diseases and have many more ingredients such as flavorings and additives.

In his 2009 book *The End of Overeating*, David Kessler, former Commissioner of the FDA and former Dean of the Yale School of Medicine, popularized the concept of "conditioned overeating" in which hyperpalatable foods designed by the food industry trigger "supernormal stimuli" via the release of the

Table 1.1 **A Comparison of Traditional and Hyperpalatable Foods**

Product	Portion Size	Type of Food	Calories	Sugar in grams	Fat in grams	Sodium in milligrams	Number of Ingredients
Apple	1 medium	Traditional	81	19	Trace	0	1
Chicken breast, roasted	3 ounces	Traditional	142	0	3	64	1
Lettuce	1 cup shredded	Traditional	7	0	Trace	5	1
Tomato	1 medium	Traditional	26	3	Trace	11	1
Tap water	8 ounces	Traditional	0	0	0	0	1
Coffee with milk and 1 teaspoon sugar	10 ounces	Traditional	80	13	1	70	3
Coca Cola	12 ounces	Hyperpalatable	140	65	0	75	7
McDonald's Big and Tasty Burger	1	Hyperpalatable	460	8	24	720	>40
Cinnamon toast crunch cereal	¾ cup (without milk)	Hyperpalatable	130	10	3	217	27
Starbucks Mocha Frappucino	Grande (16 ounces)	Hyperpalatable	400	60	15	230	13

Sources: Gebhardt S, Thomas RG. Nutritive Value of Foods. United States Department of Agriculture, Agricultural Research Service, Home and Garden Bulletin No. 72. Available at: http://www.ars.usda.gov/SP2UserFiles/Place/12354500/Data/hg72/hg72_2002.pdf. Revised October, 2002. Accessed August 8, 2012; and websites of Coca-Cola, McDonald's and Starbucks.

neurotransmitter dopamine that produces cravings. Over time, even images or the suggestion of such food products can elicit these powerful desires.[9] A food industry consultant told Kessler, "higher sugar, fat, and salt make you want to eat more." He explained that the food industry creates products to hit these "three points of the compass" in order to make their hedonic, hyperpalatable—and profitable—foods.[10]

The bakery chain Cinnabon, for example, created its signature cinnamon roll using cinnamon, brown sugar, cream cheese, high-fructose corn syrup, salt, soy oil, and 45 other ingredients[11] to create a tempting product with 880 calories, 36 grams of fat, 59 grams of sugar, 830 milligrams of sodium, and a smell that can draw customers into its 600 outlets in airports and malls.[12]

Why are hyperpalatable foods so enticing? Humans evolved in an environment of scarcity where hunger and famine were constant companions. Individuals who learned to stock up on fats, sugars, and salts when they were available were more likely to survive and reproduce than those who did not.[13] As a result, evolutionary biologists discovered, over the ages our brain circuits rewarded such binges. In the twenty-first century, the food industry has put sugar, fat, and salt within arm's reach of much of the world's population. So the hedonic impulses that once conferred survival benefits now encourage the overeating that puts people at risk of diet-related chronic diseases. Technologists now work in food industry laboratories to exploit this evolutionary lag to create products that promise continued profitability. As Harvard evolutionary biologist Daniel Lieberman put it, "The food industry has made a fortune because we retain Stone Age bodies that crave sugar but live in a Space Age world in which sugar is cheap and plentiful."[14]

Craving hyperpalatable food is different from traditional addictions to nicotine, alcohol, cocaine, or heroin in several ways. While no one needs cigarettes, beer, or crack to survive, all humans need food, including fat, sugar, and salt. And unlike traditional addictions, over-consumption of food is legitimized by culture, social convention, and aggressive advertising, rather than outlawed or punished.[15]

At the same time, a growing body of research shows that the neuroendocrine mechanisms underlying the formation of dietary habits are precisely the ones acted on by addictive drugs.[16] Laboratory rats overeating a sugar solution show changes in their brains and behaviors that are similar to those caused by addictive drugs.[17] Researchers have now integrated findings that used methods such as positron emission tomography (PET) imaging studies of dopamine's role in human drug addiction and longitudinal observations of the eating behaviors of overweight and obese individuals to show that increased body weight can increase behaviors that are common markers of addiction. Dopamine rewards the brain, thus signaling people to continue the behaviors that release it.[18] One characteristic of addiction is that it is experienced as wanting, not simply lik-ing, the addictive substance. A biopsychological research group in the United Kingdom has developed experimental methods to distinguish between explicit liking and implicit (covert) wanting.[19] Their studies found that individuals with a tendency towards binge eating reported "liking" most food types, but "want-ing" high-fat sweet foods. By hiring food and flavor chemists to design products that elicit this primal "wanting," food companies can bypass the rational pro-cesses that protect people from harming themselves.

New food-product development is a risky and expensive undertaking, with estimates that from one in six to one in twenty new products fail to make a profit.[20] So why do companies spend the money? As John Maynard Keynes observed, "The engine that drives enterprise is not thrift but profit."[21] More pro-saically, a text on new food-product development explains, "No one product has such a universal appeal that it satisfies the needs of all customers and consumers in all marketplaces. Only a battery of new products will suffice to satisfy emerg-ing market niches."[22]

Compared to other industries, the food sector has a relatively low rate of prof-itability. So new products that increase the likelihood of marketplace success are important, and products with the strongest evidence for customer appeal are most likely to win new investment. Food executives are always in quest of the blockbuster product, one that will sell itself, win over new customers, and return a generous profit.

Imagine a food company executive asked to make a choice between a new product that appeals to emerging concerns about health and the environment, or one that relies on intrinsic human cravings for sugar, fat, and salt devel-oped over the span of human evolution. The choices made by the executives at Hardee's, the corporation that operates the Hardee's and Carl Jr.'s fast-food chains, illustrate the lure of high profits. When its outlets began to lose market share of young men—a key demographic for fast food companies—the com-pany introduced its Monster Thickburgers ("audacity on a bun" according to its marketing), a jumbo-sized cheeseburger smothered in strips of steak with 1,420 calories and 107 grams of fat. Hardee's rapidly moved from lowest- to highest-ranked fast food restaurant among young male fast food customers, and its stock rose 7.7 percent over the next year.[23] Its chief executive, Andrew Puzder, told a reporter that the company's latest sandwich is "not a burger for tree-huggers. This is a burger for young hungry guys who want a really big, deli-cious, juicy, decadent burger. I hope our competitors keep promoting those healthy products, and we will keep promoting our big, juicy delicious burgers."[24] To restore profitability and increase competitiveness, Hardee's targeted young men, a demographic at high risk of diet-related heart disease, with a product whose design amplified that risk.

Conversely, if new products fail to bring in profits, CEOs and lower-level managers can expect complaints from their board and investors. In 1991, McDonald's introduced the McLean Deluxe, which it marketed as a heart-healthy alternative to other hamburgers. The burger had 310 calories and only nine grams of fat. The National Basketball Association adopted the McLean as their official sandwich. But when it failed to sell, perhaps because it was the most highly priced item on the menu, the company removed it from the menu and resumed its usual marketing of higher-fat burgers.[25]

Food companies use a variety of strategies to get more hyperpalatable food onto their customers' trays and into their shopping bags and stomachs. For example, processed food is softer than real food, making it easier to chew, which studies show leads to faster and increased consumption. Consider the different demands on the mouth that chicken nuggets and real chicken make.[26] Fast food companies also combine products that reciprocally reinforce cravings: salty french fries stimulate the thirst that sugary sodas or milkshakes can quench.

Food marketed to children is especially likely to contain high levels of sugar, fat, or salt. A study of the composition of 367 supermarket foods advertised to children found that 69 percent had high levels of sugar, 23 percent had high levels of fat, and 17 percent had high levels of salt. About 9 in 10 products had high levels of one of these three.[27] "High levels" were defined using a scale developed by the Center for Science in the Public Interest. The authors noted that 62 percent of the products with the highest levels of sugar, fat, and salt –granola bars, sweet cereals, or fruit drinks, for example—were marketed to children with health claims, serving to mis-educate them about healthy diets. Similarly, a 2012 report by the Federal Trade Commission showed that the nation's largest food companies spent more than 10 times as much money advertising fast food and other restaurants to two- to seventeen-year-olds than to advertise fruits and vegetables to children.[28] And despite increased public pressure for healthier marketing to children, the trend was in the wrong direction. Between 2006 and 2009, fruit and vegetable advertising to children 2 to 11 declined by 52 percent and to youth 12 to 17 by 19 percent.[29]

One result of the increased production of hyperpalatable foods has been dramatic growth in the volume of food that is consumed. Between 1977 and 1995, the total average caloric intake from fast food outlets for Americans quadrupled.[30] A recent study found that fast food has now become the largest contributor to caloric intake from foods consumed away from home for all children ages two to eighteen; a decade earlier, school food was the main source.[31] Americans consume about 250–300 more daily calories today than they did several decades ago. A few products account for much of this gain. Nearly half of the increase comes from drinking more sugary beverages.[32] Between 1970 and 2000, annual average consumption of caloric sweeteners increased by 23 percent, with use of the sweetener high-fructose corn syrup growing more than tenfold. Since then, consumption has fallen slightly. Total added fat and oil consumption increased by 130 percent.[33] Finally, salt consumption has also increased. More than 70 percent of the total comes from consumption of processed salty foods, not added shakes at the table. Most Americans, mostly unknowingly, now eat almost twice the recommended limit of salt each day.[34] Scientists continue to debate the precise role of salt in health and disease, but there is little doubt that many Americans consume amounts of salt that can harm their health and that our children are becoming accustomed to levels of salt far higher than those experienced when evolution created biological mechanisms for salt excretion.[35]

MARKETING MAGNIFIES EXPOSURE TO UNHEALTHY FOOD

Once food industry technologists have designed irresistible foods, the next task the company faces is to market these products. Product design and marketing are inextricably linked because designers are charged with concocting profitable products that advertisers can promote. Because hyperpalatable foods are usually high in cheap fats and sugar, they generally return more profit to the company than less-processed fruits, vegetables, and whole grains. In part, the low cost of processed food reflects federal subsidies of corn, sugar, and soy production.[36] Thus, massive advertising of these more profitable but less healthy products ensures stronger bottom lines for the food companies but wider population exposure to products that contribute to diet-related diseases.

The ingenuity of the food industry is demonstrated by its ability to simultaneously design and market new products that appeal to consumers who want both "good-for-you" and diet foods. By offering one product line that profits by producing obesity and another that generates revenues by claiming to reduce weight, food companies have found a way to have their cake and eat it, too. In these "healthier" products, food companies remove some of the calories, sugars, fats, and salt added to "fun-to-eat foods" in order to address consumers' concerns about health. Others simply add nutrients to the same unhealthy product. For example, cereal companies simply add vitamins A, C, or iron to sweetened refined-grain products, then label them as "healthy," rather than using the whole grains recommended for healthier diets. In 2009, 86 percent of cereal marketed to children contained mostly refined grain.[37]

In the United States, the market for diet-related foods and beverages is expected to grow 4.1 percent a year from 2008 to 2014.[38] In 2008, Nestlé, one of the world's largest food companies, made changes in more than 6,000 products for health and nutrition considerations.[39] Its research and development network of 3,500 scientists applied the latest findings in food science to create these new products, which marketers then touted for their health-promoting qualities.

Some of these modifications may bring modest nutritional benefits, but others are used to make deceptive claims. In 2009, the Federal Trade Commission charged that Nestlé made false claims in television, magazine, and print ads that its beverage BOOST Kid Essentials, intended for children ages one to thirteen, prevents upper respiratory tract infections in children, protects against colds and flu by strengthening the immune system, and reduces absences from daycare or school due to illness. The probiotics in BOOST Kid Essentials are embedded in a straw that comes with the drink, which was prominently featured in ads for the product. "Nestlé's claims that its probiotic product would prevent kids from getting sick or missing school just didn't stand up to scrutiny," said David Vladeck, then director of the FTC's Bureau of Consumer Protection. Nestlé agreed to drop the claims.[40]

Some big companies have made determined efforts to appeal to health-conscious consumers. In 2008, with much fanfare, Indra Nooyi, the chair and CEO of beverage and snack manufacturer PepsiCo, announced plans to double the revenues from its nutritious products by 2020, from 20 percent to 40 percent. She invested in product reformulation, increasing the research and development budget by 25 percent between 2008 and 2010, while PepsiCo's advertising emphasized images of health.[41]

When these new products failed to quickly deliver profits, the company's investors and the board of directors demanded change. Their argument was mathematical: surveys showed that while 65 percent of Americans indulge in high fat, sugar, and salt snacks, only 25 percent choose "healthy snacks."[42] PepsiCo shifted gears to refocus on its more profitable and indulgent brands. Products that PepsiCo calls "good for you" still account for only about 20 percent of revenue. The bulk of the money still comes from drinks and snacks the company dubs "fun for you," including Lay's potato chips, Doritos corn chips, and Pepsi—by far the company's single biggest seller, with about $20 billion in annual retail sales globally.[43] Sixteen of the company's 22 "billion-dollar" brands are "fun-for you" high-sugar or -fat products, and three are diet sodas,[44] products of no nutritional value that may contribute to metabolic diseases.[45] In 2011, the Wall Street Journal noted that Nooyi was "facing doubts from investors and industry insiders concerned that her push into healthier brands has distracted the company from some core products."[46] That year, PepsiCo increased its advertising budget by 40 percent, primarily to strengthen its flagging American soda business, which has lost ground to Coca-Cola.[47]

Not only do companies continue to depend heavily on the "fun-for-you" but "make you sicker quicker" foods to maintain profits, they also make exaggerated claims for the "good for you" foods.[48,49] Marion Nestle, a professor of nutrition at New York University, claims that PepsiCo only pays lip service to healthier items, not marketing them as aggressively as less-healthy core products. She believes one motivation is to prevent obesity-related lawsuits. "They're going through the motions," Nestle told the *Wall Street Journal*. "I don't think they're putting anywhere near the marketing effort into their healthier products. For me it's a philosophical issue. Is a healthier junk food a better junk food?"[50]

After food scientists and engineers have designed new products, food companies turn to their marketers to create campaigns that make customers view these items as irresistible treats. Here, too, emerging science guides their actions. In 2010, the food and beverage industry spent more than $12 billion on advertising,[51] a sum that does not include less-traditional marketing such as product placements in television and movies; most Internet advertising; special promotions; word-of-mouth marketing; and cell phone and text-messaging ads. A report by the Institute of Medicine concluded that food advertising plays a major role in shaping what children and adults eat.[52]

Much advertising is motivated by fear that, as companies' food technologists help them flood the market with new products, traditional brands will lose market share and therefore revenues will drop. For example, in recent years, the plethora of new drinks—sports drinks, vitamin water, and flavored water—has led soda makers to increase their efforts to hold on to customers. "We've got to recruit new users and hold on to users as they age," Bill Elmore, president and chief operating officer of the Coca-Cola Bottling Company told the *Wall Street Journal*.[53] This constant pressure to advertise more ensures that more people will be exposed to more messages urging them to consume more unhealthy products.

In a rare example of a food marketing executive's having second thoughts about the industry's practices, Mike Putnam, a top marketing executive at Coca-Cola from 1997 to 2000, told a meeting of health professionals in 2012 that, in his time with the company, he quickly learned that Coke's marketing had one goal: "How can we drive more ounces into more bodies more often?" The company sought to increase what it called its "share of stomach." When Putnam was able to show that sugary soda consumption had surpassed milk consumption, he remembered swelling with pride.[54]

In the 1980s and 1990s, the food industry introduced new marketing strategies such as increased portion size, fast-food value-meal bundling (a single price for several items), in-school advertising, licensing deals with entertainment companies, and child-oriented advertising, each contributing to the increases in national consumption of high fat, sugar, and salt products in this period.[55]

Increased portion size provides a good illustration of the links between marketing and obesity. Since the 1970s, the average size of portions of almost every type of food served or sold in food outlets has grown. Researchers have shown that individuals consume more calories when served larger portions. The largest increases in portion size have been in the fast food, beverage, and snack food sectors, the products that are most associated with increasing body mass.[56] Over the years, the number of calories in Coke's most common drink sold in super-markets increased from 97 (in an 8-ounce container) to 145 (12 ounces), to 242 (20 ounces). How have food companies responded to complaints about portion size? A study published in 2007 found that McDonald's had withdrawn its larg-est portion sizes, perhaps in response to the controversy generated by Morgan Spurlock's popular 2004 documentary *Super Size Me*, which showed the conse-quences of his all-McDonald's diet. However, two other major chains, Burger King and Wendy's, increased portion sizes even as public concern about obesity grew.[57]

Food advertising in schools has also increased, providing the food industry with a captive audience of millions of children ill-prepared to assess the accuracy of messages transmitted in a setting perceived to be credible. In 2009, according to the U.S. Federal Trade Commission, the major U.S. food companies spent $149 million for in-school marketing, of which 93 percent was spent on adver-tising beverages.[58] Channel One, owned by Alloy Media and Marketing, a media company that targets youth and young adults, is an in-school TV station that reaches 12,000 schools in the United States, thereby providing 38 percent of the country's middle and high school students with news—and advertising. Almost 70 percent of the commercial messages on Channel One are for fast food and junk food.[59]

Fast food and beverage companies also distribute educational materials, book covers, and branded report cards directly to schools. At the same time as PepsiCo promised to limit direct marketing of soda and unhealthy (i.e., fun-for-you) snacks to schools, it invited schools to compete for grants to support sports programs or purchase equipment.[60] A local reporter in Alton, Illinois, described how PepsiCo's philanthropy kept its brand visible in a parochial school that held an assembly to thank the company for its $25,000 grants to purchase computers. "Teachers wore turquoise shirts that read 'Every Pepsi Refreshes the World,' and the children pinned on Pepsi buttons...Father Delix Michel [a local priest] riled up the youngsters with a T-shirt toss....[He] showed a good pitching arm as he deftly threw Pepsi shirts to all areas where children were sitting."[61]

More recently, food companies have deployed higher-tech strategies, includ-ing "neuromarketing," Internet and social media marketing, and viral marketing. Neuromarketing uses clinical information about brain functions and mecha-nisms to help explain—and influence—what happens inside consumers' brains as they make decisions about what to buy. In 2003, Read Montague, a neurosci-entist at Baylor University School of Medicine, used magnetic resonance imag-ing (MRI) to find that research subjects drinking unlabeled samples of Coke and Pepsi consistently expressed a preference for Pepsi.[62] However, when Montague told other subjects that they were drinking Coke, they preferred it, and the MRIs showed activity in their prefrontal cortex, an area of the brain that controls high-level cognitive powers. He concluded that Coke drinkers' experience was shaped, not by its taste, but by the brand image, reinforcing food marketers' practice of emphasizing image over substance, and fantasy over health-related attributes.

Thomas O'Guinn, a professor of marketing at the University of Wisconsin, has shown that these "fuzzy" brand images often serve as the foundation for "brand communities," groups of people whose identity is linked to their brand preferences. By appealing to these identities, advertisers make consumers feel that by using a product, they can overcome feelings of isolation or loneliness.[63] As Robert Goizueta, a former CEO of Coca Cola, has observed, "People around the world are today connected to each other by brand-name consumer products as much as by anything else."[64] Neuromarketers help provide the specific information needed to create distinct brand community niches for advertisers to target.

Today, neuromarketers have become more sophisticated. NeuroFocus, a leading neuromarketing consulting company, explains that it "leverages ground-breaking neuroscience and expertise to measure consumer attention, engagement and memory retention through brainwave, eye-tracking and skin conductance measurements."[65] Recently acquired by Neilsen Holdings NV, a global information and marketing company that studies what consumers buy and watch, NeuroFocus works for Fortune 500 companies like McDonald's, PepsiCo, Citibank, and Microsoft.

NeuroFocus researchers use products like the Mynd, the world's first portable, wireless electroencephalogram (EEG) scanner. At a 2011 technology conference in New York City, NeuroFocus CEO and founder A. K. Pradeep explained that the Mynd fits over the brain like a skullcap, using dozens of sensors to capture synaptic waves that show how the wearer reacts to changing stimuli. By widely distributing Mynds to home panelists around the country, NeuroFocus charts consumer reactions to the commercials, products, and brands of its clients.[66]

In 2008, Frito-Lay, a division of PepsiCo, hired NeuroFocus to improve marketing for Cheetos, a junk-food favorite. After scanning the brains of a panel of customers, NeuroFocus researchers learned that the yellow-orange dust coating Cheetos evoked a powerful brain response and made the product especially attractive. Later Cheeto ads highlighted the yellow dust, winning NeuroFocus a Grand Ogilvy award for advertising research that showed "the most successful use of research in the creation of superior advertising that achieves a critical business objective."[67] More significantly, the campaign resulted in an increase in Cheetos' overall sales, and brought in an additional $47.6 million in revenues to Frito-Lay.[68]

While yellow dust might make Cheetos more attractive, the Center for Science in the Public Interest, an advocacy group, has charged that these types of artificial coloring might worsen hyperactivity in some children and asked the government to ban them. "These dyes have no purpose whatsoever other than to sell junk food," noted NYU's Marion Nestle.[69]

Proponents of neuromarketing claim it is the wave of the future, allowing companies precise, efficient, and cost-effective methods of getting inside their customers' brains. NeuroFocus's Pradeep says his company's techniques make focus groups a Cro-Magnon form of market research. Critics have called neuromarketing "hacking the brain." Two corporate-responsibility groups, the World Business Academy and Ethical Markets Media, believe that neuromarketers' deliberate attempts to influence buyers by identifying triggers to bypass evaluation processes is "manipulative and unethical."[70] By making it more difficult for consumers to make rational, informed choices, neuromarketing transforms the idealized exchange of goods and services by equally informed buyers and sellers to the more primitive "Buyer Beware." In this marketplace, corporations fail to disclose the health harms inherent in their products and appeal instead to more basic instincts, expecting to distract their customers from concerns about well-being.

Internet and cell phone marketing uses new media technologies to bring commercial messages into every nook and cranny of people's lives. Compared to traditional media like radio, television, or print, social media offer marketers the opportunity for two-way conversations in which they can elicit information from customers as well as persuade them to buy products. In recent years, food companies that target children, youth, and young adults, especially the fast food, snack food, sugary beverage, and sweetened cereal sectors, have expanded their use of advertising media such as Facebook, YouTube, mobile phone texting, and "advergames" on websites. A few statistics illustrate the scope of these forms of marketing:[71,72]

- Eleven of twelve major fast-food chains sponsor at least one Facebook account, nine of which had more than a million fans; most also used Twitter and YouTube to reach young people;[73]
- Between 2007 and 2010, General Mills, a cereal maker, tripled its investment in digital media advertising;[74]
- Eight fast food chains had smart phone telephone applications, with Pizza Hut and Dominos offering apps (applications) for ordering pizza.

Between 2006 and 2009, major U.S. food companies increased spending on New Media (e.g., on-line, mobile, and viral marketing) by 50 percent.[75] In that year, ad-supported, child-oriented websites generated more than 2.1 billion ad impressions. More than a million children averaged more than 30 minutes per month on two or more of the 73 websites operated by major food companies.[76]

Stan Sthanunathan, vice president for marketing strategy and insights for the Coca-Cola Company, told an interviewer that social media like Facebook offer a "place where we can get good, solid understanding of human condition, which can really be used for transformational business decisions"[77] He predicted that social media services could become "the biggest insights' generator of the industry." In plain English, food companies use these media to better understand how their customers think about their products, then use these insights to sell more of their most profitable products—in the case of Coca-Cola, the sugary beverages implicated in the rise of obesity, diabetes, and other diet-related diseases.[78]

Another reason companies use Internet and cell phone advertising is to gain detailed data about their customers' lives. By surreptitiously gathering online data on the demographic characteristics and purchasing behavior of customers, marketers hope to tailor advertising messages to each distinct market segment. Joseph Turow of the University of Pennsylvania wrote in his recent book *The Daily You*, an analysis of the secretive practices of online marketers, that data-mining companies working for marketers seek to "find out how to activate buying impulses so they can sell us stuff more efficiently than ever before."[79] He describes how these companies sell data characterizing the lifestyles of potential consumers within any given zip code, allowing marketers, for example, to target households that prefer "good-for-you" products separately from those that prefer "fun-for you" ones. The consequences of such precisely targeted marketing are to exacerbate existing differences in health among varying socioeconomic groups.

Marketers can purchase additional details about the lives of their consumers by hiring companies such as Nielsen, Dow Jones, and Harris Interactive to analyze email, Facebook, and Twitter messages, blogs and chat rooms to extract insights—what they call "social intelligence"—about customer behavior and attitudes. Harris promises restaurants that "our team's research aim is to attain a deep-set understanding of the restaurant customer and their patterns of behavior in decision-making to aid you in gaining an advantage in this fiercely competitive industry."[80] Harris also offers to help clients "account for other entertainment opportunities that may compete with the restaurant dollar, as well as changing social dynamics that can quickly impact consumer habits."

Companies use another technique, viral or buzz marketing, to spread commercial messages through existing social networks to increase brand awareness and product sales. Like the flu, these messages can be spread by person-to-person contact or, like computer viruses, through the Internet or other digital media. Viral marketing can employ video clips, interactive games, text messages, or paid marketers: young people who promote a product to their peers, often without disclosing their employer. McDonald's website happymeal.com includes viral marketing features that invite children to send an email message to a friend about a game or other feature on the website.

Red Bull, a pioneer in viral marketing, makes a caffeinated energy drink that it claims will increase performance, concentration, and reaction speed; improve vigilance, stimulate metabolism, and make you feel more energetic.[81] To promote the product, they sponsor sports events and competitions (e.g., a contest to build homemade, human-powered flying machines and pilot them off a 30-foot-high deck in hopes of achieving flight), and hire young people to wear a giant Red Bull can on their back and distribute free samples to their peers. In the United Kingdom, Red Bull gave free cans to club disc jockeys and asked its marketers to leave empty cans on tables in hot spots such as trendy bars, clubs, and pubs.[82]

A variety of aggressive marketing campaigns for energy drinks uses viral and other forms of edgy advertisements to promise young people that these products will enhance performance and stamina for partying and work. Between 2005 and 2009, sales increased 136 percent.[83] Isn't this just another example of entrepreneurial companies' recognizing a market opportunity and using novel promotional methods? Unfortunately, energy drinks also appear to cause heart problems, convulsions, and other serious problems. According to a 2012 Food and Drug Administration report, energy drinks have been associated with at least 13 deaths since 2008, and 13,000 emergency room visits in 2009 alone.[84]

Corporations that market unhealthy food and drinks to children and young people especially like viral marketing because it allows them to bypass parents, who may restrict the food purchases their children make in the interest of protecting their health. Since viral and online advertising is less regulated than television, radio, or print ads, it also allows companies to avoid regulatory scrutiny on misleading health claims or adherence to the voluntary standards food companies publicize. A 2011 report by investigators at the Rudd Center for Food Policy and Obesity at Yale University found a dramatic growth in the use of social media advertising by the food industry.[85]

Whatever strategy food marketers use, their messages employ two distinct approaches. The first, rapidly growing, seeks to bypass cognitive processes to create brand images associated with positive emotions (e.g., McDonald's: "I'm lovin it"; Happy Meals, "Do you believe in magic?" Coke: "Open happiness," "Life Begins Here"; Pepsi: "Refresh Everything, Every Generation Refreshes the World," "Come Alive. You're in the Pepsi Generation!")

The second approach seeks to borrow the credibility of trusted individuals or institutions such as doctors, schools, or sports or entertainment celebrities to make advertisements more credible or to overcome the resistance consumers may have to otherwise commercial messages. Among the celebrities who have sold their services to market unhealthy food to children and young people are Beyoncé, the pop star (Pepsi Cola, $50 million contract); Lebron James, the basketball player (Coca-Cola, $16 million); and the soccer player David Beckham for Burger King. Neither approach provides customers with the independent information they need to make informed decisions.

These approaches to advertising are not new, and advertisers have always used the latest technology—from newspapers, to radio, to television—to get their messages across. What is new is the pervasiveness and ubiquity of advertising, its ability to use ever more sophisticated techniques to penetrate deep into our brains and social lives, and its explicit targeting of children and young people. While these new developments raise important concerns about privacy, parents' rights, and the expanding encroachment of public space, they are especially troubling when they are used to persuade people to consume products that contribute to premature death and preventable illnesses.

A third advertising approach uses children to market to their parents. The Federal Trade Commission (FTC) report on food advertising to children cites research that testifies to the value of "pester power"—child-directed marketing designed to drive children's food requests. One restaurant chain found that 75 percent of customers bought their product for the first time because their child requested it.[86] By converting children into an unpaid sales force, food companies establish a beachhead in households across America.

RETAIL: MAKING UNHEALTHY PRODUCTS AVAILABLE EVERYWHERE

New marketing techniques have also entered the retail realm. Food companies now use technologies to gather information on their interactions with customers inside retail outlets that can then be used to persuade shoppers to buy more of their most profitable products—often cheaper, less healthy food. In 1974, grocery stores introduced barcode scanners, enabling food retailers to instantly link data on advertising with actual sales.[87] Walmart has employed emerging information technologies to become the biggest food seller in the United States, using satellites to exchange data, voice, and video messages between corporate headquarters and retail outlets around the world.[88] As Doyle Graham, then Walmart's vice-president of business systems planning, boasted to a journalist, "We can capture every transaction...the time of day, the register, whether it was paid for by check, credit card or cash, and how many of the items were at reduced prices."[89] Walmart used these data to maximize sales: if placing soda next to potato chips increased sales, that became the practice. "Everybody has a feel for what they think people like," said one Walmart information officer. "But we keep the data."[90]

Retailers also hired researchers to study how customers make decisions in a store or food outlet. Using insights from environmental psychology, ergonomics, sociology, and semiotics, these researchers have studied lighting, music, spacing of tables or shelves, width of aisles, and seating arrangements. By collecting and analyzing observational, interview, laboratory, and scanner data, stores can create selling environments.[91] Designing stores to encourage customers to buy is nothing new; hiring an army of scientists and engineers to guide the process is.

A simple way to use marketing research is to find new settings and times to entice customers with hyperpalatable food. Explaining McDonald's decision to keep some restaurants open twenty-four hours a day, CEO James Skinner said: "We've learned. We've evolved. We believe we've cracked the code in the United States."[92] The code: Americans like to eat all day long. Having won the lunch and dinner market, McDonald's now sought to take the rest of the day, keeping many outlets open around the clock.

To further increase revenues, retailers charge "slotting fees," in which food manufacturers pay for getting the store's most valuable real estate: the most visible shelf space, near cash registers, at eye level, or at the end of the aisle. For a new product, the standard price of admission to the shelves is a slotting fee of up to $25,000 per item for a regional cluster of stores.[93] For a national chain, the average slotting fee for a new product is $1.5 to $3 million, depending on its location.[94] Not surprisingly, the Big Four cereal makers—and other major food producers—can afford to pay these fees to make sure their high-sugar cereals or other unhealthy products have the prime real estate in the center aisles at eye levels visible to children and their parents. As Marion Nestle observes, the best way to find healthy supermarket cereals is to reach high or off to the side to find the less visible, less marketed products produced by companies who cannot afford the slotting fees.[95]

Retailers also provide feedback to manufacturers on packaging. One executive explained that packaging should "interrupt" shoppers on their shopping trip, and suggested that a good package should answer the questions, "Who am I? What am I? Why am I right for you?"[96] A study that showed that children as young as four years old preferred food packaged in McDonald's wrapping to the same food in plain paper showed how branded packaging can elicit favorable emotional responses.[97]

Finally, retailers use pricing to sell more food, again using real-time customer data to make the most appealing offers possible. Lower prices on super-sized portions enable shoppers to get better bargains, especially on lower cost corn- and sugar-based products where higher volume did not cut into profits. In times of economic hardship, such as the recent economic crisis, fast food chains lowered prices to offer "Value Meals." McDonald's Breakfast Value Meal contains 660 calories, 42 grams of fat, 1480 milligrams of sodium and 2 grams of sugar. This single meal has 33 percent of the calories and 65 percent of the fat and sodium recommended each day for most people.

In addition, food companies use their political clout to defeat any proposals to tax unhealthy products such as sugary beverages or high-fat food. They understand that higher prices could reduce demand for these profitable products, especially for the lowest-income populations at highest risk of diet-related disease.

Food industry concentration has facilitated its use of science and technology for product design, marketing, and retail distribution, since bigger companies are more likely to have the resources to invest in the needed experts and equipment. Between 1992 and 2009, the market share of the twenty largest U.S. food retailers increased from 39 percent to 64 percent.[98] This increasing concentration of the food industry allows the biggest companies to afford the technology that they can use to outsell their competitors. For example, Sam Walton, the founder of Walmart, the nation's largest retailer, reportedly spent half a billion dollars to deploy his satellite network,[99] an expense well out of the reach of smaller retailers.

Food producers also consolidated. By 2002, four companies produced 75 percent of breakfast cereal and snacks, 60 percent of cookies, and 50 percent of ice cream.[100] These mega-producers could afford to pay the scientists to blend their hyperpalatable products, the neuromarketers to peer inside their customers' brains, and the slotting fees to get their goods in the most desirable places in supermarkets. As a result, these companies grew and prospered, enabling them to buy up or force out of business their smaller competitors, further increasing the availability and affordability of a diet known to contribute to obesity and chronic diseases.

Tobacco Corporations: Using Lobbying and Political Clout to Override Public Health Protection

It is not news that tobacco corporations have damaged public health. In the twentieth century, tobacco caused 100 million premature deaths, and in this century it is estimated that 1 billion people will die prematurely as a result of tobacco use, making tobacco the world's leading cause of preventable deaths.[101] No product has had its harmful health consequences better documented, and no industry has had its disease-promoting practices more closely scrutinized.

But a close examination of the behavior of multinational tobacco companies in recent decades raises an important question. Why, despite the scientific evidence that its products have killed more people in the last century than all the wars combined, does the tobacco industry continue to be profitable? Why have public health authorities not been better able to protect people against the world's most important serial killer? A focus on the varied practices of the Philip Morris Company, a leading global tobacco company, may help to find an answer.

TOUGHER ENFORCEMENT IN THE UNITED STATES TOBACCO BUSINESS PUSHES PHILIP MORRIS TO GO GLOBAL

In 1999, the U.S. Department of Justice filed a racketeering lawsuit against Philip Morris, now a division of Altria, and other major U.S. tobacco companies. In 2006, U.S. District Court Judge Gladys Kessler found that the government had proved its case that the defendants had violated the Racketeer Influenced Corrupt Organizations (RICO) Act. In her decision, she wrote that cigarette makers profit from "selling a highly addictive product which causes diseases that lead to a staggering number of deaths per year, an immeasurable amount of human suffering and economic loss and a profound burden on our national health care system."[102] Five defendant companies were found to have conspired to minimize dangers, distort facts, and confuse the public about the health hazards of smoking. They were also guilty of concealing and suppressing scientific evidence that showed that nicotine is addictive, misleading people about the benefits of light and low-tar cigarette brands, and purposely marketing to young people to recruit "replacement smokers" and preserve the industry's financial future. Furthermore, they were found to have publicly denied that secondhand tobacco smoke is harmful to smokers while internally acknowledging that fact, and to have destroyed documents relevant to litigation.[103] In 2009, the U.S. Court of Appeals upheld Judge Kessler's decision.

An impartial observer might expect that a company found guilty of these offenses would suffer a penalty and be forced to change its practices in some fundamental way. And in examining the record of the tobacco industry in the last decade, it did indeed change, but not in ways that protected public health or addressed the court decisions.

In 2001, two years after the Department of Justice filed racketeering charges against Philip Morris and other tobacco companies, the company asked its shareholders to approve a change of the company's name to Altria Group, Inc. At the time, Philip Morris Companies operated Miller Brewing, Kraft General Foods, Birds Eye, and other well-known food subsidiaries in addition to its tobacco brands such as Marlboro, L&M, and Chesterfield. The primary reason for the name change, Philip Morris executives told the *New York Times*, was to "reduce the drag on the company's reputation that association with the world's most famous cigarette maker has caused."[104]

Philip Morris's decision to change its name reflected more than a decade of corporate debate about how best to respond to its public health critics.[105] In 1990, a Philip Morris executive noted that the "large number of anti-smoking activists in America" were "effective and becoming more so."[106] Another warned that it was time to "wake up to the fact that we are losing the battle" and that

many of "the enemy...really are a lot smarter than we are. It's time to comple-
ment private affairs campaigning with a major public affairs campaign."[107] The
business climate, another executive agreed, was "terrible" as a result of "25 years
of criticisms" and the "rise of public health advocacy groups."[108] This "sea change"
in the business climate, as Philip Morris CEO Michael A Miles characterized it,
called for strong measures.[109]

The Master Settlement Agreement in 1998 provided further impetus for
tobacco companies to rethink their business models. In a settlement negotiated
by state Attorneys General, U.S. tobacco companies agreed to pay 46 states $207
billion (in addition to the $36 billion settlement previously negotiated with the
four other states) in compensation for public expenditures for tobacco-related
illnesses and deaths, and to end tobacco marketing to youth. The settlement, the
outcome of a bruising political and legal battle, was a significant step in forcing
tobacco companies to pay for the health costs they had been able to impose on
government and the public.[110]

Ultimately, however, the "strong measures" Philip Morris decided to take over
the next two decades consisted of changing its image and name and creating a
new U.S.-based corporation not so identified with tobacco. Later, so as to unlock
their hidden value, Philip Morris decided to spin off its food companies—
diminished by their association with tobacco—as independent corporations. In
2008, Altria created another new offshoot company, Philip Morris International,
to exclusively manage its global tobacco businesses, the company's deepest hope
for long-term profitability.

By becoming a company that was perceived to manage popular brands,
rather than make cigarettes, Altria hoped to escape the tarnish that the
legal, legislative, and media accomplishments of tobacco-control activists had imposed. In addition, even before breaking the companies apart,
Philip Morris endorsed Food and Drug Administration (FDA) regulation of
tobacco, while the other major companies continued to vigorously oppose
it. Some cynics, arguing that FDA regulation would cement Philip Morris's
sizable market advantage, dubbed the proposed legislation the "Marlboro
Monopoly Act."[111] The company hoped that its large size and more cordial
relationship with the FDA would allow it to better prosper in the new regulatory environment than its smaller competitors. In addition, Philip Morris
preferred a single set of federal tobacco regulations to a myriad of sometimes
tougher state and local rules.

Altria's charm offensive also included new philanthropic efforts and a renewed
public relations effort on corporate social responsibility. By taking these steps,
Altria sought to show that the tobacco industry could continue to thrive in the
new environment that the tobacco-control movement had created in developed
nations such as the United States, Australia, and Europe.

How did the bottom line of Altria and other companies fare in the post–tobacco settlement era? On the domestic side, the U.S. tobacco business faces a tougher environment than in the pre–Master Settlement Agreement era. Cigarette sales are in a long-term decline as a result of the lower prevalence of smoking, which fell from 24.1 percent in 1998 to 19.8 percent in 2007.[112] The total number of cigarettes reported sold or given away decreased by 28 billion cigarettes from 2006 to 2008. Advertising and promotional expenditures also declined, falling from $12.49 billion in 2006 to $9.94 billion in 2008.[113] Altria has been able to maintain its profits by raising prices, often blaming the increases on the concurrent hikes in cigarette taxes imposed by local, state, and federal governments.

Nevertheless, for the most part, the U.S. tobacco industry continues to do nicely. Market leader Altria, with its conditional support for some government regulation, and Reynolds and Lorillard, with their continued belligerent response, have each figured out a way to maintain profits. Moreover, found Judge Kessler, "the evidence is clear and convincing—and beyond any reasonable doubt—that Defendants (the tobacco companies) have marketed to young people twenty-one and under while consistently, publicly, and falsely denying they do so." [114] In the years immediately after 1998, tobacco companies doubled the amount spent on marketing cigarettes, temporarily increased advertising in magazines reaching youth, and increased cigarette marketing in retail outlets and for other products such as smokeless tobacco, areas not restricted by the settlement.[115]

While new FDA regulations on tobacco marketing that became effective in 2010 may lead to further declines in the number of new smokers, tobacco remains one of the most profitable U.S. industries. According to one Wall Street analyst, in 2011, "revenues, earnings, and dividends are growing at a healthy pace across the industry," suggesting that investments in tobacco will continue to bring "steady returns to shareholders" for decades to come.[116] Between 2006 and 2010, Altria's average operating profit margin (the ratio of earnings to revenues after all operating costs, overhead, and taxes have been deducted from income) was about 20 percent, increasing over time; its average net profit margin (profits per dollar of sales) was about 16 percent, both high compared to other industries.'[117]

In the short and middle term, extracting higher prices from an addicted customer base that is less sensitive to price increases is a successful business strategy. By the late 1990s, however, the declining numbers of new smokers in the United States and other developed countries jeopardized future profits, since the number of new smokers failed to adequately replace dying smokers. Thus, the primary strategy that Philip Morris and other tobacco companies could use to ensure continued profitability was to find new smokers in places with fewer public health protections, weaker tobacco-control movements, and less negative public attitudes towards smoking.

TO PURSUE GLOBAL BUSINESS OPPORTUNITIES, TOBACCO INDUSTRY UNDERMINES INTERNATIONAL HEALTH TREATY

To pursue this opportunity, tobacco companies have focused on the global application of the lessons in marketing and lobbying that they had previously perfected in the United States—the same practices Judge Kessler so deplored. But here the tobacco industry faced a new obstacle: the 2003 World Health Organization's Global Framework Convention on Tobacco Control (FCTC), an international treaty now approved by 176 nations with 88 percent of the world's population.[118] The treaty mandates governments to restrict tobacco marketing, increase taxes, and limit industry involvement in setting tobacco policy. To grow markets in the emerging nations of Russia, Brazil, India, China, and Mexico, the tobacco industry would need to undermine, bypass, or weaken this treaty.

In a four-year investigation (2008–2011) of the practices of the global tobacco industry, the International Consortium of Investigative Journalists (ICIJ) revealed some of the specific ways that Philip Morris International and other tobacco companies worked to grow their businesses in countries such as Russia, Mexico, Uruguay and Indonesia.[119]

Russia. In Russia, 60 percent of adult men and 22 percent of adult women smoke cigarettes. Russia is also a leading exporter of tobacco to Eastern Europe. The rules governing tobacco use in the former Soviet nations were written in 2010 by tobacco lobbyists: two employees of Philip Morris represented Russia in the tobacco trade talks organized by the Eurasian Economic Community. Sergey Chernenko, a Philip Morris spokesman in Russia, told the ICIJ that his company's involvement in setting tobacco policy "is a natural democratic approach to legislation."[120]

Philip Morris also helped create the Council for the Development of the Tobacco Industry, a trade group that is now one of the most powerful business groups in Russia. A Russian observer of the tobacco industry observed that the multinational tobacco companies "are very effective" because they bring "a long history of promotion and diversified strategies in lobbying."[121] Among the Council's victories was its success in setting weak tobacco policies that pre-empted the more stringent safeguards mandated by the Framework Convention, which Russia did not sign until 2008.

For many years, Philip Morris and British American Tobacco, another global tobacco company, funded a Russian research institute, the Institute for the Economy in Transition, to study tobacco regulation and tax policy. Company lobbyists used the Institute's findings to argue against additional cigarette taxes. One of the study's authors, Ilya Trouin, later became head of the Russian Finance Ministry's Department of Taxes, Excises, and Custom Tariffs, the unit that wrote the rules on maximum retail prices on cigarettes. To cover all bases, Philip Morris also contributed $52,000 to a cultural charity run by the wife of the Finance Minister, the ultimate decision maker on tobacco taxes. In 2010, Russia had among the lowest cigarette taxes in the world, contributing to its high rate of smoking.[122]

In 2012, President Vladimir Putin backed curbs on smoking as part of a wider effort to stem the country's population decline and to comply with the FCTC mandate to implement its control strategies by 2015. The law he signed in 2013 calls for outlawing all cigarette advertising immediately, ending retail sales at kiosks within 18 months, and banning smoking in public buildings such as bars and restaurants in three years. Philip Morris, British American Tobacco, and Japan Tobacco immediately objected, claiming that a total ban on smoking in public places and on advertising cigarettes is too draconian, while ending kiosk sales will only end up hurting small businesses. They also argued that steep tax increases will encourage a flood of cheaper imports from neighboring countries.[123]

Until now, according to the *Wall Street Journal*, Russia has remained one of the last unfettered bastions for the industry and a major driver of profits for global players like Philip Morris International, Inc., and British American Tobacco.[124]

Russian tobacco-control activists remain concerned about implementation, however, noting the industry's influence on Putin's United Russia Party. And even if changes are enacted and enforced, the tobacco industry in Russia, including Philip Morris, has had more than a decade to recruit and addict a new generation of smokers, assuring profits for years to come.[125]

Mexico. In Mexico, 60,000 people die each year because of preventable tobacco-related diseases. While Mexico was the first Latin American nation to sign the Framework Convention and has some of the toughest tobacco-control rules, here, too, global tobacco companies such as Philip Morris have been able to delay or weaken implementation. Today, Philip Morris International controls about two-thirds of the tobacco business in Mexico; British American Tobacco has the other third.[126]

One of Philip Morris International's strongest assets in Mexico is Carlos Slim (See Fig. 1.1), ranked by Forbes as the wealthiest man in the world with a 2012 net worth of $75.5 billion. From 1997 until 2006, Slim sat on Altria's board, and now he is a member of its successor, Philip Morris International's board of directors. In 2007, he sold his Mexican tobacco company to Philip Morris for more than $1 billion. According to the ICIJ investigation, "Slim's clout in Mexico on behalf of Philip Morris, and a strong lobbying push by British American Tobacco, persuaded the government that it's better to seek deals with the industry than to fight it."[127] As one Mexican tobacco activist told ICIJ, "I think no one really wants to be in a fight with Slim in this country. In no other place is there another man who is so rich, and who has so much control over things that can affect an entire country."[128]

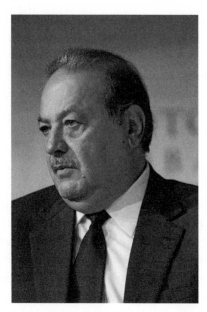

Figure 1.1 Carlos Slim, the world's wealthiest man in 2012, and a key figure in the Mexican tobacco and alcohol industries. Corbis Images.

In 2004, just three weeks after Mexico had signed the treaty, British American Tobacco's Mexico director, Carlos Slim, and Mexican Health Minister Julio Frenk (later the dean of Harvard's School of Public Health) met with then-President Vicente Fox at his official residence to make a deal on tobacco. In exchange for a $350 million fund to pay for caring for people with tobacco-related illness (to be financed by a per-pack fee to consumers), the government agreed not to make any further increases in tobacco taxes for the term of the 29-month agreement. The companies also agreed to end broadcast advertising, take down outdoor advertisements, and suspend sponsorship of public events.[129]

Both sides hailed the agreement, with one former Philip Morris executive telling ICIJ that "the agreement provided a check for three years against the increase in taxes." Tobacco-control activists, however, charged that the industry got the better deal. One Mexican public health official told ICIJ that, in his view, despite the industry concessions, the agreement "limited fiscal policy" by allowing the tobacco companies to cap taxes and "softened advertising controls. There was a clear loss of governing capacity."[130]

Philip Morris International and BAT also began lobbying Mexican legislators in hopes of weakening future legislation. They also sent selected lawmakers on international junkets and made contributions to their favorite charities.[131] In 2007, a national tobacco-control law was passed with a substantial majority, but it was much weaker than the law passed at the same time by the municipal government of Mexico City. In the ensuing years, the Ministry of Health has been slow to carry out the new law, missing deadlines for publishing its rules and sending written authorization for implementation to state governments. In addition, tobacco companies and their allies have filed thirteen lawsuits against the new rules, further delaying implementation. One of the lawsuits was filed by a restaurant chain owned by Carlos Slim.[132]

Uruguay. Uruguay hoped to set a new international standard for tobacco control. In 2006, its president, Tabare Vazquez, an oncologist, initiated a tobacco-control campaign, determined to lower his nation's 32 percent smoking rate and to comply fully with the Framework Convention. He established a ban on indoor smoking except in private homes and in 2008 required tobacco companies to put health-warning labels that covered at least half the labels on all packs. In 2009, he proposed that tobacco companies be limited to selling only one variety of each brand, to end the practice of claiming that some varieties of a brand were healthier. And in 2010, just before leaving office, Vazquez raised the taxes on cigarettes to 70 percent of the retail cost, nearly doubling the price of a pack.[133]

In 2010, however, a new Uruguayan president and health minister announced changes in the proposed tobacco rule—the result of pressure from Uruguay's domestic tobacco industry, Philip Morris International, and other global companies. Uruguayan cigarette makers complained that Philip Morris and other global companies engaged in predatory pricing, cutting sales already lowered by the tax increases. And Philip Morris International lodged an official complaint against Uruguay at the World Bank's International Center for Settlement of Investment Disputes. The company charged that the new regulations violated a 1991 bilateral investment-protection agreement between Uruguay and Switzerland, where Philip Morris International has its corporate offices.[134] These charges and counter-charges made it more difficult for Uruguay to move forward in controlling tobacco use.

Philip Morris International filed its charges against Uruguay just as the World Health Organization was set to meet in Punta del Este to establish new international standards for the enforcement of the Framework Convention. Public health advocates charged that Philip Morris International, whose 2010 annual revenues of $66 billion dollars were double Uruguay's gross domestic product, was trying to intimidate Uruguay and other small countries from taking on the deep-pocketed tobacco industry. The company also showed its ability to use trade agreements, where the rules favored multinational corporations, to override public health treaties, which lacked strong enforcement measures,[135] demonstrating its mastery of picking the most favorable venues from what one analyst has called the "spaghetti bowl" of trade agreements and bilateral agreements that global corporations have created.[136]

WHO decried Philip Morris International's trade charges; more importantly, the Bloomberg Foundation, a global philanthropic organization founded by

New York City's billionaire mayor, Michael Bloomberg, offered financial help to Uruguay in their legal battle with Philip Morris International, expected to take years and cost millions of dollars.[137] In 2011, the multinational company announced it was closing a plant in Uruguay, citing, among other things, the hostile regulatory environment.[138] In 2013, the International Centre for Settlement of Disputes, the World Bank body that settles trade disputes, agreed to consider Philip Morris's case and rejected Uruguay's request to refer the case to another trade body that would have given higher priority to public health claims.[139]

Indonesia. Indonesia is one of the few countries in the world that has not yet signed the Framework Convention Treaty. With a population of 240 million people, smoking rates of 28 percent for adults and more than 50 percent for men, and weak government regulations, Indonesia offers an example of how the tobacco industry conducts itself in the absence of government regulation.[140] Philip Morris started its operations in Indonesia in 1984, and in 2005 bought HM Sampoerna, a major local tobacco company that produced popular clove-flavored cigarettes. Philip Morris International opened its first manufacturing plant in Indonesia in 2008.[141]

After Philip Morris International acquired Sampoerna, its production volume doubled. "The acquisition was a bit of a coup," Philip Morris's Indonesian director, John Glenhill, told the *Financial Times* in 2010. "It was the only way you could get into this market correctly"; and "it has been a stunning success. It was part of the driver for growth in the last five years."[142]

After buying Sampoerna, Philip Morris rebranded its products as young, cool, and trendy. A Sampoerna billboard showed a group of attractive young people sitting around talking under the startling slogan, "Dying is better than leaving a friend. Sampoerna is a cool friend."[143] Without controls on selling tobacco to minors, Indonesian children and youth were able to buy Philip Morris products easily, further contributing to the nation's high youth smoking rate. Today, about 400,000 Indonesians die each year from tobacco-related illnesses.

South Africa. Tobacco marketing in South Africa illustrates another application of the lessons the tobacco industry learned in the United States in the previous century. In the 1920s, U.S. tobacco companies marketed cigarettes to women as "torches of freedom." In the 1960s, Virginia Slims told women, "You've come a long way, baby." Philip Morris International, which opened an office in South Africa in 2003 and is now the second-largest tobacco company in the nation, and other companies seek to bring these messages to South African women. In South Africa, tobacco ads show women using cigarettes to break racial and gender stereotypes. Tobacco marketing campaigns urge newly urbanized women to enjoy their freedom by taking up smoking.[144] Recycling themes from the United States, and adapting them to the post-apartheid moment, one tobacco company used the slogan *Liberté toujours* ("Liberty always") in its tobacco advertising to South

African women. Benson & Hedges used images featuring young black women in order to overcome cultural taboos against smoking by South African women. One advertisement showed a black woman wearing traditional headgear, accepting a cigarette from a man. The slogan "Share the feeling, share the taste" echoes the African cultural value of communalism whereby you share what you have.[145]

In 1995, population surveys in South Africa showed that 53 percent of males and 10 percent of females were daily smokers. By 2004, the rate for men had declined to 44 percent, while women's smoking rate had more than doubled to 21 percent.[146] In the coming decades, South Africa, a country hard hit by AIDS, malaria, and tuberculosis, will see rising rates of lung cancer and heart disease in women, further compromising efforts to reduce poverty and expand women's role in society and the economy.

As a result of these and other efforts, an estimated 70 million people around the world started smoking between 1998 and 2008. In 2010, the tobacco industry sold about 6 trillion cigarettes. The estimated annual cost of tobacco-related diseases was $500 billion, enough to lift more than 1 billion people a year out of extreme poverty if it were available for other purposes. By 2030, 80 percent of tobacco deaths will be in the emerging nations that Philip Morris International and other global tobacco companies are now targeting. The most promising future market is women in emerging nations. In 2009, 51 percent of men but only 2 percent of women in China smoked; in India, 26 percent of men and 4 percent of women; in Vietnam, 48 percent of men and 2 percent of women; and in Turkey, 47 percent of men and 15 percent of women were smokers.[147] If present trends continue, death rates from tobacco-related diseases can be expected to rise sharply for women, shrinking their current longevity advantage over men.

This toll raises another basic question about the coming decades: Will the world's governments and the public health community be able to apply scientific knowledge to avoid preventable illnesses and premature deaths, or will the tobacco industry continue to be able to use its power and wealth to thwart such protections? So far, despite the growing knowledge of the harmful effects of tobacco and the evidence that policies like smoking bans, tobacco taxes, and limits on tobacco marketing can reduce the health burden of tobacco, the industry has been able to stay one step ahead of public health authorities.

Alcohol Corporations: Creating New Products and Markets to Bolster Profitability

In the United States and around the world, alcohol, like high fat, sugar, and salt foods and tobacco, contributes to rising rates of chronic diseases. In addition, alcohol contributes to injuries and violence, another major cause of premature death. While many people are aware of the high death rates that tobacco and unhealthy food cause, fewer are familiar with the staggering burden of alcohol. Although some research suggests that moderate amounts of alcohol may protect against heart disease, most health researchers agree that the harm from excess alcohol use far outweighs the benefits from moderate use.[148,149] The public health goal is not prohibition but an end to policies and practices that encourage unhealthy use.

In 2010, according to the Global Burden of Disease Study, an international research effort to quantify what is known about changing causes of death, 4,860,000 deaths were attributable to alcohol, an increase of 31 percent from the 1990 toll. In those 20 years, alcohol moved from sixth place to third place in ranking as a risk factor for the global burden of disease. In 2010, alcohol contributed to more than 50 percent of the global disability-adjusted life-years (DALYs), a common measure of population health and quality of life.[150] (Since many chronic illnesses have multiple causes, alcohol interacts with tobacco, unhealthy food, and other factors to reduce longevity and worsen disability.)

Overall, alcohol accounted for 5.5 percent of the burden of global disability-adjusted life-years.[151] Another study found that alcohol contributed to more than a third of the global burden of neuropsychiatric disability (disability caused by common mental illnesses such as depression, bipolar disorder, and drug and alcohol abuse), making it the largest single contributor to this diagnosis.[152] In Russia and Eastern Europe, alcohol is the primary cause of the decline in life expectancy of middle-aged Russian men since the collapse of the Soviet Union.[153]

In the United States, excessive alcohol consumption is the third leading preventable cause of death. According to a 2012 report by the U.S. Centers for Disease Control (CDC), alcohol accounted for 80,000 deaths a year and the loss of 2.3 million years of annual productive life, a measure that recognizes the toll of alcohol on younger adults, who have more years of life to lose than older ones.[154] In 2006, the estimated economic cost of excessive drinking was $223.5 billion, or approximately $1.90 per alcoholic drink. The cost to government was $94.2 billion, which corresponds to about $0.80 per alcoholic drink consumed.[155] In 2005, alcohol use led to 1.6 million hospitalizations and 4 million emergency room visits.[156] In 2010, about 10 million young people aged twelve to twenty, 26 percent of that age group, reported drinking in the last month, and 6.5 million, about 17 percent, reported binge drinking. Each year, about 4,700 young people under age twenty-one die of alcohol-related causes.[157]

Alcohol contributes to premature death and preventable illness and injury in several ways. Alcohol consumption increases the risk for cancers of the oral cavity, pharynx, larynx, esophagus, liver, colon, rectum, and, in women, the breast.[158] Cancers account for one in five alcohol-related deaths. Heavy alcohol consumption also contributes to cardiovascular diseases accounting for another 22 percent of alcohol-related deaths. Alcohol also causes liver disease such as cirrhosis, which accounts for 16 percent of deaths.[159] Through its impairment of judgement, alcohol also contributes to motor vehicle deaths and injuries, homicide, suicide, acute alcohol poisoning, and exacerbation of psychological problems and mental illness.[160]

USING PRODUCT DESIGN, MARKETING AND RETAIL DISTRIBUTION TO RECRUIT NEW DRINKERS

Several industry practices, including marketing, product design, and retail distribution, contribute to alcohol's toll. Two of the three sectors of the industry—beer and spirits—have become highly concentrated, and wine is expected to follow suit.[161] In 2006, the ten largest beer companies in the world (corporations such as InBev in Belgium, SABMiller in the United Kingdom, and Anheuser Busch in the United States) accounted for 66 per cent market share of global sales, up from only 28 percent in 1979–1980.[162] In 2012, in a global mega-merger, Anheuser-Busch InBev (now based in Belgium) and GrupoModelo of Mexico announced that they had entered into an agreement that would create the world's largest beer company, with 2012 estimated revenues of $47 billion, operations in 24 countries, and more than 150,000 employees around the globe.[163]

In spirits, the top ten firms accounted for 59 percent of market share.[164] Concentration makes companies big enough to pour resources into marketing, which then sets off a competition among the few mega-firms for winning over the most customers. Brands and marketing know- how, rather than technological innovation, explain the growth and survival of multinational alcohol companies.[165]

In 2006, the six largest global alcohol producers spent more than $2.1 billion on advertising.[166] Exposure to alcohol advertising has been shown to contribute to drinking more,[167] and the alcohol industry targets its advertising at underage and problem drinkers, the two most reliable markets—and the populations most harmed by excess alcohol consumption.[168] This targeted marketing appears to pay off. A 2006 study estimated that the combined value of illegal underage drinking and adult pathological drinking to the alcohol industry was between $48.3 and $62.9 billion dollars, accounting for between 37.5 and 48.8 percent of consumer expenditures for alcohol.[169]

In order to expand, a company needs to develop new markets. In recent years, changing tastes in alcohol consumption, the global recession, and continuing competition from other multinationals as well as smaller national companies have created a fierce battle for recruiting new cohorts of drinkers. Two attractive markets for the alcohol industry are youth drinkers, who promise to become lifetime customers, and women, who constitute the half of the world's population, and who drink less than men.

Let's consider a campaign by Diageo, a British-based multinational company that is the world's largest producer of distilled spirits, to use its Smirnoff brand of vodka to attract the intersection of the demographic groups that can provide a new lifeline for the industry: young women.[170] In the late 1990s, Diageo was a primary developer of "alcopops," a type of alcoholic beverage that tastes like a soft drink and often contains fruit flavoring. Fruit-flavored vodka-based drinks and sweetened fruity wine coolers were conceived to compete with beer makers to win over young drinkers, especially young women, and to convert them into lifetime customers. The alcohol industry considers alcopops what one alcohol company sales manager called "the perfect bridging beverage"[171] between carbonated soft drinks and alcohol. A public health advocate has labeled them "training wheels for drinkers."[172]

After introducing alcopops, Diageo and other makers then lobbied aggressively to have this new drink regulated as a "beer," which has easier rules to follow and lower excise taxes than those for spirits. Such a designation also allowed these drinks to be sold in supermarkets and grocery convenience stores across the country, rather than as a spirit, which can be sold only in liquor stores. With this new approval, the companies invested heavily in marketing the new beverages. Measured media advertising expenditure for all alcopop brands went from $27.5 million to $196.3 million between 2000 and 2002, significantly increasing the total amount of youth exposure to alcohol advertising and contributing to a rapid growth in consumption, from 105.1 million gallons in 2000 to nearly 180.0 million gallons in 2002.[173] Diageo has seen its Smirnoff vodka sales take off, especially among young women.

One poll found that, by 2001, a majority of teens seventeen to eighteen years old (51 percent) and about a third of fourteen- to sixteen-year-olds had tried alcopops. When asked what type of alcoholic drink they would most prefer, nearly a third of teens (30 percent) said alcopops, compared to only 16 percent for beer and 16 percent for mixed drinks. Teenage girls were more likely to express a preference for alcopops than boys.[174] In 2002, according to another study, young women under the age of twenty-one were exposed to 95 percent more magazine advertising for alcopop-type beverages than legal-age women were.[175] Like fast food companies, alcohol companies also worked hard to achieve brand identification, using advertising, giveaways, and social media to promote their products. One study found that ownership of alcohol-branded merchandise was associated with underage binge drinking.[176]

In the past, young men have experienced higher rates of alcohol-related health problems than young women, but now new gender-related alcohol vulnerabilities are emerging among younger females, including suicidal ideation, osteoporosis, menstrual disorders, and some liver diseases.[177] If current trends in drinking continue, women in the coming decades might lose some of the health protections their previously lower rates of problem drinking had provided. In combination with the tobacco industry, which also seeks to increase use among women, alcohol corporations have embarked on a grand but perverse experiment to shrink disparities in longevity between women and men, not by improving the health of men, but by worsening the health of women.

In Canada and the United States, wine makers have also targeted women, particularly "moms," with new wine brands such as Mommy's Time Out, Mommy Juice, and Girl's Night Out.[178] David Jernigan, an alcohol researcher at Johns Hopkins University, explained, "In the past 25 years, there has been tremendous pressure on females to keep up with the guys. Now the industry's right there to help them. They've got their very own beverages, tailored to women. They've got their own individualized, feminized drinking culture. I'm not sure that this was what Gloria Steinem [the feminist leader of the 1960s and 1970s] had in mind."[179]

Alcohol retail practices have also been shown to influence health. Living in an area with more outlets where individuals can buy alcohol is associated with higher rates of alcohol problems.[180] For this reason, the industry's success in creating more times and places where a person can purchase or drink alcohol—grocery and convenience stores, on the Internet, airports and airplanes, outdoor cafes, and public festivals as well as liquor stores, bars, and restaurants—has contributed to more problem drinking.[181]

Lower prices for alcohol enable producers to sell more to low-income customers, the populations with higher rates of alcohol-related health problems. Thus, the industry opposes any effort to increase the price of alcohol through the raising of excise taxes that have been shown to discourage youth and problem drinking.[182] Alcohol companies also look to evade corporate taxes, leaving more revenue for profit and enabling them to keep prices low. According to a global watchdog organization's estimate, SAB Miller, a multinational London-based brewing conglomerate and maker of such beer brands as Coors Light, Miller's High Life, and Carling's Black Label, uses transfer pricing to avoid paying taxes in many countries.[183] Through a network of sixty-five tax-haven companies, SAB Miller uses tax-avoidance strategies to reduce the company's global tax bill by as much as 20 percent, giving the company an advantage over local competitors who do pay national taxes, while depriving national governments of needed revenue. SAB Miller's tax planning strategies have lost the treasuries of developing nations up to $33 million, enough to put a quarter of a million children in school. They also put lower-priced alcohol into the hands of drinkers in emerging nations.

WEAKENING GOVERNMENT OVERSIGHT OF ALCOHOL

Another strategy alcohol companies use to advance their business is to weaken and co-opt government's regulatory apparatus. For their part, government leaders in business-friendly nations are often eager to help. In New Zealand, for example, in 2011, the government appointed Katherine Rich, CEO of the Food and Grocery Council, to the health advisory group that sets alcohol marketing standards—an inherent conflict in light of her professional interest in selling more alcohol.[184] In the United Kingdom, the Conservative-Liberal coalition government initiated the "Public Health Responsibility Deal for Alcohol," an industry–public partnership that seeks to "foster a culture of responsible drinking" by negotiating voluntary pledges from participating corporations. According to the Global Alcohol Policy Alliance, the pledges "are not based on evidence of what works, and were largely written by Government and industry officials before the health community was invited to join the proceedings."[185] Not surprisingly, many health and advocacy organizations have refused to participate in the process.

Finally, the alcohol industry contributes to alcohol-related health problems by promoting and sponsoring ineffective "responsible drinking" campaigns that compete with under-funded independent but more effective approaches. These efforts reduce the pressure on government to develop more aggressive campaigns to lower problem drinking and its associated health burden.[186] Some industry-sponsored "Drink Responsibly" campaigns, for example, use "strategic ambiguity" to create messages that mean one thing to young people (e.g., "don't drink too much") and another to their parents ("don't drink if you're under 21").[187] By telling each group what they want to hear, these advertisements offer alcohol companies positive publicity without jeopardizing market share or the recruitment of new customers.

Are the world's alcohol-related health problems likely to increase in coming decades? The mixed evidence offers a shot glass of optimism but a magnum of worries. According to the World Health Organization, worldwide recorded per capita consumption has remained stable at around 4.3–4.7 liters of pure alcohol since 1990.[188] Levels of consumption vary greatly by national income level, with average per capita consumption in high income countries more than 3.5 times higher than in low income countries. In general, higher levels of consumption are associated with higher levels of alcohol-related health problems. However, in the United States and other high-consumption countries, alcohol consumption has declined since 1970.[189] In the last two decades, the proportion of U.S. high school seniors who reported drinking in the last month declined from 54 percent to 40 percent.[190] Just over half the world's adult population does not drink alcohol, reports WHO, with abstention rates higher in poorer countries and among poorer people within countries. However, rates of abstention have declined in many places, and further declines are predicted. In the coming years, WHO predicts that alcohol consumption will increase most in low- and middle-income countries, the nations with the least capacity to regulate alcohol and with populations whose other health problems put them at risk of alcohol-related harm.[191]

As we have seen with the tobacco industry, global alcohol corporations are modifying their practices as their previous prime market, male drinkers in high-income countries, reaches the saturation point and as governments in high-income nations take more effective regulatory actions. Around the world, the alcohol industry has increased marketing to the untapped markets that represent its hope for the future: young people, women, problem drinkers, and most importantly, drinkers in emerging nations, each a reliable source for new and lifetime customers.[192,193,194]

At a trade meeting, Martin Riley, the chief marketing officer for the French-based multinational wine and spirits corporation Pernod Ricard Group, explained the attraction of the Chinese market. Alcohol plays a major role in Chinese society, he said, because it is:

> involved in the majority of food occasions, and the Chinese drink 11.6 liters per head a year of beer, wines and spirits...the Chinese like the idea of luxury and are keen to associate drinking good quality alcohol with success.[195]

As the global alcohol industry becomes concentrated in a handful of multinational companies, these leading corporations successfully compete with the small, nationally based producers that still constitute an important part of the market in emerging nations. By lowering prices, expanding their retail network, buying up smaller companies, and advertising aggressively, the multinationals recruit new drinkers and increase their bottom line—at the cost of rising rates of alcohol-related health problems.

The Rise of the Corporate Consumption Complex

The recent history of these three very different industries—food, tobacco, and alcohol—show how everyday business decisions in product design, marketing, and distribution, combined with corporate lobbying, campaign contributions, and business-friendly trade agreements, have led to increases in avoidable illness and preventable deaths. It is certainly not news that companies are trying to make a buck or get a bigger return on their investments, even if this sometimes means cutting a corner or two. And it is hardly news that corporations are powerful players in today's world.

What is new is the vast and unprecedented array of scientific, technical, marketing, economic, legal, and political powers that modern corporations have accumulated. By harnessing the discoveries of the modern period to their power to realize their economic and political objectives, modern corporations have become the dominant influence on the foods we eat, our use of alcohol and tobacco, and on the wider social and physical environments that shape health. Never before in human history has any single social institution been able to influence so many of the determinants of health for so many of the world's people.

And in the last three decades, a network of corporations; trade associations; and law, lobbying, and public relations firms that produce and market consumer goods have joined with corporate-sponsored elected officials, scientists, and journalists to form what I call the *corporate consumption complex*. As the stories of the food, tobacco, and alcohol industries show, this corporate consumption complex promotes hyperconsumption, a way of living directly linked to premature mortality and avoidable illness or injury. The organizations that constitute the complex share resources, learn from each other, and mold our political systems to fit their needs.

Part of corporations' new power to shape health comes from the public health successes of earlier generations. Until the beginning of the last century, infectious diseases like cholera, smallpox, and influenza were the main causes of death in both developed and developing nations. As governments learned to apply technology and their political power to improving water, sanitation, food, and public health services in the late nineteenth and early twentieth centuries, these causes of death declined, first in the developed world and then everywhere. But as I describe in the next chapter, new killers have emerged, and to control these causes of death will require new approaches to changing the business practices described here.

Today and in the coming decades, corporations are largely responsible for the most serious emerging health problems that people face, and they alone have the global power, reach, and authority to change the fundamental causes of our these conditions. What they lack is the motivation to make such changes a priority; indeed, current economic and political conditions often serve as disincentives to change. This accumulation of corporate power has made it much more difficult to challenge the health-related business and political practices of the corporate consumption complex.

Despite the current asymmetrical balance of power between promoters of health and promoters of disease, history provides some hope. During the twentieth century, industrialization and urbanization catalyzed reform movements that led to spectacular advances in public health: food, drugs, and automobiles became safer; children and workers were protected from social and occupational hazards; air and water pollution were reduced. As a result, infectious diseases and injuries declined, longevity increased, and premature deaths fell. In this century, globalization, new technologies, the growing power of corporations, and the undermining of government's role in protecting health and safety, have again created new threats to health.

Once again, reformers, health professionals, researchers, and social movements have reached a turning point. One path, business as usual, leads to continuing increases in premature deaths and preventable illnesses and injuries. The other can take us to a place where we can finally close the gap between the potential for human well-being that our collective knowledge and ingenuity now promise and the sober reality of persistent inequalities, needless suffering, and avoidable costs. Never before in human history has humanity had both the knowledge and the resources to close this gap. With what we know today, changing the practices of a few hundred corporations has the potential to prevent millions of premature deaths and tens of millions of avoidable illnesses and injuries. In the chapters that follow, I examine the rationale for choosing to act on this historic opportunity.

2

The Public Health Evidence

How Corporate Practices Contribute
to Global Epidemics of Chronic
Disease and Injuries

In September 2011, more than 30 heads of state and at least 100 other senior ministers and experts gathered in the cavernous, wood-paneled General Assembly Hall at the United Nations in New York City for the first-ever UN High-Level Meeting on Non-Communicable Diseases (NCDs).[1] Also attending were representatives of hundreds of civil society groups working to control NCDs and representatives of business including the International Federation of Pharmaceutical Manufacturers and Associations, the International Food and Beverage Alliance, GlaxoSmithKline, Diageo, and SAB Miller (alcohol companies), and PepsiCo.[2]

What brought these disparate groups together was a growing concern about high and rising global rates of NCDs. In 2008, an estimated 36 million of the 57 million deaths in the world were due to these chronic conditions, including cardiovascular ailments, cancers, chronic respiratory diseases, and diabetes. Nearly 80 percent of those deaths occur in developing countries and one quarter among people younger than 60 years of age.[3] By 2030, NCDs will cause more than three quarters of all deaths in the world, and their cost to the world economy over the next two decades is estimated at $47 trillion (in 2012 dollars).[4]

As Dr. Margaret Chan, director general of the World Health Organization, told the delegates to the UN meeting, "noncommunicable diseases deliver a two-punch blow to development. They cause billions of dollars in losses of national income, and they push millions of people below the poverty line, each and every year."[5]

Leaders of emerging nations such as Brazil, India, and China recognize that although largely preventable, NCDs threaten sustainable development, deepen social inequities, hinder human development, and undermine the fight against poverty and hunger. The World Economic Forum has also described NCDs as one of the top threats to worldwide development, driving up healthcare costs, disabling workers, and imposing debilitating financial burdens on households.[6]

In developed countries, the growth of NCDs is the driving force in increasing healthcare costs. In the United States (where NCDs are usually called *chronic diseases*, as I will call them here), 44 percent of all Americans had at least one chronic disease in 2005, and 13 percent had three or more. Between 1999 and 2010, the number of 45- to 64-year-olds in the United States with two or more chronic conditions increased by an alarming 30 percent.[7] By 2020, it is predicted that 157 million people—almost one out of every two adult U.S. residents—will have one or more chronic diseases.[8] Many experts believe that unless the United States comes up with better ways to prevent and manage chronic diseases, its healthcare system will become increasingly unaffordable and unsustainable.[9] Today, treating chronic conditions accounts for more than 75 percent of U.S. healthcare costs.[10]

On a human level, the unfolding consequences of the rise in these diseases will be devastating. As WHO's Dr. Margaret Chan explained:

> The impact of NCDs comes in waves. What we are seeing now in much of the developing world is a first wave. This is marked by growing numbers of people with raised blood pressure, raised cholesterol, and the early stages of diabetes. The growing prevalence of obesity and overweight, seen nearly everywhere, is the warning signal that big trouble is on its way. The second wave, which is yet to come, will be much more horrific. One statistic tells the story. Of the estimated 346 million people worldwide who suffer from diabetes, more than half are unaware of their disease status. For many of these people, the first contact with the health services will come when they start to go blind, need a limb amputation, experience renal failure, or have a heart attack.[11]

The grim predictions that permeated the UN NCD meeting were a departure from earlier optimism about improving the health of the world's population. In many ways, the twentieth century was a time of unprecedented public health triumphs. By 2003, average lifespan in the United States jumped from 49.2 years in 1900 to 77.5 years, a 57-percent increase. In the same period, infant mortality fell from 100 deaths per 1,000 births to fewer than 7 per 1,000 births. Life spans also increased in developing nations. In India, for example, life expectancy increased from 20 years in 1900 to 59 years in 2000, an even larger proportional increase than in the United States. These improvements were primarily due to improved living conditions, cleaner water, better sanitation, and a more plentiful food supply; the medical advances that extended life came later.

Based on these improvements, in 1978, the World Health Organization declared that "a main social target of governments, international organizations and the whole world community in the coming decades should be the attainment of all the people of the world by the year 2000 of a level of health that will permit them to lead a socially and economically productive life," a goal embodied in the slogan "Health for All by 2000."[12] In 1999, the United States Department of Health and Human Services announced the goal of eliminating by the year 2010 racial/ethnic disparities in health,[13] the stark differences in death rates and disease between whites on one hand, and blacks, Latinos, some Asian groups, and Native Americans on the other.

Several decades later, these goals are unachieved, and confidence about progress has faded. Several recent trends undermine earlier accomplishments and contribute to a growing burden of ill health and preventable deaths. If we want to match last century's progress in improving health, we need to understand what is causing today's health problems, then devise strategies to address those causes that can put us back on track to these more ambitious goals.

Let's look at some of the warning signs. First, since 1980, the rate of obesity among U.S. children and adolescents has almost tripled; for adults the rates have doubled. Today more than two-thirds of adults and one third of U.S. children and adolescents are overweight or obese.[14,15] Weighing too much has become the new normal. If current trends continue, one in two adults will be obese by 2030.[16] And as CDC Director Tom Freiden has observed, "diabetes follows obesity like night follows day."[17] Today almost 26 million people in the United States (8.3 percent of the population) have diabetes. Of these, 7.0 million have undiagnosed diabetes. If these trends persist, one out of three U.S. adults will have diabetes by 2050.[18] Over the twentieth century, progress in extending life span in the United States slowed. In the first half of the twentieth century, the average American lifespan increased by almost 19 years; in the second half, by less than 10 years. As more Americans are diagnosed with more chronic conditions, these improvements in health may end. In fact, researchers have estimated that if increases in obesity and diabetes persist, our children and grandchildren will have shorter lifespans than the current generation, reversing more than a century of public health progress.[19] While some recent reports suggest that child obesity rates may have plateaued,[20,21] few experts are optimistic that current efforts will succeed in returning obesity rates to the healthier levels of 25 years ago.

Another global health warning sign is the increasing number of deaths due to injuries. While injuries account for a much smaller portion of mortality than chronic conditions, they raise concern for other reasons. First, around the world, deaths and disability from automobiles and self-inflicted and violent injuries are expected to rise in the coming decades and account for a larger proportion of deaths.[22] Global annual road traffic crash deaths are projected to increase from 1.2 million in 2002 to 2.1 million in 2030, primarily due to increased motor vehicle fatalities associated with economic growth in low- and middle-income countries.[23] In addition, road crashes injure up to 50 million people a year.[24]

Injuries also raise concern because of their growing impact on younger populations. In the second half of the twentieth century, violence and suicide became increasingly important causes of death in young people, contributing between a quarter and a third of deaths in young men aged 10 to 24 in all regions of the world.[25] By the early twenty-first century, injuries were the dominant cause of deaths among young men and women in most parts of the world.

In the United States, motor-vehicle crashes caused 32,885 deaths in 2010; unintentional injuries were the single most important cause of death for children aged 2 to 14. Guns are another cause of injuries that kill: almost 10,000 young people aged 15–24 died in 2010 as a result of suicide or homicide, most commonly caused by a firearm.[26]

Despite the improvements of the twentieth century, health inequalities between poor people and the better-off and between blacks and Latinos and whites, persist. In some cases, they are even widening. In the United States, in 2003, white women lived 4.5 years longer on average than black women and white men lived 6.3 years longer than black men.[27] After some declines in the gap in the first half of the century, the gap in death rates between blacks and whites was as large five years ago as it was 50 years ago.[28] Only a few chronic diseases account for almost half the difference in early deaths between whites and blacks: cardiovascular diseases, cancer, diabetes, and kidney disease.[29] For diabetes, the fastest growing chronic disease, the gap in death rates between whites and blacks is actually increasing, and the death rate from diabetes for blacks is now twice as high as for whites. A report by the CDC found that in 2009–2010, the proportion of U.S. blacks aged 45–64 with two or more chronic conditions was 35% higher than for whites. Rates of those with two or more chronic diseases had increased significantly for whites, blacks, and Hispanics since 1999.[30] Absent changes in policy, these trends suggest stagnant or growing health inequalities in the United States, despite more than 25 years of government pronouncements that eliminating such inequalities was a top priority.

In some cases, the health status of Americans is actually worsening. A recent study found that women's longevity declined in the past decade, with life expectancy for women falling or stagnating in one of five counties. The researchers identified obesity, smoking and stress—risk factors for many chronic diseases— as the main causes.[31]

As the UN NCD meeting showed, other nations also face rising rates of chronic disease, yet no nation in the world spends more on healthcare than the United States—17.6 percent of its gross domestic product in 2009 and an estimated almost 20 percent by 2020.[32] And no other wealthy nation gets such consistently disappointing results in life expectancy, infant mortality, self-reported well-being, or days lost to disability.[33,34] While improvements in healthcare organization and quality may contribute to somewhat better outcomes, most researchers do not believe that changes in healthcare alone can reverse the chronic disease trends that threaten our future. In sum, today, the United States is paying more for healthcare, getting less, and appears unable to meet the health goals it sets for itself. The national debates about healthcare reform and the implementation of the 2010 Affordable Care Act are vitally important for the future of the U.S. healthcare system and economy. Yet in many ways these conflicts have distracted national attention from a deeper question: How can we prevent rather than simply treat the new threats to health that are causing so many Americans to die prematurely or to suffer preventable illness or injury?

Chronic Diseases and Injuries Become Main Killers Around the World

Not only the United States and other developed nations, but emerging and low-income nations around the world are also experiencing a large and growing burden of preventable premature deaths and ill health from NCDs and injuries. Public health researchers and policymakers offer three main explanations for these disturbing trends.

The first explanation for rising rates of chronic diseases is, "You gotta die of something." In this view, increases in chronic diseases and injuries are the inevitable result of declines in infectious diseases. If infectious diseases don't kill you, then chronic conditions or injuries are the logical and inevitable alternative.

The second explanation is that increases in chronic-disease deaths are the unavoidable consequence of population aging. Between 2000 and 2030, the portion of the U.S. population over the age of 65 will nearly double, from 12.4 percent to 19 percent; a similar doubling is expected in the global population over 65. Average life expectancy in the United States now exceeds age 77, an all-time high. Improvements in living conditions over the twentieth century have allowed many more people to survive into their seventh and eight decades, making them vulnerable to the chronic conditions that often take decades to develop. In this view, the increase in chronic diseases is the price of our success in extending life.

The third explanation for the increase is the global changes in lifestyle observed over the last century or so. More people are smoking, drinking too much alcohol, moving too little, and eating too much food high in fat, sugar, and salt. Given the associations between consumption of alcohol, unhealthy food, and tobacco and increases in heart disease, cancer, stroke, and diabetes, these increases are attributed to modern lifestyles. Similarly, more driving and more people owning cars and guns contribute to rising global rates of injury-related deaths. As these lifestyles spread to vast emerging nations like China, India, and Brazil, their impact on global morality increases significantly. In this view, increases in chronic diseases and injuries are the collateral damage of the patterns of consumption associated with economic development and global progress.

Each of these arguments has elements of truth and helps explain some of the shifting patterns of illness and death. But these explanations fail to account for several disturbing facts. First, NCD deaths are increasing even in the countries in Africa and Asia that still have high rates of infectious diseases. Many sub-Saharan African countries now have a quadruple burden of infectious diseases, including HIV, malaria, and tuberculosis; childhood illnesses due to contaminated water, insufficient food, and inadequate sanitation; injuries and violence; and emerging chronic diseases. If deaths from chronic diseases simply replaced deaths from infectious diseases, then the rise in chronic diseases would always follow the decline in infectious disease deaths, not accompany it. Yet in nations like India, Liberia, and Rwanda, infectious disease mortality continues to be high even as deaths from cancer and heart disease are also rising.

Second, in the past few decades, more people are being diagnosed with chronic diseases at earlier ages. As I noted, a quarter of the annual global deaths from NCDs strike people under age 60. Growing evidence finds the early signs of these diseases in children and young adults. According to Dr. David Katz, a public health researcher at Yale University, in the span of less than a generation, Type 2 diabetes has been transformed from a chronic disease of the midlife years into a rather routine pediatric diagnosis, mostly as a result of rising rates of child obesity.[35] Several recent studies have documented an alarming rise of difficult-to-treat Type 2 diabetes and serious liver disease in 10- to 20-year-olds, a trend that flatly contradicts the theory that rising rates of chronic disease are the result of increases only in the middle-aged and elderly.[36,37] If the increase in chronic conditions were simply a consequence of aging, one would expect to see the increased death rates only among older people, not among adults under 60. One would not expect to see growing signs of these conditions among children and younger adults. In addition, more people are now being diagnosed with multiple chronic conditions, suggesting the possibility of some new exposure to a more dangerous environment.

A further blow to the theory that only aging populations account for increasing chronic diseases comes from the work of David Stuckler, a medical sociologist at the University of Cambridge, England. He compared demographic, health, and economic information from 56 developed and developing nations for which comparable data were available. He found that relationships between national chronic disease death rates and social indicators such as market integration, foreign direct investment, and urbanization rates were three time stronger than the relationship to population aging.[38] In other words, social factors like the role of corporations in a nation's economy and politics and the pace of urbanization were stronger predictors of that country's chronic disease rates than the proportion of people over the age of 65.

Finally, while the health-related behaviors that have come to define the Western lifestyle do of course play a role in the proliferation of chronic diseases, simply noting the association raises the question, *Why* these changes now? Nothing we know about human genetics or biology indicates that people have become greedier or more biologically susceptible to addiction over the last few decades. Nor has anyone presented evidence that human nature has rapidly changed in some fundamental way that brings about these changes in health. Rather, the most plausible explanation is profound changes in our social landscape and environment, a subject to which I will soon return. The argument that changes in lifestyle are the main cause for increases in chronic diseases and injuries confuses the *symptoms* of a changed environment, i.e., rises in unhealthy behavior, for the *causes* of those changes. In public health as in medicine, treating symptoms rather than causes rarely leads to lasting improvements in health.

The conventional explanations for why more illness and deaths are now caused by chronic disease and injuries are inadequate for another reason. They offer little guidance for action and therefore make these trends seem inevitable, simply—the results of bad choices by individuals, not of large-scale social and political decisions. The vanquishing of infectious diseases, increased life expectancy, and the economic development that supports more comfortable lives are some of the greatest successes of the last two centuries. Reversing these trends is unthinkable. After all, the purpose of public health analysis is to inform action to improve population health. If the best it can offer is to document allegedly immutable trends, then researchers come to resemble the medieval monks who described the unfolding of the epidemic of Black Death in Europe, while praying for salvation in another world.

Another Explanation

So who or what is the culprit responsible for today's most serious health problems? One suspect stands out, both because it is a leading cause of chronic diseases and injuries and because over the last few decades it has been touching the lives of more people in more pervasive ways. That suspect is the products and practices of the industries that define the modern global consumer economy. Let's look at the ways that three more industries—automobiles, firearms, and pharmaceuticals—contribute to the previously described toll from the industries that make food and beverages, tobacco, and alcohol. The auto industry is a major contributor to both chronic diseases and injuries, firearms are a main cause of injuries and deaths around the world, and the pharmaceutical industry causes illness and death as a result of unintended side effects, inappropriate use, and industry practices that value profit more highly than improved population health.

Automobile Corporations: Manufacturers of Modern Life, Chronic Diseases, and Injuries

Automobiles transformed life in the twentieth century and provided many people previously unattainable freedoms. But motor vehicles contribute to poor health directly in three ways—increased air pollution, traffic-related injuries and deaths, and discouraging the physical activity that promotes health. In addition, motor vehicles are a major contributor to human-induced climate change, a growing threat to global health. Already by the year 2000, scientists estimated that 150,000 people died each year because of climate change, mostly poor people in low-income countries.[39] In developed nations, motor vehicles contribute about one-fifth of the carbon dioxide emissions that cause human-induced global warming.

Air pollution causes both chronic and acute health conditions. Long-term exposure to air pollution contributes to inflammation, stroke, atherosclerosis, and increased risk of heart disease, the leading cause of death around the world. Recent research has found that traffic-related pollution in particular is associated with early signs of heart disease, such as systemic inflammation and with incidence of coronary heart disease and cardiovascular mortality.[40] For most people, the risks associated with air pollution exposure are small, but given the pervasive exposure, the public health consequences are large.[41] Ambient particulate matter air pollution is estimated to be the ninth-leading cause of global mortality, responsible for 3,223,540 deaths in 2010.[42] Urban air pollution, largely the result of motor vehicles, is alone responsible for about 700,000 annual deaths from car-diopulmonary disease.[43] In the United Kingdom, exposure to fine particulate pol-lution from automobiles now causes more annual premature deaths than motor vehicle crashes.[44] Despite the significant progress that has been made in reduc-ing motor vehicle emissions in the United States, cars and trucks continue to be a primary cause of air pollution. In most cities, motor vehicles are a significant contributor to urban smog, a trigger for asthma and other health conditions.

Motor vehicles also cause traffic injuries and deaths. In the United States, 32,885 people died in motor vehicle crashes in 2010, the lowest number of deaths since 1949. Among the factors contributing to the decline were reduc-tions in drunk driving, increased seatbelt use, improved roadways, and better design and safety-related vehicle features.[45] These improvements show that focused government regulation can prevent automobile deaths. But on the global front, traffic injuries and deaths are expected to almost double, to more than 2 million deaths a year by 2030, due to the increased number of vehicles on the roads in Africa, Asia, and Latin America where design standards and enforcement are more lax than in wealthy nations.[46] In 2010, automobile colli-sions killed an estimated 1.3 million people and caused non-fatal injuries to an additional 20 to 50 million more people.[47]

Finally, a society that has come to depend on motor vehicles for most trans-portation contributes to poor health by changing physical and social environ-ments. Cars and highways discourage walking and biking, thus contributing to obesity[48] and reducing the demand for cleaner, more active, and safer public transportation.[49] A growing body of evidence points to physical inactivity as a major cause of premature mortality.[50] Cars also contribute to road rage and other psychological problems and isolate people from social interactions that promote health.[51]

As with the other industries described here, the automobile industry has pur-sued business and political strategies that increase the harm they cause. From the 1960s through the 1980s, the automobile industry initially opposed standard seatbelts, airbags, better brakes, and better emission standards.[52] Throughout the 1990s and into the next decade, the U.S. auto industry heavily promoted sport utility vehicles, despite evidence that these vehicles were more dangerous and polluting than other vehicles. SUVs' simple design—and the fact that as "trucks" they did not need to meet many of the safety and environmental regulations imposed on cars—led to unit profits 10 to 12 times higher than from conven-tional sedans. In 1998, Ford's Michigan truck factory became the most profit-able factory in the world, turning out $11 billion worth of Ford Expeditions and Lincoln Navigators.[53]

In the 1990s, the U.S. auto industry, the nation's largest advertiser, spent $9 billion on advertising to make SUVs its best-selling and most profitable vehicles, doubling their market share between 1980 and 2000.[54] Chrysler employed a medical anthropologist to help them design SUVs and the advertising to sell them. He suggested that Chrysler design a vehicle that appealed to customers' unconscious "reptilian instincts" for survival and reproduction and to advertise SUVs as both protection against crime and unsafe drivers and as a means to escape from civilization.[55] Unfortunately, these SUVs pollute 47 percent more than do conventional sedans, and have higher rates of roll-overs and pedestrian and driver deaths.[56] SUVs contribute to an estimated 3,000 preventable excess deaths in the United States a year.[57]

After the 2008 financial crisis, the U.S. federal government and taxpayers bailed out the auto industry, rescuing it from its failure to compete effectively with European and Asian auto companies that had designed smaller, more fuel-efficient cars. At the insistence of the federal government, the auto industry did design and bring to market less polluting and safer cars, a rare example in this period of the federal government using its clout to insist on health improvements in a product. But Detroit's "Big Three" could not wean themselves from the higher profits that SUVs and pickup trucks brought in, so they continued to aggressively market these polluting and unsafe vehicles. By the end of 2011, reported the *Wall Street Journal*, for many U.S. automakers, sales of huge 4x4 pickup trucks and SUVs again surpassed car sales,[58] a trend that continued through 2013.

Over the years, the auto industry has consistently opposed every safety feature—seatbelts, airbags, improved brakes, and better fuel efficiency, to name a few—for as long as possible, arguing that mandatory installation of these measures would jeopardize the viability of a quintessentially American industry. As a result, innovations that could have saved thousands of lives were delayed, often for decades. For example, for more than 15 years, the U.S. auto industry successfully opposed regulations to require either airbags or automatically-closing seat belts in automobiles. Finally, in 1986 the U.S. Supreme Court ordered the National Highway Transportation Safety Administration to implement the rules. By one estimate, this delay contributed to at least 40,000 deaths and 1 million injuries at a cost to society of more than $17 billion.[59] This resistance to regulation continues to this day. In 2013, Chrysler refused a National Highway Traffic Safety Administration request to recall 2.7 million Jeeps, one of its most popular and profitable brands. The NHTSA contended a manufacturing defect made Jeeps prone to fire in the event of a rear-impact collision.[60]

Earlier, the auto industry also lobbied for generous federal subsidies for highway construction, creating a transportation system that made cars essential for many kinds of travel. The industry's opposition to federal support for public transport ensures that this less polluting and more active form of transit remains out of reach for most Americans and most municipalities.

The largest threat that automobiles pose to world health will come from the decisions that global auto corporations make in emerging nations. In recent years, China has become the world's fastest growing automotive producer, surpassing the United States in 2009. China's annual vehicle output has increased from fewer than 2 million vehicles to more than 10 million in 2011. Since 2000, China's growth has been led by an increase in passenger cars, which now account for more than 65% of its vehicle production.[61] Many Western automakers are forging partnerships with Chinese companies. How the Chinese government—and economy—choose to manage auto industry growth will have an important effect on China's already significant problems of air pollution, motor vehicle injuries, and sedentary behavior.[62]

High rates of auto industry growth are also expected in Brazil, whose auto manufacturers sell to consumers throughout Latin American. Per capita car ownership on that continent has more than doubled over the last decade and is predicted to do so again over the next ten years, in part due to expanded access to consumer credit.[63] Similar trends have been reported in India[64] and Russia.

Among the growing victims of increased car sales are children. In Brazil, the death rate for children under 10 from motor vehicles increased 20 percent between 1997 and 2005.[65] While some of the increases are due to urban density and lax enforcement of traffic rules, shoddy manufacturing standards may also contribute. A 2013 report by the New Car Assessment Programme, a consumer safety group, found that General Motors, Renault-Nissan, and Suzuki are manufacturing car models in Latin America that score much lower on global safety standards than equivalent models made in Europe and America.[66]

Firearms: Making Lethal Products Available on Every Street Corner

Since 1960, more than 1 million people in the United States have been killed by guns, and more than 2 million more have suffered non-fatal gun injuries. In this period, 13 times more Americans have been killed by firearms in the United States than by the wars in Vietnam, Iraq, and Afghanistan combined.[67] Every day, 1,500 people die in armed conflicts around the world, one person every minute. The weapons that stoke these clashes are used to force tens of thousands of children into armed conflict and to rape women and girls in conflict zones.[68] An examination of the role of the gun industry's business and political practices in these injuries and deaths provides additional evidence on how corporate decisions shape our country's health profile.

In 1968, amid a rise in urban gun violence and after the assassinations of John F. Kennedy, Martin Luther King, and Robert F. Kennedy, President Lyndon Johnson overcame traditional opposition to a federal role in gun safety by persuading Congress to pass the Gun Control Act of 1968. One of the goals of this legislation was to reduce the availability of "Saturday night specials"—the cheap, poorly designed, and easy-to-conceal handguns that contributed to high rates of gun deaths and injuries.[69]

The new law achieved its goal by restricting interstate commerce of guns; denying firearms to felons, minors, fugitives, drug addicts, and the mentally ill; and banning the import of handguns that did not meet strict new design and performance standards. It was the strongest gun control legislation in decades. These measures reduced the supply of the cheap weapons favored by low-level criminals and abusive jealous men.

However, due to opposition from the gun industry and the National Rifle Association, Congress did not require domestic gun manufacturers to meet these new standards. As one firearm company executive said, the law was "designed to protect the U.S. firearms industry from unfair competition."[70] Thus, the new rules created a new business opportunity for domestic gun makers: making and marketing cheap handguns in the United States.

In a familiar story for lethal but legal products, falling demand for firearms triggered gun makers to promote their products more aggressively. Prior to the 1960s, the gun industry had lost business as fewer people hunted or collected guns, causing sales of rifles and shotguns to plummet. Handguns—pistols and revolvers—became the industry's hope for renewed profitability. In order to realize this goal, handgun producers had to make handguns affordable, and they had to convince more people that they needed the protection a handgun offered.

New companies emerged determined to find ways to produce and distribute affordable handguns. In 1970, George Jennings founded Raven Arms, Inc., a company that manufactured cheap handguns. Over the next several years, Jennings and his family and friends created several more companies surrounding the city of Los Angeles, later dubbed the "Ring of Fire" companies. These companies cut costs by using cheap metals and fewer moving parts; dropping traditional safety features such as firing pin blocks that help prevent accidental discharge; and scrimping on plant security. It cost Raven $13 to make a gun it could sell wholesale for $30, a gross margin of more than 100 percent.[71]

One of the Ring of Fire companies was Lorcin Engineering of Mira Loma, California. James Waldorf, its founder and a friend of Jennings, told a *Frontline* TV interviewer that his goal was to make the "world's most affordable handguns.... We consider ourself the blue-collar gun of America."[72] Waldorf also noted that "There are more poor people than rich people. Cheap is synonymous with volume."[73] Between 1990 and 1992, Ring of Fire companies increased their production of handguns 24 percent a year, while production by other gun companies declined. By the mid-1990s, Ring of Fire companies sold as many handguns as Smith & Wesson, Colt, and Ruger, the largest national companies.[74]

The second part of increasing profits was to expand the customer base. Several Ring of Fire companies targeted women. One Lorcin ad showed three of its pistols, including one with a pearl-handled grip and another with a pink grip. The caption read, "Three little ladies that get the job done."[75] The companies created a network of wholesalers that sold to pawn shops and licensed firearm dealers, and priced its products to make them attractive starter guns for "the fearful, the criminal, and increasingly, the very young."[76] Lorcin also offered to cover firearm distributors and retailers under their own company's liability policy, an attractive promise on which it was ultimately unable to deliver.[77] In California in the 1990s, for every 10,000 cheap handguns sold each year, roughly 2,200 showed up in crimes, an explosion that caught even veteran law enforcement officers by surprise.[78]

In 1993, Lorcin Engineering sold half the .38 caliber handguns in the United States. According to Waldorf, "80 percent of Americans in the United States that own handguns own one of our products."[79] The low prices that Lorcin and other Ring of Fire companies charged—$60 to $100 retail and as little as $50 on the street—led established gun makers like Smith & Wesson to lower their costs and prices, creating a race to the bottom on prices and quality—and an overall increase in handgun sales. As one violence-prevention advocate put it shortly before the Los Angeles Rodney King riots broke out in April 1992, killing 53 people and injuring thousands more, "We have a fire burning, and these companies are throwing gasoline on it. These people know what the inner-city gun buyer wants."[80]

Data from the U.S. Bureau of Alcohol, Tobacco, and Firearms showed that for several years in the late 1990s, Lorcin's L380 pistol was the gun most often traced at crime scenes.[81] Waldorf rejected the charge that his company's products were more likely to be involved in crime, arguing it was like saying "there are more Chevrolets involved in accidents than Mercedes."[82] But BATF data suggest otherwise: in 1999, seven of the top ten handguns recovered from persons under the age of 18, and five of the ten from those aged 18 to 24, were inexpensive semiautomatic pistols made by Ring of Fire companies.[83] In addition, lax security at Lorcin led to a steady flow of guns into the illegal market. A BATF investigation found that two Lorcin employees sold thousands of handguns made at the plant, which at the time employed no security guards.[84]

By the late 1990s, a combination of factors undermined the Ring of Fire business model. Increasing competition among these companies and from outside companies made it harder to make a profit. Lawsuits from gun owners injured by the shoddy products and from municipalities concerned with rising rates of gun violence scared investors, and tougher state and municipal legislation required big new investments in production and security.[85] Lorcin tried briefly to follow the tobacco model by going overseas to find less regulated markets. In 1997, Lorcin sold 25,000 handguns in South Africa, where rising crime rates and fears of crime created a lucrative market.[86] But by the new century, Lorcin, Raven, and three other of the six Ring of Fire companies had declared bankruptcy or gone out of business.[87]

On one hand, the Ring of Fire story is as American as cherry pie. New companies are created as a market opportunity arises, and after initial success, many of these companies fail, not tough enough or well-financed enough to survive and prosper. Some make shoddy products or use unscrupulous marketing. As early as 1992, based on a five-month investigation, the *Wall Street Journal* described the Ring of Fire companies as "an empire that built itself on the mundane details of low-cost manufacturing and high volume distribution and thrives on the advantages of government protectionism and de facto oligopoly." On the other hand, as the *Journal* went on to observe, "In many ways this is such a typical business that it's easy to lose sight of the product's main feature: It kills."[88]

As is often the case with lethal but legal products, the failed businesses left a long shadow. Millions of cheap guns remained in circulation, contributing to crime, accidental injuries, homicides, and suicides. For many young people, Ring of Fire companies had provided their starter gun. Tom Diaz, a gun control advocate and former senior staff member for the House Judiciary Committee's Subcommittee on Crime, has charged that the gun industry deliberately marketed increasingly lethal pistols to promote repeat sales to a customer base that had become saturated with less-powerful weapons.[89]

After 2000, new handguns have been super-sized to make them deadlier than the Ring of Fire weapons. The Glock 19 nine-millimeter semiautomatic pistol can fire 30 shots in seven seconds. It was advertised in the magazine *Soldier of Fortune* and elsewhere, enjoyed product placements on the popular television serial *Law and Order* and in rap songs and movies, contributing to the dubious distinction of becoming the firearm of choice of police, gun enthusiasts, gangsters, and mass murders.[90] Unlike the Ring of Fire companies, which operated on the margins, Glock is a respected multinational corporation based in Austria with operations in Hong Kong, Uruguay, the United Arab Emirates, and America, and customers in more than 100 countries. Its biggest customers are U.S. law enforcement agencies, but Glock's other customers have included accused mass murderers Jared Loughner, who shot U.S. Congresswomen Gabrielle Giffords and more than a dozen others in Tucson, Arizona, and James Holmes, who allegedly fired on a movie theater in Aurora, Colorado, killing 12 and wounding 58 people. A decade earlier, in a court deposition, an attorney had asked Paul Jannuzzo, Glock's chief operating officer at the time, whether the company had ever considered not selling high-capacity magazines for its guns. "Not for one half a second, no sir," he replied and called the 1994 law that temporarily banned such magazines "ridiculous," a "feel good" measure.[91]

Even after their extinction, the Ring of Fire companies continue to influence the gun business by showing the potential profit in widely marketing low-cost weapons and targeting advertising to women, the young, and the fearful. Today the U.S. firearms industry is a $3 billion-a-year business that includes about 200 companies. It produces 3 millions guns a year, of which 40 percent are handguns. The industry is now highly concentrated, with five companies controlling 55 percent of the pistol market and 72 percent of the rifle market. Three companies control 86 per cent of the shotgun market, and just two, Smith & Wesson and Sturm Ruger, control 80 percent of the revolver market.[92,93]

While the food industry embraced science and technology in order to design and market more irresistible products, gun makers have for the most part rejected technologies that could make guns safer, fearing that added safety features might raise the cost for a price-sensitive market—or that its largest customer base didn't care much about safety. Among the new technologies that have been proposed but not brought to market on any wide scale are trigger locks, "smart guns" that fire only when operated by the owner, magazine safeties that prevent firing once the clip has been removed, and childproofing.[94,95]

A new entry in the gun business is the Freedom Group, Inc., a corporation created in 2007 by the private investment firm Cerberus Capital Management[96] (named after the three-headed dog of Greek mythology that guards the gates of Hades). Freedom Group sells guns and gun supplies under 10 brand names, including Remington, Marlin, and Bushmaster. Cerberus, led by Wall Street buyout king Stephen Feinberg, now manages more than $20 billion in capital, with additional subsidiary revenues in the range of $40 billion annually—a very different stratum of American business than the hard-scrabble Ring of Fire companies.[97]

Cerberus first came to national attention in 2007 when it bought Chrysler. Feinberg hopes that Cerberus can cut costs and raise profits at the handful of small, struggling gun companies he has bought in the last five years, and take them public, making a single big and profitable company. The Freedom Group released an initial public offering (IPO) to go public in 2009 but later put off the action because financial markets seemed turbulent.

In 2011, the company had sales of $775 million, according to its Annual Report, and sold 1.1 million rifles and 2 billion rounds of ammunition, making Freedom Group the largest gun and ammo maker in the United States.[98] In 2012, its profits increased by 20 percent and its sales reached $932 million. One part of its business plan is to sell more weapons to the military, a task facilitated by a board that includes former Vice-President Dan Quayle and two retired generals.[99] While Freedom Group has so far focused on rifles and shotguns, some analysts believe it may enter the handgun business to diversify its offerings. One of its companies, Remington, recently introduced its first pistol in decades, the Remington 1911 R1.[100] In the last few years, in order to sell more guns and ammunition to more people, Freedom Group expanded its business with Walmarts, which in 2011 accounted for 15 percent of the gun makers' total sales.[101]

On December 14, 2012, Adam Lanza, a 20-year-old, used an AR-15 .223-caliber rifle made by the Freedom Group to kill 27 people, including 20 first graders and his mother. Lanza also carried a 9mm Sig-Sauer pistol and a 10mm Glock pistol, which he used to kill himself after police arrived.[102] Ten days later, William Spengler, Jr., also used a Bushmaster AR-15.223-caliber rifle (as well as a Mossberg 12-gauge shotgun and a.38-caliber Smith & Wesson pistol) to kill two volunteer firefighters and wound two others who came to extinguish a fire he had set in his upstate New York house.[103]

In his eulogy for the Newtown victims, President Obama observed that:

> This job of keeping our children safe and teaching them well is something we can only do together, with the help of friends and neighbors, the help of a community and the help of a nation. This is our first task, caring for our children. It's our first job. If we don't get that right, we don't get anything right. That's how, as a society, we will be judged. And by that measure, can we truly say, as a nation, that we're meeting our obligations? . . . Are we really prepared to say that we're powerless in the face of such carnage, that the politics that the politics are too hard?[104]

Around the same time, Freedom Group founder Stephen Feinberg discussed his company's responsibilities in a different way. "We do not believe that Freedom Group or any single company or individual can prevent senseless violence or the illegal use or procurement of firearms and ammunition," the company said. In a statement released four days after the Newtown shooting, Feinberg's Cerberus Capital Management wrote:

> As a Firm, we are investors, not statesmen or policy makers . . . It is not our role to take positions, or attempt to shape or influence the gun control policy debate. That is the job of our federal and state legislators. There are, however, actions that we as a firm can take. Accordingly, we have determined to immediately engage in a formal process to sell our investment in Freedom Group. We believe that this decision allows us to meet our obligations to the investors whose interests we are entrusted to protect without being drawn into the national debate that is more properly pursued by those with the formal charter and public responsibility to do so.[105]

Joe Nocera noted in the *New York Times* that Freedom Group's newfound reluctance to enter the national debate seemed somewhat hypocritical. Its chief executive, George Kollitides, has run for the board of the National Rifle Association and serves on several N.R.A. committees, and the N.R.A. has described company executives as "strong supporters of the Second Amendment."[106] Its advertisement for the Bushmaster (Figure 2.1) shows little reluctance to influence attitudes towards guns.

According to one industry analyst, by the end of 2011, Cerberus had already realized profits of nearly $100 million on Freedom Group, and sale of the company was likely to triple its gross investment.[107] Cerberus, the mythical three-headed dog after whom Feinberg's company was named, has one head to stare into Hell to make sure nobody escapes, another to look back at the world of the living, and the third to peer into the future. For Cerberus, that future may not include firearms. But like the fly-by-night Saturday night special makers of Los Angeles, the millions of guns that the Freedom Group leaves behind and the regulatory environment the company helped to create ensures that its legacy will include more deaths and injuries. And as gun ownership continues to decline—the number of American households with firearms fell from an average of 50 percent in the 1970s to 35 percent in this decade[108], gunmakers and

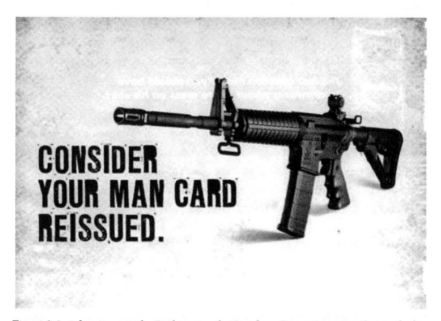

Figure 2.1 Advertisement by Bushmaster, the Freedom Group Company that made the weapon Adam Lanza allegedly used in Newtown, Connecticut. Appeared in *Huffington Post* on Dec. 17, 2012, at http://www.huffingtonpost.com/emma-gray/bushmaster-rifle-ad-masculinity-gun-violence-newtown-adam-lanza_b_2317924.html.

their allies can be expected to continue to use their political power to resist any effort to enact public health measures that jeopardize their profits.

Pharmaceutical Corporations: Misrepresenting Risk, Selling Sickness, and Co-opting Doctors to Make a Profit

Modern drugs have saved hundreds of thousands of lives, and no patient or physician would want to do without the many effective products that the pharmaceutical industry has developed. But the fact that the drug industry has helped many people is no reason to ignore or excuse its products or practices that harm health. A variety of evidence shows that pharmaceutical products cost lives as well as save them, and that the pharmaceutical industry consistently engages in practices that threaten the health of the public. Some of these cause unintended injuries or side effects, while others represent missed opportunities to use our collective pharmacological wisdom to prevent or treat diseases rather than produce profit for the industry.

According to the U.S. Food and Drug Administration, each year, prescribed medications cause hundreds of thousands of injuries and deaths, making prescription drug mortality a leading cause of death in the United States and generating billions of dollars in additional healthcare costs. A 1998 study reported that 2,216,000 hospitalized patients in the United States had serious adverse drug reactions, and 106,000 had fatal reactions.[109] Adverse events from prescription drug use result in more than 4 million annual visits to emergency departments, doctors' offices, or other outpatient settings, and 117,000 hospitalizations each year. One in ten residents of long-term care facilities experience an adverse drug event every month, and between two and six of every 100 hospitalized patients experience adverse drug events.[110] A recent review of studies from around the world concluded that 17 percent of hospitalized patients experience an adverse drug reaction.[111]

Many factors play a role in these injuries and deaths, including the behavior of patients and the practices of healthcare providers and healthcare institutions. The pharmaceutical industry contributes by heavily promoting inadequately tested drugs to manage chronic conditions, both directly to consumers and to physicians. Since many people suffer from these conditions and are often required to take these drugs for extended periods of time, these drugs are highly profitable. For the same reasons, the public health impact of overzealous marketing and inadequate testing can be significant. For example, in 1999, Merck Pharmaceuticals obtained FDA approval to market the pain killer Vioxx (generic name, rofecoxib) to treat arthritis, migraine, and other causes of pain and inflammation. Five years later, after more than $10 billion in sales, Merck withdrew Vioxx from the market because of a study that showed it doubled the risk of heart attacks and strokes in long-term users.[112] By then, more than 20 million people had taken the drug, and thousands may have experienced adverse events, including deaths, attributable to Vioxx.[113] Late in 2007, Merck agreed to pay $4.85 billion to settle 27,000 lawsuits by people who claimed that they or their family members suffered injury or died after taking the drug. Analysts considered the settlement a victory for Merck, limiting its future liability and allowing it to focus on other priorities.[114]

Vioxx's harm was amplified by deceptive advertising. Merck marketing promised that Vioxx would bring pain relief to people with arthritis without the gastrointestinal side effects associated with other medications. Over six years, Merck spent more than $500 million advertising Vioxx to consumers, and in 2003 alone, more than $500 million on Vioxx ads to physicians,[115,116] promoting the message of fewer side effects than similar drugs.[117] In 2009, however, the Massachusetts researcher who had authored the studies used to justify this claim admitted that the data in some or all of his 21 journal articles reporting these results had been fabricated.[118]

In 2010, GlaxoSmithKline's diabetes drug Avandia (generic name, rosiglitazone) was taken off the market in Europe because the European Medicines Agency determined the "benefits no longer outweigh the risks." One study published in the *New England Journal of Medicine* found that Avandia increased patients' chance of heart attack by 43 percent and cardiac-related death by 64 percent.[119] Nevertheless, 60 million prescriptions for Avandia had been written between 1999 and 2007. In 2012, Glaxo agreed to plead guilty to criminal charges and pay $3 billion in fines for failing to report safety data about Avandia to the FDA and for promoting its best-selling antidepressants for unapproved uses. The agreement also includes civil penalties for improper marketing of a half-dozen other drugs.[120] The Justice Department charged the company with unlawfully promoting antidepressants to children and for weight loss, helping to prepare misleading medical journal articles to support its case, and entertaining doctors with ski trips and pheasant hunts.[121] In 2013, Glaxo agreed to pay $229 million to settle lawsuits in which several U.S. states accused the drug maker of deceptively marketing Avandia.[122] Despite these continuing setbacks, a month earlier an FDA panel voted to ease the restrictions on Avandia, partially reversing its 2010 vote. Dr. Steven Nissen, the lead author of the *New England Journal of Medicine* study that led to the 2010 action, attributed the partial reversal to "a bureaucracy that never wants to admit it made a mistake. It is tragic for public health that the people who approve the drug in the first place (the FDA) remain to act against the drug. It's like a parent admitting their child is ugly."[123]

As Table 2.1 shows, other pharmaceutical companies paid large fines for improper marketing of drugs, suggesting a calculation that the profits from

Table 2.1 Largest Settlements Reached Between the United States Department of Justice and Pharmaceutical Companies from 2001 to 2012

Company	Settlement	Violation(s)	Year	Product(s)	Laws allegedly violated
GlaxoSmithKline	$3 billion	Off-label promotion/ failure to disclose safety data	2012	Avandia/Wellbutrin/ Paxil	FCA/FDCA
Abbott Laboratories	$1.5 billion	Off-label promotion	2012	Depakote	FCA/FDCA
Amgen	$762 million	Off-label promotion/kickbacks	2012	Aranesp	FCA/FDCA
GlaxoSmithKline	$750 million	Poor manufacturing practices	2010	Kytril/Bactroban/ Paxil CR/ Avandamet	FCA/FDCA
Allergan	$600 million	Off-label promotion	2010	Botox	FCA/FDCA
Novartis	$423 million	Off-label promotion/kickbacks	2010	Trileptal	FCA/FDCA
AstraZeneca	$520 million	Off-label promotion/kickbacks	2010	Seroquel	FCA
Eli Lilly	$1.4 billion	Off-label promotion	2009	Zyprexa	FCA/FDCA
Pfizer	$2.3 billion	Off-label promotion/kickbacks	2009	Bextra/Geodon/ Zyvox/Lyrica	FCA/FDCA
Merck	$650 million	Medicare fraud/kickbacks	2008	Zocor/Vioxx/ Pepsid	FCA/Medicaid Rebate Statute
Cephalon	$425 million	Off-label promotion	2008	Actiq/Gabitril/ Provigil	FCA/FDCA
Purdue Pharma	$601 million	Off-label promotion	2007	Oxycontin	FCA

Company	Amount	Violation	Year	Drug(s)	Statute
Bristol-Myers Squibb	$515 million	Off-label promotion/kickbacks/Medicare fraud	2007	Abilify/Serzone	FCA/FDCA
Schering-Plough	$435 million	Off-label promotion/kickbacks/Medicare fraud	2006	Temodar/Intron A/K-Dur/Claritin RediTabs	FCA/FDCA
Serono	$704 million	Off-label promotion/kickbacks/monopoly practices	2005	Serostim	FCA
Pfizer	$430 million	Off-label promotion	2004	Neurontin	FCA/FDCA
Schering-Plough	$345 million	Medicare fraud/kickbacks	2004	Claritin	FCA/Anti-Kickback Statute
AstraZeneca	$355 million	Medicare fraud	2003	Zoladex	Prescription Drug Marketing Act
Schering-Plough	$500 million	Poor manufacturing practices	2002	Claritin	FDA Current Good Manufacturing Practices
TAP Pharmaceutical Products	$875 million	Medicare fraud/kickbacks	2001	Lupron	FCA/ Prescription Drug Marketing Act

Notes: FCA = False Claims Act; FDCA = federal Food, Drug, and Cosmetic Act.

Sources: "Abbott Labs to pay $1.5 billion to resolve criminal and civil investigations of off-label promotion of Depakote." Justice.gov. May 7, 2012. Available at: http://www.justice-gov/opa/pr/2012/May/12-civ-585.html. Accessed on April 28, 2013.

Almashat S, Preston C, Waterman T, Wolfe S. Rapidly Increasing Criminal and Civil Monetary Penalties Against the Pharmaceutical Industry: 1991–2010, Public Citizen's Health Research Group, December 16, 2010. Available at: http://www.citizen.org/documents/rapidlyincreasingcriminalandcivilpenalties.pdf. Last accessed on April 27, 2013.

"Amgen Inc. pleads guilty to federal charge in Brooklyn, NY; Pays $762 Million to Resolve Criminal Liability and False Claims Act Allegations." Justice.gov. December 19, 2012. http://www.justice.gov/opa/pr/2012/December/12-civ-1523.html. Accessed on April 28, 2013.

Goldacre B. *Bad Pharma: How Drug Companies Mislead Doctors and Harm Patients.* New York, Faber & Faber, 2013.

Thomas K, Schmidt MS. "Glaxo agrees to pay $3 Billion in fraud settlement." *New York Times*, July 3, 2012, p. A1.

illegal marketing make such fines an acceptable cost of business. "What we're learning is that money doesn't deter corporate malfeasance," observed Eliot Spitzer, who, as New York's Attorney General, sued GlaxoSmithKline in 2004 over similar accusations involving Paxil. "The only thing that will work in my view is C.E.O.'s and officials being forced to resign and individual culpability being enforced."[124]

Other drugs withdrawn from the market because of safety concerns include Eli Lilly's Darvon, a painkiller pulled because of concerns about heart toxicity,[125] and Abbott's Cylert (pemoline) a medication used to treat attention-deficit hyperactivity disorder (ADHD) pulled in 2005 due to concerns about its contribution to deaths from liver failure.[126] In these cases, the drug industry's desire to get or keep profitable products on the market led them to inadequate pre- or post-marketing testing.

As Table 2.1 shows, several drug companies encouraged doctors to use their drugs for purposes other than those approved by the FDA, a potentially dangerous—and illegal—practice. For example, in 2004, Warner Lambert, then a division of Pfizer, pled guilty to criminal charges and agreed to pay $430 million to settle the charges that it had illegally promoted Neurotonin (gabapentin), a drug approved by the FDA for control of certain types of seizures in people who have epilepsy.[127] Among the conditions for which the manufacturer encouraged doctors to prescribe Neurotonin were bipolar disorder, peripheral neuropathy, diabetic neuropathy, complex regional pain syndrome, attention deficit disorder, restless legs syndrome, trigeminal neuralgia, periodic limb movement disorder of sleep, migraine headaches, and alcohol withdrawal syndrome, none supported by the literature. A year later, the U.S. Department of Justice official testified before Congress that it had begun 180 separate investigations of off-label marketing by drug companies.[128]

The drug industry's pervasive misrepresentation of scientific evidence on drug efficacy and widespread marketing of drugs for off-label use harms not only the patients and their providers who end up misusing these drugs, but also the public at large. As one major drug company after another pleads guilty to these illegal practices or settles court cases with penalties of hundreds of millions or billions of dollars, it becomes harder for patients and doctors to trust even the drugs that are effective. Doubts about treatment efficacy or pharmaceutical industry integrity can increase non-compliance, putting patients at risk of inadequate treatment for many conditions.

Non-compliance with prescribed medications has been estimated to cost $100 to $300 billion a year and to contribute to 125,000 deaths annually.[129] Some portion of these human and financial costs are another example of an industry willing to sacrifice its credibility by breaking the law and then transferring the costs of its harmful practices onto taxpayers and the general public.

Pharmaceutical companies can also contribute to avoidable illnesses by their pricing practices. In the United States, millions of people cannot afford the high prices for prescription drugs for their asthma, diabetes, heart disease, or cancer, leading to under-treatment and missed opportunities for prevention and early intervention and thus higher costs for chronic disease care. In 2012, prescription drug prices surged 13 percent, far higher than the increase in inflation. In that same year, 45 percent of people under age 65 who do not have insurance coverage for prescriptions said they had not filled a prescription in the last year because of the cost, almost double the rate of those reporting this problem the previous year.[130] By one estimate, 150 million prescriptions a year go unfilled because of cost,[131,132] a clear sign of a market failure to meet a social need.

The revenues from popular patent-protected drugs constitute the lifeblood of pharmaceutical profits, so the industry looks to maintain this flow by charging exorbitant prices for needed medications and discouraging or preventing the release of more affordable generic drugs. Drug companies often justify the high prices they charge by claiming high research and development costs, but in fact many drugs are developed by federally funded, university-based researchers,[133] and many of the costs they call "research" are in fact marketing. And at least until the current economic crisis, drug companies reported among the highest profit levels of any industry sector.

Whatever the cause, high prices put life-saving drugs out of the reach of people who need them, especially in the developing world. As we have seen, high prices also contribute to patients' not taking prescribed medicines, a practice that contributes to worsening of chronic diseases such as diabetes or hypertension, especially among lower-income patients, and to drug-resistance to treatments of infectious diseases.

Another industry practice that contributes to unnecessary or harmful drug use is to define a common social problem as a medical problem, publicize and exaggerate its seriousness, then market a drug that can "solve" this problem, a process described as "disease-mongering."[134] Examples include male pattern baldness (treated by Rogaine), social anxiety disorders (treated by Paxil or Zoloft), and female sexual dysfunction (treated by various hormone therapies, including a testosterone patch).[135,136] These new drugs divert pharmaceutical companies' research and development from other drugs that could help control ailments that truly jeopardize global health—malaria and tuberculosis, for example—to ones that promise generous profits from wealthier consumers for treating problems of modern living.

Some of these drugs also have side effects. After GlaxoSmithKline obtained FDA approval to market Paxil for the new condition "social anxiety disorder," it immediately hired a public relations firm, Cohn & Wolfe, to "educate" the public about this condition. A year later, the PR firm boasted of generating 1.1 billion media impressions for the conditions and its treatment in just one year.[137] Unfortunately, it later turned out that as many as one in four Paxil users suffered withdrawal from the drug when they tried to stop its use.[138]

In recent years, drug companies have found new ways to extend the patent protections that allow them to charge higher prices. In her book *The Truth about Drug Companies*, Dr. Marcia Angell, former editor of the *New England Journal of Medicine*, describes how drug companies have used various strategies to extend their exclusive marketing rights on profitable drugs. These include making minor changes in the formulation to get extra years of protection, filing for multiple patents to extend protection or generate lawsuits that can delay the end of protection, or testing the drug in children, which extends patent protection, whether or not children are likely to benefit from a drug.[139] They have also engaged in "pay for delay," whereby a big drug company will pay a generic maker or smaller company not to release a generic brand for several years, allowing the original patent holder to keep prices high for longer. The Congressional Budget Office estimated in 2011 that making pay for delay illegal could save the government almost $5 billion over 10 years and lower drug costs in the United States by $11 billion.[140]

In 2012, in a case that involved a drug manufactured by the Schering-Plough Corporation, a federal court in Philadelphia ruled that pay for delay was inherently anti-competitive. Eleanor M. Fox, an antitrust expert and professor at the New York University Law School told the *New York Times* that the court's finding that agreements between generic and branded drug manufacturers "are cases of competitor collaboration, which the Supreme Court has called 'the supreme evil of antitrust.' "[141] In 2013, the U.S. Supreme Court ruled that pharmaceutical companies can be sued for paying rivals not to release lower-cost drugs.[142]

Around the world, the pharmaceutical industry is growing, albeit more slowly after the 2008 financial crisis than before. Spending for prescription drugs in the United States was six times higher in 2008 than in 1990, making it one of the fastest growing components of the nation's healthcare costs.[143] Between 2010 and 2019, retail sales of prescription drugs in the United States are expected to increase by 176 percent.[144] Between 2010 and 2015, the revenues from the global over-the-counter pharmaceutical industry are expected to increase by 20 percent,[145] while in the same period, the global pharmaceuticals, biotechnology, and life sciences industries are expected to increase in market value by 40 percent.[146] These trends, combined with the increasing rates of chronic conditions that require long-term pharmaceutical treatment, suggest that the problems associated with increased pharmaceutical use will continue to grow. As in the case of other industries, the increased consolidation of the global pharmaceutical industry will give it the resources needed to continue aggressive marketing and lobbying to thwart or delay more stringent global regulation that could reduce its most harmful practices.

Defenders of Big Pharma argue that any effort to regulate its practices more closely risks strangling the goose that lays the golden life-saving eggs that global health requires. This argument that society needs to choose between risky business as usual and jeopardizing human progress, a favorite of producers of legal but lethal products, ignores that the status quo is the result of political decisions that humans made—and can unmake.

From Evidence to Action: Reducing the Harm from Business Practices

The practices of the food, tobacco, alcohol, automobile, firearms, and pharmaceutical industries sicken, injure, and kill people prematurely in different ways. Clearly, the products themselves play very different roles in our lives. Food and pharmaceuticals enhance health and are essential for modern living. In moderation, automobiles and alcohol can make our lives easier and less stressful, making them an important part of everyday life for people around the world. Tobacco and firearms, on the other hand, kill people if used as directed, although firearms have other uses such as for hunting and crime deterrence, and are sanctioned for some types of killing, such as in war, state killing, and self-defense.

Yet these six industries share two common characteristics. First, all contribute substantially to the rising global burden of chronic diseases and injuries, as summarized in the table below. Table 2.2 shows that the products of these industries contribute annually to several hundred thousand premature deaths in the United States and to several million deaths globally. Of course, not all these deaths are directly attributable to corporate practices—consumer behavior, government policy, and other factors also play a role. But the magnitude of the carnage makes it imperative to consider the role of corporations, the prime source of these lethal products.

Moreover, the relatively small number of multinational corporations makes the task of changing their products and practices at least theoretically feasible. Another important reason for changing corporate practices in order to improve health is their dominant role in another major cause of the twenty-first-century epidemics. Public health researchers have identified growing income inequality and the widening gap between the power and status of the wealthiest one percent of the population and everyone else as major causes of global ill health.[147,148] Finding the links between these two defining characteristics of modern capitalism—risky products and business practices and growing income and

Table 2.2 **Annual U.S. and Global Deaths Attributable to Products and Practices of Selected Consumer Industries[a]**

Industry	Main Health Conditions Related to Products and Practices	Estimated Annual US Deaths in 2005[b]	Estimated Global Annual Deaths, 2010 Source: [c unless otherwise noted]
Tobacco	Heart disease, lung and other cancers, respiratory diseases	467,000	6,297,287 (includes exposure to second-hand smoke)
Food and beverages	Obesity, diabetes, heart disease, some cancers	216,000 deaths attributed to overweight/ obesity	3,371,232 (attributed to high Body Mass Index)[d]
Alcohol	Accidents, homicides, liver cancer, cirrhosis	64,000	4,860,168
Motor vehicles	Injuries, respiratory diseases including cancer, heart disease	43,667[e]	1,300,000 (from collision injuries)[f] 3,223,540 (from particulate matter air pollution, of which motor vehicles are largest contributor)
Firearms	Homicide, suicide, unin- tended injuries	30,694[b]	500,000, of which 300,000 are conflict-related and 200,000 homicides, suicides and accidents[g] (2000)
Pharma- ceuticals	Over and under medication	128,000 deaths from fatal drug reactions in 2011[h]	Not available

[a]US estimates come from reports from the US Centers for Disease Control and the global ones from the World Health Organization, unless otherwise noted. Missing data and the difficulties of attributing cause to a particular product contribute to some uncertainty. Some observers believe some of these estimates exaggerate the specified death toll (e.g., Kopel DB, Gallant P, Eisen JD. Global deaths from firearms: Searching for plausible estimates. *Texas Review of Law & Politics.* 2003;8(1):113–141), but most believe that the uncertainties lead to underestimates of the impact.

[b]Danaei G, Ding EL, Mozaffarian D, Taylor B, Rehm J, et al. The Preventable Causes of Death in the United States: Comparative Risk Assessment of Dietary, Lifestyle, and Metabolic Risk Factors. *PLoS Med.* 2009;6(4):e1000058. doi:10.1371/journal.pmed.1000058

[c]Lim SS, Vos T, Flaxman AD, Danaei G, Shibuya K, Adair-Rohani H, et al. A comparative risk assessment of burden of disease and injury attributable to 67 risk factors and risk factor clusters in 21 regions, 1990–2010: a systematic analysis for the Global Burden of Disease Study 2010. *Lancet.* 2013;380(9859):2224–2260.

[d]Does not include deaths attributed to high sodium diet (3,104,308 deaths); high sugar sweetened beverage consumption (299,521 deaths); or high trans fatty acid consumption (515,260 deaths).

[e]Kung HC, Hoyert DL, Xu JQ, Murphy SL. Deaths: Final data for 2005. *National Vital Statistics Reports.* 2008;56(10). Hyattsville, MD: National Center for Health Statistics.

[f]Mathers CD, Boerma T, Fat DM. Global and regional causes of death. *British Medical Bulletin.* 2009;92:7–32.

[g]Cukier W. *Small Arms and Light Weapons: A Public Health Approach. World Aff.* 2002(9):261:263.

[h]QuarterWatch: Monitoring FDA MedWatch Reports. Institute for Safe Medicine Practices. Available at: http://www.ismp.org/quarterwatch/pdfs/2011Q4.pdf. Published May 31, 2012. Accessed August 14. 2012.

power inequalities—has the potential to inform the policies and politics that can overcome rising rates of premature deaths and preventable illnesses and injuries.

A second common characteristic of all six industries is that they have used many of the same strategies to advance their business interests at the expense of public health. They use modern science and technology to seek profits in ways that harm health. They design and aggressively promote products without adequately testing their impact on health They make false or misleading claims about the health benefits of their products and minimize the known harms or seek to obfuscate the science that demonstrates this harm. They price unhealthy products cheaply to maximize their market penetration, but charge high prices that put healthy products out of reach of many who need them. They transfer—externalize—the costs of their harmful practices onto consumers and taxpayers, allowing the companies to keep their prices low and profits high, but bankrupting the governments and families who need to pay for health care or environmental cleanups. They encourage lifestyles and patterns of consumption known to harm population health, especially to vulnerable populations such as children. They elicit brand loyalty for risky blockbuster products by appealing to customers' fears, insecurities and addictions. They undermine regulations and standards designed to protect public health or the environment when these protections are perceived to jeopardize profits or market share. And they distort democracy by using campaign contributions and lobbying to overcome popular support for stronger public health protections.

In pursuing these strategies, these industries are following not the rules of the Better Business Bureau but the playbook written over the twentieth century by tobacco corporations and their allies, the pariah industry that has killed more people than any dictator or war in history. These common strategies of the corporate consumption complex now challenge the ability of the United States, other nations, and the World Health Organization to respond effectively to emerging threats to health and to achieve the health goals they have promulgated.

At the conclusion of the 2011 UN High-Level Meeting on Non-Communicable Diseases, many participants celebrated the progress. One WHO official said the meeting was a "great achievement" because it succeeded in "elevating NCD prevention from a health priority to a development priority."[149] An Australian public health researcher observed,

> Overall, the UN meeting has consolidated steadily growing global concern about NCDs and articulated what is known and the kinds of action that must be taken. The huge increase in interest in these conditions by governments, health agencies, non-government organizations and academia in the past seven years is deeply encouraging, especially when competing worries such as climate change and economic

instability could have easily displaced NCDs from both national and international agendas.[150]

But underneath the hopeful sound bites, some participants sounded more pessimistic. Some delegates objected to the substantial industry presence in the planning process and at the meeting. In a letter to the *Lancet*, a coalition of 140 health groups warned, "there are clear conflicts for the corporations that contribute to and profit from the sales of alcohol beverages, foods with high fat, sugar and salt content, and tobacco products—all of which are important causes of NCDs." They warned that "failure to address these concerns will undermine the development of competent policy…and the confidence of the global community and the public at large have in the UN's and the WHO's ability to govern and advance public health."[151]

In a speech to the delegates, Dr. Margaret Chan, the WHO director general, used unusually strong language: "I call on heads of state and heads of government to stand rock-hard against the despicable efforts of the tobacco industry to subvert this treaty. We must stand firm against their open and extremely aggressive tactics."[152] Ann Keeling, then chair of the NCD Alliance, a coalition of more than 2,000 civil society groups from 170 countries, called the meeting declaration "a great disappointment."[153]

This disappointment was triggered in part by the revelation that, even before the meeting, industry lobbyists and their government supporters had watered down the declaration that the delegates would consider. As revealed by investigations by *Lancet* and the *British Medical Journal,* government and industry representatives from the European Union, the United States, Canada, and Australia had "systematically deleted, diluted and downgraded" stronger commitments and replaced them with vague intentions to "consider" and "work towards change."[154,155]

A few specific debates about the wording of the declaration illustrate the power of corporate interests, even at an international meeting of heads of state and top health officials. The health experts who drafted the final declaration proposed to use the word "epidemic" to describe the skyrocketing rates of increase of NCDs around the world—a seemingly routine use of a well-accepted public health and medical concept, frequently applied to both communicable and non-communicable diseases. But for pharmaceutical companies, that word is not just a word. In 2001, the Doha Declaration, the World Trade Organization's agreement on intellectual property rights, ruled that a poor country could force pharmaceutical companies to let its domestic manufacturers make generic drugs for use in low-income countries in exchange for a smaller royalty, even if that drug still had patent protection.[156] This option enabled governments in countries like Brazil and South Africa to get affordable anti-retroviral HIV medications to their people, an important step in containing the epidemic in these and other countries.

The Doha Declaration allowed suspension of patent protection in the case of HIV, tuberculosis, malaria, and "other epidemics." Now pharmaceutical and other corporations worried that the suspension of patent protection in the case of "epidemics" of NCDs could be a precedent, applying not only to the production and marketing of profitable medicines for diabetes, heart disease, and cancer, but perhaps to other types of trade agreements that protect marketing of food, alcohol, and tobacco against public-health regulation. Corporate interests thus successfully argued against including the single word that could have alerted the world to the magnitude of the crisis from NCDs and also given governments in low-income and emerging nations new tools to combat NCDs. Ultimately, in a Newspeak compromise that would have delighted George Orwell, the negotiators reached agreement to describe NCDs as "a challenge of epidemic proportions."[157]

In another issue related to the declaration's proposals for international regulation of advertising, the developed countries opposed new international restrictions on tobacco advertising. Keeling from the NCD Alliance observed, "I think it is completely immoral that (these countries are) arguing against this for the rest of the world when they have done this to safeguard their own population."[158]

Participants also debated about how to describe the food industry. Was it a target of action, part of the problem, like the tobacco industry, or a partner in deciding the rules? One meeting participant, a longtime health activist, told a *Washington Post* reporter, "Our position is that 'partnership' isn't the right word. It implies trust and respect. The allegiance of the food companies is to create profits. Their voluntary commitments are only good for as long as they want to keep them."[159] Ultimately, the word "partner" stayed in the declaration.

Finally, the health experts wanted to set targets for reducing the prevalence of NCDs and mandate consumer corporations to take specific actions— reformulating food products, setting mandatory standards for advertising, and using taxation to encourage health. Several developed-country delegates, more concerned about protecting their industries than the health of their public, opposed these measures, preferring voluntary partnerships and a more general call for action. They favored this approach both because it did not require specific commitment of resources (a challenge during a time of perceived austerity), and because it ensured that neither governments nor corporations would have any specific accountability for taking action to reduce NCDs. The final declaration did not include any targets and encouraged, but did not mandate, adoption of the evidence-based recommendations for NCD prevention.[160] Later WHO follow-up meetings added targets but did not allocate resources to reach them.

The fact that representatives of the tobacco, food, alcohol, and pharmaceutical industries were able to win major concessions in a global public health agreement that was a statement of principles, not a formal, binding treaty that addressed the world's most serious and expensive public health problem, illustrates the power of corporations to protect their own interests at the expense of public health.

Choosing Strategies to Promote Public Health

To select a strategy for public health improvement, the strategy must meet two criteria. First, it must reduce an important cause of ill health; second, it has to be feasible in the real world. As we have seen, substantial evidence shows that the business and political practices of the major consumer corporations are a significant cause of the health conditions that now threaten world health. Before considering the feasibility of making changes in corporate practices that harm health, let's examine two other approaches to improving health: biomedicine and lifestyle modification. These are the alternatives favored by corporate interests—and by most policymakers.

BIOMEDICINE'S ROLE IN IMPROVING HEALTH

Biomedicine seeks to improve health by changing genetic, biochemical, or structural characteristics of individuals. Lifestyle modification promotes health by encouraging individuals to abandon unhealthy behavior and take up healthier habits. Clearly both of these strategies can play an important role in disease prevention and treatment, but a closer examination shows the limits of their effectiveness and feasibility—and suggests the importance of the third alternative, changing corporate practices.

Biomedical approaches to treating illness are now the dominant way that the United States addresses its health problems. Of the almost $2.6 trillion of public and private health expenditures in the United States in 2010, only about 3 percent was spent on prevention and public health, showing the priority we place on treatment.[161,162,163] This disproportionate spending on treatment has achieved some impressive results: survival rates for many cancers have increased significantly, and improvements in cardiac care have saved millions of lives. One influential study estimates that about half the decline in U.S. deaths from coronary heart disease from 1980 through 2000—a drop that resulted in 341,745 fewer deaths in 2000 than if the 1980 rate had persisted—can be attributed to medical therapies.[164] While almost 15 percent of Americans lacked health insurance in 2012—and thus access to state-of-the art treatment, many insured and better-off Americans benefit from some of the world's best medical care.

But biomedicine has its limitations. Despite advances in molecular and genomic medicine, few observers expect the huge investments we have made in these areas to result in improvements in population health anytime soon. Francis Collins, now the head of the National Institutes of Health and formerly the leader of the publicly funded gene-sequencing efforts, recently noted that ten years after scientists deciphered the human genome, its "consequences for clinical medicine...have thus far been modest...the Human Genome Project has not yet directly affected the health care of most individuals."[165] Some new pharmacotherapies have dramatically improved outcomes for conditions like AIDS and tuberculosis, but most make only modest contributions, and several, as we have seen, have imposed substantial harm. Even when new discoveries do prove effective, it has been difficult to bring these benefits to all who need them. An unintended consequence of some discoveries is the exacerbation of health inequalities, since advances in biomedicine most often go to the better-off who can afford them.

And biomedicine is extraordinarily expensive. According to the National Institute of Health, a single gastric-bypass surgery costs between $12,000 and $35,000, with millions of people worldwide suffering from the extreme obesity that warrants the procedure.[166] In 2006, lung cancer care in the United States cost more than $10 billion; global tobacco-related deaths are expected to be ten times higher in the twenty-first century than in the twentieth.[167] In poor countries and rich ones, healthcare systems now and for the near future lack the science, technology, and operational capacity to genetically engineer, perform surgery, or medicate to reduce the growing human and economic burden of chronic diseases and injuries.

ROLE OF LIFESTYLE-MODIFICATION IN IMPROVING HEALTH

The second strategy that policymakers and researchers advocate is to modify the lifestyles of people who eat, drink, or smoke too much, or pursue other unhealthy habits. Throughout the world, lifestyle change is the dominant public health approach to reducing NCDs. The Political Declaration approved by the UN General Assembly at the NCD meeting recognized "the critical importance of...strengthening the capacity of individuals and populations to make healthier choices and follow lifestyle patterns that foster good health" and vowed to "engage...the private sector and civil society, in collaborative partnerships to promote health and to reduce non-communicable disease risk factors, including through building community capacity in promoting healthy diets and lifestyles."[168]

This strategy has the advantages of preventing illness, rather than waiting for it to develop, and has empirically proven to be an effective tool in making health progress in the last 50 years. The decline in smoking in the United States, a result of prolonged and intensive educational campaigns as well as policy changes like smoking bans and tax increases, illustrates the benefits of comprehensive approaches to behavior change.

But relying on lifestyle change as the primary strategy to reduce the incidence of chronic diseases and injuries has three flaws: it doesn't work very well, it blames the victims rather than the perpetrators of unhealthy lifestyles, and it is profoundly inefficient.

Numerous scientific reviews of the thousands of behavior change studies that researchers have evaluated over the last several decades show that intensive behavioral interventions can bring about changes in diet, physical activity, alcohol use, and risky driving.[169,170,171] However, these often costly programs usually benefit only the fraction of motivated volunteers who actively participate, are difficult to translate from research study into practice, and rarely end up having a measurable impact on overall health. In the relatively successful effort to reduce smoking in the United States, it took more than 40 years to cut the 1965 smoking rate in half. If this pace of change applied to other countries and other chronic diseases, it will doom tens of millions of people to premature and preventable deaths and illnesses.

Corporations claim that individuals choose their unhealthy products and that by producing lethal but legal products they are simply addressing market demands. But as the accounts in this chapter have shown, these companies aggressively market their products based on their customers' fears, insecurities, addictions, and primitive and precognitive urges (e.g., the "reptilian instincts" SUV marketers appeal to).In addition, public or consumer-funded lifestyle modification programs require ordinary people to pay twice: first for treatment of their product-related illnesses, and second, through taxes, for the health education programs to undo or prevent the damage from marketing unhealthy products. It's like being forced to pay the shady auto dealer to repair the lemon car he sold you.

The third and most serious problem with the attempting to change consumers' lifestyles is its inefficiency. Each year, the industries described here spend billions of dollars to persuade people to buy their unhealthy products. Those marketing costs are tax-deductible, recognized by the Internal Revenue Service as legitimate business expenses. And each year, billions of people around the world take up smoking, grow overweight or obese, buy a handgun, or an SUV, or use an inadequately tested but heavily marketed prescription drug.

A public policy that requires government and civil society to persuade each of these billions of individuals to quit smoking, eat or drink less, or avoid risky gun use or driving is literally insane, the irrational act of a society incapable of thinking clearly. To spend billions of dollars each year to persuade people to consume unhealthy products, then to spend a fraction of that to undo the damage that the world's most sophisticated persuaders have wrought is a public health strategy doomed to failure. This approach requires health professionals to become Sisyphus, as shown in Figure 2.2, rolling billions of people with unhealthy lifestyles up the steep hill of behavior change, knowing that

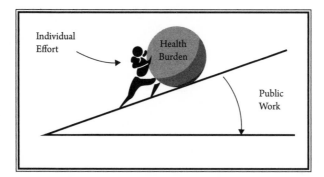

Figure 2.2 Modified from Milstein B. Hygeia's constellation: navigating health futures in a dynamic and democratic world. (Doctoral dissertation.) Cincinnati, OH: Graduate College of Interdisciplinary Arts and Sciences, Union Institute and University; 2006.

only a small fraction will succeed and that an army of new recruits to tobacco, alcohol, and unhealthy food await at the bottom. Even classic capitalist theory recognizes that to allow corporations to externalize their costs contributes to market inefficiencies and unfairly burdens consumers. In a sane world, making behavior change easy by changing the policies and environments that promote disease would be common sense.

ROLE OF CHANGING CORPORATE PRACTICES IN IMPROVING HEALTH

Biomedicine and lifestyle change will always be part of the solution to the growing burden of NCDs and injuries, but each has such severe constraints on effectiveness and cost that it cannot serve as the primary strategy to reverse these twenty-first-century epidemics. This brings us back to the question of the political feasibility of the third strategy: changing corporate practices.

In theory, changing the practice of the few hundred corporations that produce and market most of the world's unhealthy products should not be so difficult. Shouldn't they be able to find ways to make money on healthier products? Shouldn't governments be able to use the same tools they used in the last century to safeguard public health against special interests? Shouldn't social movements and popular outrage force both corporations and governments to take stronger action to prevent premature death and avoidable illnesses?

Sadly, in the last few decades the answers to these questions have been mostly "no." Few societies make a high priority of requiring companies to make healthier choices. For most public officials, this strategy seems too hard, too time-consuming, or too risky. To understand why this promising and effective strategy for improving world health remains a naïve or idealistic aspiration, we need to step back and examine the recent history of multinational corporations.

3

Corporations Take Control

A New Political and Economic Order Emerges

The Powell Memo: Battle Plan for Corporations to Take Back America

On August 23, 1971, Lewis Powell sent a confidential memo to his friend Eugene Sydnor, Jr., the director of the U.S. Chamber of Commerce. The memo was both a call to arms and a battle plan for a business response to its growing legion of opponents. Powell was a corporate lawyer, a former president of the American Bar Association, and a board member of eleven corporations, including Philip Morris and the Ethyl Corporation, a company that made the lead for leaded gasoline. Powell had also represented the Tobacco Institute, the research arm of the tobacco industry, and various tobacco companies.[1] Later that year, President Richard Nixon would nominate Powell to sit on the U.S. Supreme Court, where he served for fifteen years.

Powell's memo serves as a useful starting point for understanding how the transformation of the corporate system that began in the 1970s set the stage for today's global health problems. "No thoughtful person can question that the American economic system is under broad attack," wrote Powell. "The assault on the enterprise system is broadly based and consistently pursued. It is gaining momentum and converts."[2] "One of the bewildering paradoxes of our time," Powell continued, "is the extent to which the enterprise system tolerates, if not participates in, its own destruction." He enumerated the system's enemies: well-meaning liberals, government officials intent on regulating business, news media, student activists, and an emerging environmental and consumer movement—especially its most visible leader, Ralph Nader (Figure 3.1), in Powell's view "the single most effective antagonist of American business."[3]

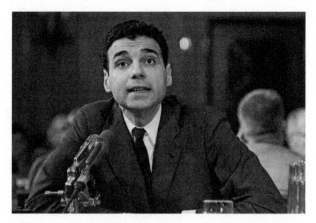

Figure 3.1 Ralph Nader Testifying Before the Senate, 1967. Corbis Images.

Powell called on business, especially the Chamber of Commerce, to end its "appeasement" of its critics and launch an aggressive and systematic counter-assault. The memo warned that "independent and uncoordinated activity by individual corporations, as important as this is, will not be sufficient. Strength lies in organization, in careful long-range planning and implementation, in consistency of action over an indefinite period of years ... and in the political power available only though united action and national organizations."[4]

Powell urged new, well-funded public media campaigns to support the free enterprise system, the creation of think tanks and institutes to develop policy proposals and "direct political action" in legislative and judicial arenas. "It is time," he argued, for "American business ... to apply their great talents vigorously to the preservation of the system itself."[5] Powell's "confidential" memo was first circulated within the Chamber of Commerce, then released in 1972 by investigative reporter Jack Anderson during the Powell Supreme Court confirmation hearings. While the document may not have been the blueprint for the rise of the Republican right that some analysts claim,[6] its real value is as the articulation of the corporate prescription for capitalism's ills.

Today, more than forty years after business took up Powell's appeal, its success in achieving the goals he laid out makes it hard to fathom the depth of his concern. But the early 1970s were a high point for several public-interest movements that personified and amplified a growing opposition to business dominance. In addition, the recent victories of the civil rights and antiwar movements, coupled with the emergence of the women's and environmental movements, meant change was in the air. Millions of Americans had shown their willingness to protest, demonstrate, and oppose corporate consumerism, so corporate leaders were understandably worried about their future.

Table 3.1 **National Legislation and New Agencies Created on Environmental, Occupational, and Consumer Protection, 1960–1980**

President John F Kennedy 1960–1963, 4 laws

Federal Hazardous Substances Act, 1960

Color Additive Amendment, 1960

Kefauver-Harris Drug Amendments to the Pure Food and Drug Act of 1906, 1962

Air Pollution Control Act, 1962

President Lyndon Johnson 1963–1968, 14 laws and 2 agencies

Water Quality Act, 1965

Noise Control Act, 1965

Solid Waste Disposal Act, 1965

National Traffic and Motor Vehicle Safety Act, 1966

Highway Safety Bureau, 1966

Fair Packaging and Labeling Act, 1966

Child Protection Act, 1966

Wholesome Meat Act, 1967

Flammable Fabrics Act, 1967

Air Quality Act, 1967

National Commission on Product Safety, 1967

Fire Research and Safety Act, 1968

Natural Gas Pipeline Safety Act, 1968

Consumer Credit Protection Act, 1968

Gun Control Act, 1968

Interstate Land Sales Full Disclosure Act, 1968

President Richard Nixon 1969–1974, 19 laws and 5 agencies

Coal Miners' Health and Safety Act, 1969

Child Protection and Toy Safety Act, 1969

Consumer Product Safety Act, 1970

Fair Credit Reporting Act, 1970

Water Pollution Control Act, 1970

Truth in Lending Act Amendments, 1970

Poison Prevention Packaging Act, 1970

Clean Air Act, 1970

National Environmental Policy Act, 1970

Environmental Protection Agency, 1970

Council on Environmental Quality, 1970

National Oceanic and Atmospheric Administration, 1970

Occupational Safety and Health Administration, 1970

Marine Protection, Research, and Sanctuaries Act, 1972

Water Pollution Control Act Amendments, 1972

(*continued*)

Table 3.1 (**Continued**)

Coastal Zone Management Act, 1972;

Insecticide, Fungicide, Rodenticide Act, 1972

Consumer Product Safety Commission, 1972

Endangered Species Act of, 1973

Safe Drinking Water Act, 1974

Equal Credit Opportunity Act, 1974

Fair Credit Billing Act, 1974

Freedom of Information Act, 1974

Magnuson-Moss Warranty Act, 1974

President Gerald Ford 1974–1976, 4 laws

Federal Trade Commission Improvement Act, 1975

Hazardous Waste Transportation Act, 1975

Resource Conservation and Recovery Act, 1976

Toxic Substances Control Act, 1976

President Jimmy Carter 1977–1980, 8 laws

Water Pollution Control Act Amendments (Clean Water Act), 1977

Soil and Water Conservation Act, 1977

Surface Mining Control and Reclamation Act, 1977

Fair Debt Collection Practices Act, 1977

National Energy Act, 1978

Endangered American Wilderness Act, 1978

Antarctic Conservation Act, 1978

Comprehensive Environmental Response, Compensation, and Liability Act, commonly known as the Superfund Act (1980)

Sources for table: Cohen LA. *A Consumers' Republic: The Politics of Mass Consumption in Postwar America.* New York: Vintage Books; 2003, p. 360; and William Kovarik's *Environmental History Timeline,* available at http://www.environmentalhistory.org./.

These fears were amplified by legislative action. Between 1960 and 1980, as shown in Table 3.1, under three Democratic and two Republican presidents, Congress passed an astonishing forty-nine laws that gave consumers, workers, and the environment new protection. These new laws, and the agencies that implemented them, governed the practices of the auto, alcohol, firearms, food, pharmaceutical, and tobacco industries, discussed previously, as well as every other industry in America. While each law had limitations, and many were inadequately enforced, together they constituted a sea change in government and corporate relations and signaled the willingness of both Republicans and Democrats to expand the rights and protections of consumers. After 1980, new regulations were of course still promulgated, but at a much slower pace, and many of the new laws limited or rolled back those passed in the previous two decades.

New organizations, such as Common Cause and Friends of the Earth, emerged to bring middle-class opposition to harmful business practices to Washington. Ralph Nader, Powell's nemesis, founded a myriad of groups, including the Center for Auto Safety, the Corporate Accountability Project, the Center for Responsive Law, and the Public Citizen Litigation Group—all to create what Mark Green, a Nader protégé, called "a government in exile" that "waged a crusade against official malfeasance, consumer fraud and environmental degradation."[7] Nader's 1965 book, *Unsafe at Any Speed*, an exposé of the auto industry, and Rachel Carson's 1962 *Silent Spring*, a critique of pesticide use, alerted millions of Americans to the harmful health consequences of certain corporate practices.

Powell's memo emphasized the domestic threats to corporate America, but abroad, even more pervasive challenges to United States–based corporate control were emerging. First, following the devastation of World War II, Japan and Germany had rebuilt their economies. Between 1950 and 1980, real annual per capita growth in gross national product went up by 7.4 percent in Japan and 4.9 percent in West Germany—but only by 2 percent in the United States.[8] Fueled by this rapid growth, Japanese, German, and other European corporations began to compete with U.S. companies for global markets and profits. In the auto industry, for example, in 1953, the United States made 70 percent of the world's motor vehicles; by 1968, this share was down to 38 percent.[9]

Over the next four decades, the increasing globalization of multinational corporations forced U.S. companies to develop new strategies for increasing profits. This globalization of capital also changed how U.S. companies interacted with the U.S. government, ultimately diminishing government influence on companies. By 2008, shortly before the start of the economic crisis, *Business Week* observed that, "in effect, U.S. multinationals have been decoupling from the U.S. economy in the last decade. They still have their headquarters in America, they're still listed on U.S. stock exchanges and most of their shareholders are still American. But their expansion has been mainly overseas."[10] As economic pressures forced corporate managers to let go of patriotism that may have motivated earlier decisions, their concern for the well-being of the American people and its economy declined.

The early 1970s also brought the first of several energy crises, precipitated by declines in energy production in the United States and by the growing power of oil-producing states to set energy prices. Rising oil prices contributed to a global economic downturn, ending two decades of American prosperity during which U.S. national income had nearly doubled and the size of the middle class had expanded significantly. A stock market crash in 1973–1974 further contributed to a global economic downturn, alarming investors and corporate owners.

It was in response to these national and international threats that corporate America devised a new game plan, designed to restore corporations' ability to advance their political and economic agendas. No single individual or organization had the power to shape this response, but Powell's memo clearly laid out a comprehensive agenda that could mobilize American business to take on its challengers.

Corporations' Rise to Dominance: From the Early Years to the 1970s and 1980s

Responding to changing economic and political conditions was nothing new for corporations; they had long been an essential component of American society and had learned how to adapt to modifications in the political climate. Corporations were first created in the late seventeenth century in Holland, Great Britain, and elsewhere to mobilize capital for public development projects such as railroads or shipping canals that were too big for individual investors, and for colonization. In the mid–nineteenth century, they played an important role in creating the infrastructures for American industrialization, and by the late nineteenth century, they had become central players in the American economy. Later, through federal legislation, they received additional legal protections such as limited liability, constitutional protections, and extended lifespan. By the end of the twentieth century, most observers across the political spectrum agreed that corporations dominated the global economy and served as the principal agents for modern capitalism.[11,12,13,14]

In some periods, corporations and their allies were more successful in achieving their business and political objectives than others. In the 1880s, for example, the "robber barons"—the corporate leaders of the steel, oil, and railroad industries—were able to win new government protection for trusts; and in the 1920s, prior to the Great Depression, business persuaded the federal government to keep taxes low, tariffs high, and regulation weak. At other times, popular movements won important victories from business, including the creation of the Food and Drug Administration in 1906, the right for workers to organize labor unions, and, during the New Deal, the creation of new regulatory agencies such as the Securities and Exchange Commission and the Federal Communications Commission. In 1936, campaigning for reelection, Franklin D. Roosevelt articulated this populist theme, "We now know that government by organized money is just as dangerous as government by organized mob."[15] Even in these more populist moments, however, corporate leaders were able to play major roles in structuring reforms and government regulations to ensure that their long-term interests were not sacrificed.

On one hand, the orchestrated corporate response to the domestic and global political and economic crises of the 1970s was simply corporations taking care of business as usual. Different were the concurrent changes in the economy, technology, and politics, which gave corporations powerful new tools to bring to their counter-offensive. New discoveries in information and communications such as computers, mobile phones, and later the Internet, made it easier to plan and coordinate national and global campaigns and to move capital and production around the world. Air transport and containerized shipping created the conditions for global consumer markets. Professions such as public relations, advertising, and lobbying developed sophisticated new techniques that enabled corporations to mobilize support for their economic and political goals.

At the same time, many of the countervailing powers that had in earlier times challenged corporate advances were in decline. Changes in family structure and job opportunities allowed corporations to take over what had been family responsibilities: McDonald's replaced Mom's cooking, TV became the new baby sitter, and Hollywood and Madison Avenue taught children about food, shopping, sex, and relationships.

Other institutions also lost influence to corporations. Patients learned about new drugs from advertisements rather than from their family doctor or local pharmacist. Churches and faith organizations, which had been an arena for social interactions, and sometimes offered critiques of unrestrained markets, lost parishioners to the mall, or decided to endorse wealth as the new virtue. Labor unions declined in membership and political influence. In the mid-1950s, more than a third of U.S. private sector workers belonged to labor unions; by 2005 this had declined to less than 10 percent.[16] Political parties, in the past a limited avenue for popular participation in politics, became increasingly professionalized and subject to the influence of wealthy campaign contributors and lobbyists.

The mass media, at times a powerful critic of corporate excess, also came under the control of big business. Large media conglomerates such as Disney, National Amusements, Time Warner, Viacom, News Corp., Bertelsmann AG, Sony, and General Electric took over television, radio, book publishing, movies, music, and other media and often shared directors or owners with other companies, reducing any impetus for journalistic investigations of harmful corporate practices.[17] Later, the Internet, increasingly dominated by big corporations and advertisers, replaced more intimate and face-to-face forms of communication.

Together, these changes helped clear the playing field for the amplified corporate voice that Lewis Powell had urged in his memo. As the public-interest movements that had alarmed Powell and his allies waned in the late 1970s and especially after the election of Ronald Reagan in 1980, big business again became the dominant voice in social and economic policy and politics, as it had been in the 1880s and 1920s.

In the short term, the Powell memo and the point of view it represented led to rapid changes. The Chamber of Commerce soon "doubled its membership, tripled its budget and stepped up its lobbying efforts"[18] in Washington, where it became the dominant corporate voice. In 1971, the National Association of Manufacturers, the voice of corporate producers, moved from Cincinnati to Washington, D.C., where it, too, played a growing role in public policy. In 1971, 175 companies had registered lobbyists in the capital; by 1982, the number had increased to almost 2,500. Between 1976 and the mid-1980s, the number of corporate political action committees (PACs) increased from 300 to more than 1,200.

Several new business-friendly think tanks were established, including the Heritage Foundation and the Cato Institute, and during the 1970s, the American Enterprise Institute, another Washington-based business-friendly organization, increased its staff from ten to 125 and its budget from $1 million to $8 million. Business leaders also created more activist organizations designed expressly to change policy, including the Business Roundtable and the American Legislative Exchange Council.[19] As journalist Bill Moyers wrote in 2011, these responses to Powell's call "triggered an economic transformation that would in time touch every aspect of our lives."[20]

How Economic Change Led to Changes in Health

From their inception, the primary objective of corporations was to make money for their investors. Until the changes that began in the 1970s, however, social, political, and economic factors constrained corporations and limited their impact on people's day-to-day lives outside the factory gates. Several key developments set the stage for this transformation.

SHORT-TERMISM

"Short-termism" describes the emphasis on investors' getting a return on investment quickly—in a few quarters or years rather than in decades. As capital became more mobile and companies extended their global reach, investors had more opportunities to look for higher rates of return. "Shareholder value" became the new mantra for corporate managers, and executives who failed to meet earnings goals had their salaries docked or lost their jobs. Managers were forced to focus on cost-cutting, quarterly returns, and short-term quick fixes to boost revenues. For the corporation itself, too many disappointing quarters led to a loss of investors and fears of takeover.

In an oft-quoted 1981 speech, General Electric CEO Jack Welch laid out the principles. The questions companies need to ask during what he called "slow growth" periods, he told financial analysts meeting at the Pierre Hotel in New York City, were "how big and how fast" a company could grow. "Management and companies that hang on to losers for whatever reason, tradition, sentiment, their own management weaknesses, won't be around in 1990." "Neutron Jack" practiced what he preached: each year he fired the managers with the lowest returns, ensuring a sharp focus on the bottom line.[21] This focus often had an impact on health: the Big Three auto companies chose to invest heavily in polluting SUVs because these vehicles produced windfall profits that kept investors happy— even as they contributed to the longer term decline of the auto industry. In this environment, concerns about the long-term safety of new products or the sustainability of a production practice inevitably lost precedence to profitability.

FINANCIALIZATION

"Financialization" has been defined as a "pattern of accumulation in which profit making occurs increasingly through financial channels rather than through trade and commodity production."[22] As investor demand for profit increased, the returns on investments in mortgages, derivatives, or commodities futures were higher than for those in industries that produced goods or services. This increased the demand for short-term results in the traditional industries and contributed to rapid acquisition and selling of companies. Increased use of leveraged buyouts, junk bonds, and hedge funds were among the consequences of the increasing financialization of corporate America. Between 1990 and 2010, the financial sector's share of total corporate profits doubled in the United States, reaching as high as 44 per cent in 2002.[23] The fast growth and high profits in this sector exacerbated the pressure on consumer corporations to match these returns or risk losing capital to these more promising investments. Over time, companies that made products to sell to consumers lost ground to companies that bought and sold risk, depending on these new financial firms for investment and loans. Maximizing shareholder value often trumped holding on to long-term customers, leading to more volatile markets and ever more urgent quests for blockbuster products that would please investors even if they harmed consumers.

The story of the leveraged buyout of RJR Nabisco, a leading tobacco and food company, told by Bryan Burrough and John Helyar in their book *Barbarians at the Gate*, shows how companies became more concerned with making deals than with making products. In 1988, Henry Kravis, one of the originators and a master of leveraged buyouts, took on RJR Nabisco CEO Ross Johnson in a battle for control of the corporation that had made its fortune from selling tobacco (Camel and Winston), alcohol (Heublein Spirits, maker of Smirnoff vodka and Don Q Rum) and processed food (Oreos and Mallomars). The drama featured a cast of more than a dozen other leading companies, banks, and law firms: Shearson Lehman Hutton, American Express, Dillon Read, Drexel Burnham Lambert, The First Boston Group, Forstman Little, Goldman Sachs, Lazard Frères, Morgan Stanley, Salomon Brothers, Skadden Arps, and Wasserstein Perella. In the end, Kravis signed a $31.4 billion deal for one of America's premier companies—at the time, the highest price ever paid for a corporation.[24]

Since the deal was financed with debt, it heightened the pressure on RJR to produce profits by any means necessary. In the musical-chairs game leading up to the deal, businesses involved in the negotiations included corporate giants such as Kellogg's, Pepsi, Philip Morris, and Pillsbury.[25] During the hostile-takeover boom of the 1980s, nearly one-third of the largest U.S. manufacturers were acquired or merged.[26] If companies were being traded like baseball cards, what executive had to worry about the long-term liability of the company's products or practices?

DEREGULATION

"Deregulation" is the dismantling of existing regulations or their lax enforcement. Beginning in the 1970s, businesses argued that government regulations, not changes in the global economy, were a main cause of lower profits, and therefore these regulations should be suspended or "reformed."[27] In his successful 1980 campaign for president, Ronald Reagan promised business audiences that he would "turn you loose again to do the things I know you can do so well,"[28] and delivered on his promise for regulatory relief by withdrawing, relaxing, or not enforcing dozens of regulations, including many of those passed in the previous two decades.[29] One of Reagan's contributions was to centralize regulatory oversight in the White House. As James Miller, the head of the newly created Vice-President's Task Force on Regulatory Relief (and an alumnus of the business think tank the American Enterprise Institute) put it, by claiming direct oversight, the president "would not have guerrilla warfare from agencies that don't want to follow Reagan's prescription for regulatory relaxation."[30] In other words, politics, not science, was to inform regulatory decisions.

One example of this deregulation helps explain the growth of marketing of unhealthy food to children described in Chapter 1. In 1984, the Federal Communications Commission lifted restrictions on television advertising to children that had been in place since the 1970s, opening the door to a flood of ads for fast food, soda, sweetened cereals, and candy targeting young children.[31]

That decade marked the beginning of the dramatic rise in child obesity. After the 2008 financial crisis, corporations renewed their war on regulation, charging that it (not their risky speculation) was preventing a return to economic growth.

Two other examples show how deregulation can harm health. In 1994, as a result of intense lobbying by vitamin and food supplement makers, the U.S. Congress passed the Dietary Supplement Health and Education Act (DSHEA), which limited the Food and Drug Administration's authority to regulate supplements. Under the new Act, as long as manufacturers made no claims about their products' treating, preventing, or curing diseases, the FDA had to prove they were harmful rather than the industry having the prior obligation to prove they were safe. *Consumer Reports* judged that "the law has left consumers without the protections surrounding the manufacture and marketing of over-the-counter or prescription medication."[32] Supplement manufacturers were now able to launch products without any testing at all, just by sending the FDA a copy of the language on the label. In 2010, a Government Accountability Office (GAO) report on FDA oversight of dietary supplements found that nearly all of the herbal dietary supplements that the GAO tested contained trace amounts of lead and other contaminants, and 16 of the 40 supplements tested contained pesticide residues that appeared to exceed legal limits. Among the illegal claims that supplementary makers made were that a product containing ginkgo biloba was a treatment for Alzheimer's disease, and a product containing ginseng could prevent diabetes and cancer.[33] The deregulation instituted by DSHEA endangered the health of consumers and provided misleading and deceptive health education. This further complicated the task of nutrition educators accountable to the public rather than corporations. These educators now needed, not only to give people the facts they needed to make informed food choices, but also to counteract the better funded misinformation campaigns that industry sponsored.

A study of alcohol regulation in the United Kingdom concluded that the deregulation of alcohol marketing that began in the 1960s and continues to the present has significantly increased the health-related harms caused by alcohol. Repealing laws that limited the hours and places of sales, and the pricing and marketing of beer, wine, and liquor contributed to increases in deaths from cirrhosis of the liver, hospital admissions for alcoholic liver disease and acute intoxication, and binge drinking among teenage girls.[34] Compared to the United States, which still has more robust state and local alcohol regulations in place, the United Kingdom has higher rates of alcohol consumption, fewer alcohol abstainers, and a youth and childhood drinking rate more than twice the American rate.[35] In 2013, bowing to pressure from the alcohol industry, the United Kingdom again missed an opportunity to remedy these problems by rejecting a proposal to institute regulations that would have used alcohol pricing to discourage excess use, a decision decried by public health advocates.[36]

TAX RELIEF

Another plank of the business plan for restoring profitability is tax relief. Although U.S. businesses paid lower corporate taxes than in Europe and Japan, American businesses insisted that high taxes were a deterrent to economic growth and a drag on the U.S. economy. Beginning in 1980 with the Reagan tax cuts and continuing for the next three decades, U.S. corporations saw their tax rates fall. Between 1955 and 2010, the percentage of federal revenues generated by corporate taxes fell from 27.3 percent to 8.9 percent. In the same period, the percentage of the gross domestic product that came from corporate taxes fell from 4.3 percent to 1.3 percent. By 2010, compared to other nations, U.S. corporate taxes constituted a smaller percentage of the GDP (1.8 percent) than those in Australia (5.9 percent), Japan (3.9 percent), or Great Britain (3.6 percent).[37] In 1978, Congress passed and President Carter signed a tax bill that cut the top rate of capital gains taxes from 48 percent to 28 percent,[38] thus also reducing the taxes on the private investors who supplied corporations with the capital needed for expansion, including expansion of the industries that promoted hyperconsumption. By 2012, the effective corporate tax rate in the United States had dropped to 17.8 percent, about 40 percent of the 1960 rate.[39]

Many loopholes that businesses won in the tax code further reduced corporate taxes. A 2008 Government Accountability Office study found that 55 percent of United States companies paid no federal income taxes during at least one year in a seven-year period it studied.[40] It also found that from 1998 through 2005, two out of every three United States corporations paid no federal income taxes. One favored strategy for avoiding taxes is to shift profits to countries with low tax rates. According to a 2013 Congressional Research Service report, United States corporations operating in the top five tax havens (the Netherlands, Ireland, Bermuda, Switzerland and Luxembourg) generated 43 percent of their profits in these countries but employed only four percent of their foreign employees and seven percent of their foreign investment in these locations.[41]

Lower corporate taxes, combined with lower taxes on the wealthy, contributed to government deficits and provided ammunition for the conservative argument that the United States could no longer afford a government that provided extensive services or took on ambitious regulatory efforts to protect public health or the environment. In fact, as President Reagan put it, government became the problem, not the solution. This represents an amazing bait-and-switch by big-business–minded leaders in the United States: by failing to tax businesses, they rob other government programs of the tax income needed to carry out their social functions. Then, when the government's bottom line looks bleak due to the dearth of tax revenues, it's the social programs, not the free-wheeling corporations, that get the blame and suffer the budget axe. The political support that corporate leaders have generated for this austerity program, despite its devastating impact on public health and poverty reduction,[42] is one of their greatest triumphs.

In summary, lower rates for corporate taxes and capital gains taxes, combined with the lower personal income taxes for the wealthy inaugurated by President George W. Bush in 2001 and 2003 hurt the health of the public in three important ways. The tax cuts increased income inequality,[43] a powerful contributor to health inequality.[44] They deprived the government of revenues needed to maintain strong public health and other safety net programs.[45] And, by freeing capital for investment, they fueled the growth of the corporate practices that encouraged hyperconsumption with its attendant increase in chronic diseases and injuries.

PRIVATIZATION

"Privatization" is the transfer of services from the public to the private sector. Throughout the 1980s and 1990s, federal, state, and local governments sought to privatize public services, such as education, healthcare, and policing. Such privatization creates new profit opportunities for the businesses that provide these services but also reduces public accountability and oversight. Also privatized were the enforcements of public health and environmental regulations. The rationale for such privatization was that businesses were better equipped to set and enforce their own rules than government, and that private enforcement was more efficient than public. Thus, many local health departments privatized environmental health services;[46] some states privatized regulation of the retail alcohol industry;[47] and national regulators such as the Occupational Safety and Health Administration (OSHA) and the USDA turned over responsibility for some safety inspections to the companies being inspected.[48] Another rationale for privatization of enforcement was that national governments often lacked the mandate or expertise to monitor increasingly global exchanges, leading them to delegate such responsibility to private international organizations, often controlled by the industry to be regulated.[49]

How does privatization affect public health? While the specific impact depends on the details, among the consistent relevant scholarly criticisms of privatization are a loss of regulatory capacity,[50] an increased share of costs shifted to profit,[51] diminished oversight of privatized services, a tendency to allocate services based on cost rather than need, and the vulnerability of privatized services to market volatility.[52,53] In general, privatization of regulatory or service functions reduces the power of government and increases the power of corporations. A study of privatization of tobacco companies in the former Soviet-bloc nations and other countries suggests that the process leads to increases in tobacco consumption.[54] A review of privatization of water supplies in Latin America concluded that "privatization marked a troubling shift away from the conception of water as a 'social good' and toward the conception of water—and water management services—as commodities" and reduced access to clean water.[55]

Threats from privatization continue. In 2013, the Obama Administration proposed new rules to protect the safety of food imported from other countries. Each year 130,000 Americans are hospitalized and 3,000 die from contaminated food. About 15 percent of the food comes from abroad, often from countries with limited capacity to monitor food safety. Yet the FDA inspects only one to two percent of all food imports. Acknowledging the political reality that corporations and their conservative allies were unlikely to fund regulations that required independent oversight of the food industry, the FDA instead proposed that private companies like Walmart and Cargill inspect their own imports, thus delegating a core public health function to private industry.[56] A pernicious long-term effect of privatization is that it further diminishes the public sector, the only actor with the capacity and resources to make protecting public health a priority.

MARKET CONCENTRATION

"Market concentration" is the tendency for the number of companies producing specific goods or services to decrease, with the resulting firms becoming bigger and controlling more of the market, often driving smaller companies out of business. In theory, capitalism promotes competition, but in practice, markets often concentrate, reducing competition. In the 1970s and beyond, many major industries become increasingly concentrated, both nationally and globally. For example, between 1970 and 2002, the proportion of food-processing sales in the United States accounted for by the fifty biggest companies increased by 39 percent.[57] In the alcohol industry, concentration was even more pronounced. Between 1979 and 2006, the ten largest global beer makers more than doubled their global market share, from 28 percent to 70 percent.[58] This concentration left business decisions about what to produce in the hands of a few major corporations, diminishing the power of governments and consumers to shape markets.

As we saw in previous chapters, it also made it easier for the remaining few big corporations to afford the most advanced technological, marketing, and research and development expertise and to compete successfully with smaller companies on price. Lower prices for unhealthy products result in greater population exposure and risk. These competitive advantages led to further concentration, giving the biggest global corporations an even stronger voice in shaping the economy, politics, and the environments in which individuals made consumption decisions. In systems theory, this is a "positive feedback loop" that amplifies a problem rather than corrects it. Since most economists predict further concentration of the global consumer industries, absent intervention, the health problems associated with market concentration can be expected to grow.

Changing Corporate Political Practices Increase Their Clout

These economic changes led to dramatic changes in corporations' *business* practices, but Powell's memo emphasized that corporations needed to launch a *political* campaign against their opponents. After 1971, corporations moved to occupy Washington, D.C., making it the headquarters of their counter-offensive.

The trickle of lobbyists flowing into Washington in the 1970s turned into a flood that all but drowned out the voices of citizens. By 1998, according to the Center for Responsive Politics, special-interest groups had accumulated more than thirty-eight registered lobbyists and $2.7 million in lobbying expenditures for every member of Congress.[59] Between 2000 and 2005 alone, the number of registered lobbyists in Washington, D.C., more than doubled, from 16,342 to 34,785, and annual spending on federal lobbying reached $2 billion.[60]

To reinforce its Washington messages, corporations also beefed up lobbying at the state and local levels of government. After losing several key state battles, for example, the tobacco industry began hiring lobbyists in state capitals; by 1994, according to one study, at least 450 state-level lobbyists were working to resist tobacco-related legislation.[61] In 2006, the Center for Public Integrity, an investigative journalism outlet, reported that companies and other organizations spent almost $1.3 billion to lobby state legislators, a 10 percent increase from the previous year.[62] The 40,000 registered state lobbyists outnumbered state legislators five to one, and total spending on lobbying averaged $200,000 per legislator.[63]

Campaign contributions provide another route to influence legislators. In 1971, in response to public pressure, Congress passed the Federal Elections Campaign Act, which required disclosure of campaign financing. After the Watergate scandal, Congress strengthened the Act in 1974 by creating a comprehensive system of regulation and enforcement, including public financing of presidential campaigns and the establishment of a central enforcement agency, the Federal Election Commission. In 1976, however, in the *Buckley vs. Valeo* decision, the U.S. Supreme Court (including Lewis Powell) struck down most limits on candidate expenditures and certain other limits on spending, calling such rules unconstitutional infringements of free speech.[64] This and subsequent court decisions opened the door for a growing corporate role in election financing.

Thirty years later, in the 2006 congressional elections, corporate political action groups contributed $120 million to congressional candidates, a 33 percent increase from the 2002 elections.[65] As the electoral winds shifted towards the Democrats that year, so did corporate contributions. The pharmaceutical, tobacco, and insurance companies that had previously heavily favored Republican candidates began to hedge their bets, increasing their contributions to Democratic candidates. "Our approach to our political contributions," David Howard, a spokesman for Reynolds American Tobacco Company, told the *Wall Street Journal*, "is that we support those who will support us or will give us an ear."[66]

By 2012, another record year in campaign spending, outside corporate and PAC contributions became a primary source of funding for both Democratic and Republican congressional and presidential candidates, as shown in Table 3.2. Total reported spending exceeded $4 billion, probably an underestimate. The U.S. Chamber of Commerce, which describes itself as the world's largest business association, reported independent spending of $32,676,075 in the 2012 election cycle. However, according to the Sunlight Foundation, an independent monitor of campaign spending, only 6.9 percent of the Chamber's spending supported winning candidates.[67] The day after the election, Gregory Casey, head of the Business Industry Political Action Committee, a Chamber-rival organization that encourages political participation by corporations, told the *Washington Post*, "We learned you cannot address the fiscal and cultural differences in our society by throwing money at political dogmas that may have outlived their usefulness."[68]

A year later this Wednesday-morning quarterbacking seemed to have been forgotten. In a 2013 speech to small businessmen, Thomas Donahue, the President of the Chamber of Commerce, sounded like he was channeling Lewis Powell. He exhorted the audience to "defend and advance a free-enterprise system" whenever it "comes under attack" and to give politicians in Washington a piece of their minds. "It's about time," he thundered, "that our leaders in Washington start making the tough decisions that we pay them to make!"

Corporations had long used the revolving door between the corporate suite and government offices in Washington to shape policy by sending top executives to advise presidents, and offering corporate jobs to departing public officials. In 1953, for example, General Motors president Charles Erwin Wilson became Eisenhower's Secretary of Defense. Wilson's famous quote, "What's good for the

Table 3.2 **2012 Campaign Spending**

Campaign Spending Reported to Federal Elections Commission

Category	Democrats	Republicans	Total	Percent from PACs
House of Representatives	$482,321,522	$619,413,257	$1,111,705,043	32
Senate	$302,953,666	$378,229,388	$699,206,755	11
President	$732,741,988	$620,187,082	$1,357,487,680	NA
Total	$1,518,017,176	$1,617,829,727	$3,168,399,478	NA

Outside Campaign Spending

Funded by	Amount
Super PACS	$641,836,709
Political Parties	$245,103,933
Others (Corporations, Unions, Individual People, Other Groups, etc):	$422,387,597
Total	$1,309,328,239

Reported Spending by Selected Industries

Sector	Total	From Organizations	From Individuals	To Liberal Candidates	To Conservative Candidates
Pharmaceuticals/ Health Products	$9,528,246	$113,500	$9,414,746	$4,283,000	$5,233,528
Automotive	$5,008,292	$2,805,518	$2,202,774	$9,250	$4,998,042
Food Processing & Sales	$3,962,163	$2,675,300	$1,286,863	$86,700	$3,868,916
Tobacco	$275,600	$88,500	$187,100	$23,500	$10,300

This table includes donations to the outside spending groups that can accept unlimited contributions. This includes "Super PACs," earmarked donations that are reported by 501c nonprofit organizations, and earmarked donations reported by "527" organizations that use the contributions explicitly for electioneering communications or independent expenditures. This page does not include donations to political action committees. Source for table: Center for Responsive Politics. *Open Secrets.* Available at: Accessed December 29, 2012, from http://www.opensecrets.org/overview/index.php.

country is good for General Motors, and vice versa," demonstrated the belief that there was no conflict between the interests of the country and of a corporation. Later, Ford president Robert McNamara left Detroit to become John F. Kennedy's Secretary of Defense.

What changed in the 1970s was the extent to which politics and business interests became entangled. In 1973, in an example that symbolized the revolving door, President Nixon appointed Earl Butz (Figure 3.2), then a director of Ralston Purina, a major company that produced food for people and animals, as Secretary of Agriculture, replacing Clifford Hardin, who then became head of Ralston Purina.[69] Nixon, and later President Ford, gave the new Secretary Butz two explicitly political tasks: first, to help resuscitate a declining economy in order to win farm-state support for Nixon, and later, to bring down the rising cost of food to increase Gerald Ford's popularity.

Butz took on these tasks with enthusiasm. But his political chores gave him the opportunity to take on a grander task: making government not the protector of farmers and consumers, but the expeditor for agribusiness, helping it become the dominant force shaping the production and distribution of the world's food. Butz negotiated a deal to sell U.S. grains to the Soviets, leading to record rates of inflation of food prices in the United States but assuring profits for food companies.[70] By 1975, six major corporations controlled 90 percent of the world's $11 billion a year grain-export business.[71] Subsequently, Butz used federal policy to favor large farms at the expense of smaller ones (his advice: "Get big or get

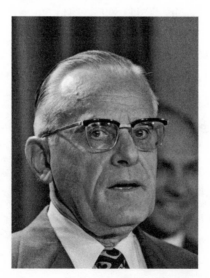

Figure 3.2 Agriculture Secretary Earl Butz in 1973. Corbis Images.

out") and to support subsidized production of corn, soy, and wheat, the staples of the industrial food system.

Over time, as Butz's policies increased production, prices fell. Cheap corn, which the food writer Michael Pollan has called "the dubious legacy of Earl Butz," became the building block of fast food, along with high-fructose corn syrup, and super-sized sodas.[72] By allowing market forces to drive farm policy, Butz planted the seeds of the food system that is causing the current crop of diet-related chronic diseases. As it turned out, what was good for Ralston Purina and other big food companies was not so good for global health.

Public relations firms and law firms also grew enormously in this period in both number and size, largely as a result of corporate clients. The art of public relations first emerged in the 1920s. Using new insights from psychology, one of PR's founders, Edward Bernay, a nephew of Sigmund Freud, helped corporate clients mold mass opinion. As Bernay recounts in his autobiography, George Washington Hill, the president of American Tobacco Company, asked Bernay in 1929, "How can we get women to smoke on the street? They're smoking indoors but damn it, if they spend half the time outdoors, we'll damn near double our female market. Do something. Act!"[73] Bernay obliged by setting out to identify and then modify the beliefs that prevented women from smoking in public. Acting behind the scenes, he persuaded a feminist leader to invite women to march in the 1929 Easter Parade under the slogan "Women! Light another torch from freedom! Fight another sex taboo." Young women marched down Fifth Avenue puffing Lucky Strikes, attracting wide newspaper coverage.[74] Bernays had offered corporations a tool to manufacture, not new products, but the demand for them.

In his work for Beechnut Packing Company, a leading pork producer, Bernay had the opportunity to contribute to another twentieth-century epidemic, heart disease. To convince Americans that a heavy breakfast of bacon, a Beechnut product, and eggs, promoted health, Bernays conducted a survey of 5,000 doctors, asking them if heavy breakfasts supported health. In a national advertising campaign with the headline, "Physicians urge heavy breakfasts to improve health," he presented their favorable positive response as if it were a scientific study, a technique of third-party endorsement later used by other industries to promote unhealthy products. Sales of bacon soared.[75]

From 1980 to 2000, the number of public relations specialists increased by 56 percent, with the largest number working in the corporate sector.[76] Many new hires went to the mega-PR firms that emerged. WPP, founded in 1985, calls itself the world's largest communications services group, employs 153,000 people working in 2,400 offices in 107 countries. Burson Marsteller, established in 1953, became the world's largest public relations firm by 1983. Edelman, the largest independent PR company, employed 3,600 staff in 53 cities around the world. Some companies became to go-to source for corporations with a health-related image problem. Hill & Knowlton has been employed by 50 percent of global Fortune 500 companies and has helped the tobacco, infant formula, lead, vinyl chloride, and other industries fight off government regulations of products associated with health harms.[77]

Increasingly, these companies became communications supermarkets, with the ability to provide corporations with help on lobbying, crisis management, and strategic planning, as well as more traditional public relations. Working on similar issues for multiple clients enabled these PR companies to gain the expertise needed to master the common tasks their clients expect: creating favorable opinion for a new product or brand, resisting government regulation, managing a crisis due a safety threat, or turning back a new tax. As government downsized, the corporate capacity to manipulate government super-sized, further tilting the asymmetrical power relationship.

Businesses also expanded existing trade associations, like the Chamber of Commerce and the National Association of Manufacturers, while creating new ones to bring the corporate policy agenda to elected officials. In the 1960s, according to business historian David Vogel, trade associations were "under-staffed, relatively unsophisticated, and were held in little regard by either the companies that belonged to them or the legislators whose views they were supposed to influence."[78] By 1980, more than 2,000 trade organizations, employing 42,000 staff, had their headquarters in Washington, D.C.[79] For the first time since the 1920s, when Secretary of Commerce Herbert Hoover pushed for the establishment and growth of trade associations, the total number of people working for private businesses such as trade associations and lobbying, law, and PR firms exceeded the number of federal employees in the Washington metropolitan area.[80]

A New Environment for Health Decisions

By the 1980s, these changes in business and politics had transformed the environment in which investors and corporate managers made decisions, narrowing their options for satisfying Wall Street, while widening their opportunities for using their political clout to overcome opposition to their business plans.

On the business side, corporate managers really had only a few choices that allowed them to satisfy investors' growing thirst for quick and steady returns on investment. They could create blockbuster products that produced windfall profits for at least a few quarters or years. They could dramatically increase market share by finding new populations of customers or by driving competitors out of business. They could buy and sell companies, hoping to profit by selling off assets or acquiring fast-growing businesses. Finally, companies could increase profits by firing workers, cutting benefits, or using their political muscle to lower taxes or resist or weaken regulations, thereby leaving more revenue as profit. On the political front, corporations expanded each of these opportunities by deploying their new armies of lawyers, lobbyists, public relations staff, and trade associations.

Each of these options had health consequences, but two, the marketing of blockbuster products and the relentless efforts to develop new markets, have had direct and particularly harmful results for people's health. It is the growth of these corporate practices that set the stage for the global epidemics of chronic diseases and injuries.

Blockbusters satisfy investors, who then reward the managers who have brought them to market. But as the stories of Saturday night specials, SUVs, and Vioxx show, new products often have flaws or unintended consequences, and the massive advertising and retail distribution needed to achieve blockbuster status mean that millions of people can be exposed to a product before the hazard becomes apparent. In addition, given the benefits that blockbusters bring, managers feel justified in cutting corners, resisting safety regulations, exaggerating the benefits, or minimizing the harms. After all, given that chronic conditions take years to develop and that faulty product design may be difficult to detect without counting bodies, it is likely that managers will have moved on and companies changed hands before problems are identified.

A second option for corporate managers who are expected to produce positive quarterly returns is to find new markets where rapid expansion is possible. As we have seen, the tobacco industry discovered women as new recruits for tobacco use in the 1920s. After the 1990s, the industry turned its attention to women and young people in Africa, Asia, and Latin America. In this situation, an industry took an existing product and marketed it to new customers. The marketing of alcopops and guns to young women and unhealthy foods to blacks and Latinos in the United States are other examples of this strategy.

Common Roots of Epidemics and 2008 Economic Crisis

The deeper economic changes that magnified corporations' contributions to epidemics of chronic diseases and injuries also helped to precipitate the world economic crisis of 2008, which in turn jeopardized health in other ways. Financialization of the world economy, combined with deregulation of the financial industry in the 1980s and 1990s, led to the creation of sub-prime mortgages, housing derivatives, and other financial instruments—basically, financial constructs meant to facilitate immediate profit. By providing easy credit, these new tools for speculation inflated the housing bubble in the United States and elsewhere. When it burst, first in the United States and later in many European countries, the world economy was thrown into recession. By the end of 2011, more than 14 million Americans had homes in foreclosure, were delinquent on their mortgages, or owed more than their houses were worth.[81] The housing crisis, the resulting freeze in credit, and the reluctance of corporations to use their cash reserves to create new jobs to produce more goods contributed to record rates of homelessness, loss of health insurance, unemployment, and poverty. As the crisis spread, similar problems emerged in Europe and later China, India, and Brazil, albeit with variations due to the different roles that government played.

As the housing collapse forced investors to find new arenas for speculation, commodities like energy and food became attractive, leading to skyrocketing prices in these sectors. The World Bank has estimated that, since 2008, more than 170 million people around the world have been pushed into extreme poverty by increases in the cost of basic commodities such as food and energy, triggered by multiple factors, including speculation.[82, 83]

The economic crisis also encouraged corporations to spend cash on buying back stock, rather than avoiding layoffs, hiring new workers, investing in new products, or testing them more carefully. In 2011, U.S. companies spent more than $445 billion, the most since 2007, in buying back stock so they could return more to investors and pay executives more. "It's a symptom of a deeper problem," said William W. George, a Harvard Business School professor and former corporate CEO. "If we're not investing in research, innovation and entrepreneurship, we're going to be a slow growth country for a decade."[84] Pfizer's decision to spend more than $39 billion on stock buybacks in between 2011 and 2013 illustrates the consequences of this type of short-termism.[85] By choosing to cut back research and development and lay off workers in order to buy back more stock, Pfizer missed an opportunity to use these resources to create new drugs that could better address the world's most serious health problems.

Deregulation of financial services and tax cuts for the wealthy also contributed to massive income redistribution. Between 1996 and 2006, according to an analysis of tax returns by the Congressional Research Service, the poorest 20 percent of tax filers experienced a 6 percent reduction in income, while the top 0.1 percent of tax filers saw their income almost double. The wealthy also got more of their income from investments than from work. During this period, the top 0.1 percent increased the proportion of their income that came from capital from 64 percent to 70 percent.[86] Given the contribution of inequality to poor health,[87] this growing income and wealth inequality bodes ill for the health of America. It's directly connected to our concern about chronic diseases and injuries, because the increasing proportion of people living in poverty are more vulnerable to these conditions.

Finally, the growing political power of corporations, financial institutions, and their allies led to the undermining of democracy. Increasingly, while citizens still have votes, multinational corporations often have vetoes over policy directions that threaten profitability. The U.S. Supreme Court became the most corporate-friendly ever. According to an analysis by the *New York Times*, in its first five terms, the Roberts Court ruled for business interests 61 percent of the time, compared with 46 percent in the last five years of the Court led by Chief Justice William H. Rehnquist, himself a conservative, who died in 2005; and 42 percent by all Supreme Courts since 1953.[88] Today the Supreme Court is more concerned about protecting corporations from litigation than consumers from harmful business practices, a sad commentary on the changes in its priorities.

The Court's 2010 *Citizens United* decision threw out regulations that prohibited corporations from buying campaign commercials that explicitly advocate the election or defeat of candidates, thus for the first time extending constitutional protection to corporate political as well as commercial speech. The decision opened the floodgates for massive, unregulated, and often secret corporate contributions into political campaigns. For corporations, Citizens United provided unprecedented new opportunities to influence the policies that shaped health, lifestyle, and the environment.[89]

Some analysts credit Chief Justice Roberts's 2012 vote to uphold the constitutionality of the Affordable Care Act as a conciliatory gesture designed to restore the credibility of the Court as a defender of justice rather than corporations. Others, however, expressed worry that Roberts's opinion sets the stage for future limitations on government regulation of corporate practices.[90] Roberts and the majority decided that Congress can regulate *existing* interstate commercial activity, but it cannot force people to enter into a market. "The power to *regulate* commerce," he wrote, "presupposes the existence of commercial activity to be regulated."[91] Yale law professor Akhil Reed Amar suggested that the decision signals that the Court is moving in a still more conservative direction. "The underlying logic here is they're considerably more skeptical of innovative or ancillary uses of federal power," Amar said. "It's about reading federal powers more skeptically than a year ago."[92]

Like Supreme Court justices, elected officials, too, came to resemble the wealthiest Americans, further pushing the government to favor the wealthy. In part, that was who enabled them to get into office. In 2010, nearly 25 percent of all money spent on elections came from the top .01 percent of the population; this top group of American earners spent on average more money on political campaigns than the average American earned in income.[93] And increasingly, those whom we send to Congress are the wealthy. Between 1984 and 2009, when the average net worth of American families decreased by about 1 percent, members of Congress, on average, enjoyed an increase in their worth of about 159 percent.[94] With legislators concentrated in the top layer of the economic hierarchy, the likelihood that they will be the motors for change seems low.

The 2011 Occupy Wall Street demonstrations and the 2012 presidential election made income inequality a topic for national discussion, if not yet action. The 2012 Republican presidential candidate Mitt Romney's response to a heckler that "Corporations are people, my friend," and his claim that the 47 percent of the population "who are dependent upon government, who believe that they are victims, who believe the government has a responsibility to care for them, who believe that they are entitled to health care, to food, to housing, to you-name-it" are "takers not makers," sparked further debate about the roles of government and corporations in reducing inequality.[95]

The shared causes for the world's health, social, and economic problems suggest both trouble and hope for those who believe another world is possible. On one hand, the common problem is an increasingly concentrated global economic system in which those at the very top of the hierarchy have acquired the power and skill needed to run the world to benefit themselves, often at the expense of the rest of the world's population. Never in history has such a small group controlled so many domains of human existence, nor had at its disposal such a panoply of wealth, technology, and ideology. In addition, the current corporate system now undermines health via three distinct but synergistic pathways: by encouraging consumption of unhealthy products, by widening inequality and pushing more people into poverty, and by imposing austerity on governments, rolling back safety net programs and the regulations and standards that protect public health.

On the other hand, the hope is that never before have so many people had a common interest in transforming the world. Never before has the potential to use knowledge and technology to create healthy, sustainable societies that will allow humanity to survive and prosper been greater. In the final two chapters, I will consider how we can find the paths to this transformation.

4

The Corporate Consumption Complex

In January 1961, three days before he was to leave office, President Dwight D. Eisenhower gave a speech in which he warned the nation that a "military-industrial complex" had emerged from World War II and the Cold War.

> We have been compelled to create a permanent armaments industry of vast proportions. Added to this, three and a half million men and women are directly engaged in the defense establishment.... This conjunction of an immense military establishment and a large arms industry is new in the American experience. The total influence—economic, political, even spiritual—is felt in every city, every State house, every office of the Federal government.... Our toil, resources and livelihood are all involved; so is the very structure of our society.... In the councils of government, we must guard against the acquisition of unwarranted influence, whether sought or unsought, by the military industrial complex. The potential for the disastrous rise of misplaced power exists and will persist. We must never let the weight of this combination endanger our liberties or democratic processes.[1]

Today a new complex has emerged: the corporate consumption complex. The complex is a web of organizations that include the global corporations that produce the goods of the modern consumer economy, the retail conglomerates that sell their products, and the trade associations that represent them in the political arena. Key actors are the banks, hedge funds, and investment firms that lend these corporations money, and, increasingly, dictate their priorities. It includes the law firms, advertising agencies, public relations firms, and lobbying groups that cater to them. Elected officials and government regulatory agencies these industries have captured through the revolving-door or campaign contributions, the think tanks and university-based researchers that conduct studies for them, the "astroturf" citizens groups they create to advance their policy aims, and the media outlets and journalists who help promote their goals are also participants in the complex. Figure 4.1 provides a schematic illustration of the complex: the corporations that produce products for the global consumer economy are at the center, with supporting organizations radiating out. The strands of the web serve as communications networks to exchange intelligence, money, goods and services, and political lessons. And like the military industrial complex, this new complex endangers not only our democratic processes, but it also, as we have seen, the current and future health of humanity.

Before proceeding, let me be clear about what the corporate consumption complex is not. It is not a cabal, a conspiracy that meets in secret to plan new strategies to undermine global health. Some corporate executives have been found to withhold harmful information from the public and plot ways to maintain profits at the expense of public health; e.g., tobacco industry leaders. But for the most part, the complex operates in public and we can read about many of its activities in the *Wall Street Journal* or on the Internet every day.

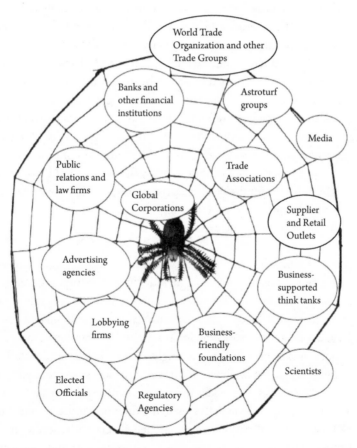

Figure 4.1 The Corporate Consumption Complex.

For the most part, it's not an organization of evil men, some latter-day SMERSH, the nemesis of Ian Fleming's James Bond. Many of its participants are ordinary people who love their children, donate to charity, and hope for a better world, choosing to put aside any moral qualms about the harmful consequences of their actions. And it is not a single unified organization whose participants agree on every point or speak in a single voice.

But these caveats should not disguise what the corporate consumption complex is. It has become the most powerful influence on the health of the world's population and on the environment that sustains life. It is the primary modifiable cause of today's major causes of premature death and preventable illnesses and injuries, contributing directly and indirectly to the rising rates of chronic diseases and injuries. It operates at the local, national, and global levels to influence the values, behaviors, and lifestyles of consumers and citizens; our physical and social environment; the legal, executive, and legislative decisions of government; and the activities of the media, scientists, and philanthropy. Its principal goals are to create a world where the largest multinational corporations can maximize their profits and preempt or remove any threat to their current dominance. Since its activities threaten the well-being of so many sectors of society, it also seeks to undermine the democratic processes that could diminish its power to profit at the expense of world health.

From a health perspective, the most problematic activity of this complex is its promotion of hyperconsumption, a term I use to describe patterns of consumption associated with premature death and preventable illnesses and injuries. In itself, consumption is a vital human activity, neither good nor bad. In theory, a free market economy could emphasize production, marketing, and distribution practices that support human health, contributing to a virtuous circle where more and more people choose healthy products, leading to greater profits and more widespread availability of these goods. And for the decades after World War II, corporations did contribute to improving the standard of living and in some cases the health of the world's growing middle-class population.

Today, however, the economic and political changes described in the previous chapter discourage the corporate consumption complex from this virtuous cycle. Instead, consumer corporations are engaged in a race to the bottom, where companies compete to sell ever more of products known to cause health problems or damage the environment. Short-termism—investor insistence on a rapid return on investment—leads corporations to promote blockbuster products, often without adequate testing. Our legal system allows industries to externalize the adverse health consequences of harmful products, forcing consumers and tax payers to pay the costs for health or environmental damage, further encouraging unhealthy practices. Deregulation has weakened or removed the safeguards that can protect the public, reducing the risk that corporations will have to pay more for violating health or environmental safeguards than the profits their unhealthy practices generate. Finally, the concentration of market share by a handful of global companies produces asymmetrical power and information—where one side, producers, has more political power and information than the other, consumers. This inequality contradicts the basic assumption of free market theory, in which producers and consumers have equal power and information to make free exchanges.

These dynamics serve to distort the market in favor of health-imperiling products I have described—sports utility vehicles; drugs like Vioxx, Celebrex, and Avandia; unhealthy foods like Coke and Pepsi, McDonald's Big Macs, and Oreos; youth-targeted addictive substances like alcopops and tobacco; and mass market weapons like Saturday night specials, Bushmaster AR-15s, and Glocks. These dynamics also make these products much more profitable than healthier counterparts such as mass transit buses and subway cars, non-pharmacological treatments for common chronic diseases, fresh fruits and vegetables, or stress-reducing alternatives to tobacco, alcohol, or handguns.

Today, the corporate consumption complex has the power to maintain a political and economic system that allows companies to produce and market lethal but legal products and to promote unhealthy lifestyles and unsustainable practices at the expense of healthier alternatives. This power constitutes the most significant threat to improved health and reduced healthcare costs. For those who seek to improve health, a closer examination of the operations, strengths, and vulnerabilities of this complex is now a priority.

Let's begin with a look at the size of the consumer economy in the United States and globally. In the United States, for the last decade, the consumer economy—that part of the economy driven by consumer spending—accounts for about 70 percent of the gross domestic product, up from about 60 percent in the early 1950s.[2] According to the U.S. Bureau of Labor Statistics, in 2010, America's 121 million households spent $5.83 trillion dollars.[3] Table 4.1 shows total spending for various consumer goods. It shows that the five categories of consumer spending listed in the table account for more than a quarter of all household expenditures. This consumer spending is the magnet that attracts the corporate consumption complex to find new ways to increase its share of this wealth.

Note that tobacco and alcohol spending account for less than two percent of annual household spending, yet tobacco use is estimated to generate $96 billion in direct medical costs (about 5 percent of all healthcare expenditures),[4] and alcohol $24.6 billion in direct healthcare costs and a total of $223.5 billion in all costs.[5] The economic burdens these products impose illustrate the power of the corporate consumption complex to protect its markets.

Total global consumer spending is now more than $18 trillion a year. In the last few years, the United States has accounted for about 16 percent of global consumer

Table 4.1 **U.S. Consumer Expenditures on Selected Products, 2010**

Category	Average spending per household $	Total spending in billions $
Food	6,129	742
Food at home	3,624	439
Food away from home	2,505	303
Alcoholic beverages	412	50
Car and truck purchases—new and used	2,588	313
Healthcare	3,157	382
Drugs	485	59
Medical supplies	119	14
Tobacco and tobacco supplies	362	44
All expenditures	48,109	5.83 trillion

Source: Average annual expenditures and characteristics of all consumer units, Consumer Expenditure Survey, 2006–2010. U.S. Bureau of Labor Statistics; 2011. Available at: http://www.bls.gov/cex/2010/standard/multiyr.pdf. Accessed August 21, 2012.

spending (as a proportion of world GDP), Western Europe for about 15 percent, and the BRIC countries (Brazil, Russia, India, and China) for about 8 percent, a proportion that is expected to increase significantly in the coming decade.[6]

For most of the last century, maintaining high levels of consumption in order to promote economic growth was a central goal of developed nations, an aim achieved through economic policies that encouraged debt and discouraged savings, thus contributing to the 2008 economic crisis. Although some analysts have correctly noted the growing power of the financial sector, it is worth noting that consumption remains the fuel that drives the world economy. And growing consumption remains the policy choice of politicians and businesses on both the political left and the right, even if they disagree on how to achieve this aim.

In the coming decades, some emerging nations also want consumption to play a greater role in their economies. For instance, the Indian government is trying to stimulate consumption by attempting to open up its domestic market to foreign multi-brand retail stores, and the Chinese government wants domestic consumption to play a stronger role in its economy rather than to continue to rely so heavily on exports and investment to stimulate growth. As one business analyst noted, these trends and the "rise of the middle class in China, India, and Brazil is having a clear impact on consumption patterns, providing more opportunities for consumer-oriented multinational corporations to increase their revenues and profitability."[7] Regional or global business cycles can accelerate or slow down this growth, but few economists doubt that in this century, consumer spending will continue to be the engine for economic growth.

A report on consumer spending commissioned by MasterCard provides another look at the value of emerging markets. MasterCard predicts that, for the period from 2012–2016, emerging markets will add an average of $1.2 trillion of consumer spending to the global economy per year, whereas developed markets will add only around $700 billion annually, and the transitional markets in former Soviet States will add another $95 billion.[8] By 2020, spending on food, alcohol and tobacco, healthcare, and transport will account for 40 percent of consumer spending in the 25 largest emerging economies of the world.[9] These predictions explain why consumer corporations see their future profits in these emerging nations.

But, should these nations follow the consumption patterns that multinational corporations promoted in developed nations, they can expect a similar rise in premature mortality and preventable illnesses from chronic diseases and injuries, a trend that we have seen has already begun. The organizations and networks that constitute the corporate consumption complex are also linked to broader business and political groupings, the U.S. Chamber of Commerce, for example, or the two major U.S. political parties. At the global level, the complex interacts with the World Trade Organization and other international organizations. These larger entities may have broader policy agendas or its various sectors may differ on some issues. For example, the insurance industry has been an active proponent of car safety, often to the consternation of the automobile industry. The distinct perspective of the corporate consumption complex is its insistence that more consumption is the solution to all problems.

To get a clearer view of the unique anatomy and physiology of the corporation consumption complex, I profile two leading organizations and their allies in the complex: McDonald's, a fast food corporation, and the Pharmaceutical Research and Manufacturers of America, a trade association. These profiles illustrate how the strands of the web bind together these and other actors to extend their power to shape lifestyles, public policy, and politics, and to maximize profits by promoting hyperconsumption.

McDonald's: A Franchise for Super-sizing Children Around the World

With 33,510 restaurants serving more than 68 million people in 119 countries every day, McDonald's is the second-largest fast food company in the world, topped only by Subway. It has also become an international symbol of modern consumption. The company is the single largest global purchaser of beef, pork, potatoes, and apples. In 2012, total revenue was $27.6 billion, of which $8.8 billion came from the United States and $10.8 billion from Europe.[10] Its gross profit in 2011 was $2.7 billion, and the net profit margin was 20.38 percent.[11] McDonald's employs 1.2 million people worldwide. In the United States, the company employs 673,000 workers at its 14,000 domestic outlets; half of these are under the age of twenty-one. About 8 percent of Americans eat a meal at McDonald's on an average day, and 96 percent eat there at least yearly.[12] In a recent national survey, 84 percent of parents reported taking their child to a fast food restaurant at least once in the past week; 66 percent reported going to McDonald's.[13] No other organization feeds more children daily.

McDonald's spends more than $2 billion on global marketing and brand-building each year. Nearly $888 million is spent for U.S. measured media alone.[14] In part as a result, McDonald's is ranked as the fourth-most-valuable brand on the planet, with an estimated brand value of $81 billion in 2011, up 23 percent from 2010.[15] This translates into near-universal brand recognition. A poll by Sponsorship Research International in six countries found that 88 percent of the respondents could identify the golden arches, but only 54 percent could name the Christian cross.[16]

But, as the *Wall Street Journal* has noted, "to build a brand is to create a hostage,"[17] and McDonald's hires a retinue of public relations and advertising firms to protect the Golden Arches, Ronald McDonald, and other branded icons.

Among its advertising agencies are Omnicon's DDB Worldwide Communications Group and its German affiliate Heye & Partner, the designer of the global "I'm lovin' it" campaign. Another global powerhouse ad agency, Publicis Groupe's Leo Burnett, designed the Happy Meals ad campaign.[18] In 2013, Omnicon Group and Publicis Group decided to merge to create the world's largest family of agencies, with a stock market value of more than $35 billion. If approved by governments, this merger will allow the megafirm to compete with companies like Google in processing Big Data to better target their clients' consumers with tailored advertising campaigns. Among the other clients the merger will serve are Coca-Cola, Walmart, Nestlé and PepsiCo, other stalwart promoters of hyperconsumption.[19]

Since its founding in the 1950s, McDonald's has developed a business model that viewed children as its most reliable customers. Ray Kroc, one of its founders, recommended that if a company had $1 to spend on marketing, it should spend it on kids, because they bring Mom and Dad. He also noted that "A child who loves our TV commercials and brings her grandparents to a McDonald's gives us two more customers."[20] In the early years of the chain's growth, Kroc flew in a Cessna plane scouting for new sites near schools.[21]

To attract its target demographic, McDonald's has developed creative ways to entice children through the Golden Arches. The company operates more than 8,000 "playlands" around the United States, more playgrounds than any other private corporation, and far more than any municipality. It also gives away toys to children who buy its products. According to the U.S. Federal Trade Commission, in 2009, the food industry spent $393 million purchasing toys and other premiums, making McDonald's the world's largest toy distributor. Fast food outlets sold more than 1 billion children's meals with toys to children ages twelve and under, about 18 percent of all child customers.[22]

Like other fast food companies, McDonald's advertises heavily (See Figure 4.2). In 2009, all U.S. fast food corporations spent $4.2 billion on advertising their products, of which 16 percent was spent on ads targeting children.[23] According to the Nielsen Company, a rater of advertising exposure, the average American child saw 368 McDonald's television ads in 2009, more than one a day, and almost twice as many as its nearest competitor, Burger King.[24] In 2008, American children aged two to eleven saw on average 1,106 commercials for fast food outlets on television, and adolescents saw on average 1,684 such ads. Adults saw on average 1,905 ads.[25]

In addition, McDonald's uses social and other media to reach children and teens. Its corporate websites attract 365,000 unique visitors aged twelve or younger per month and 249,000 teen visitors.

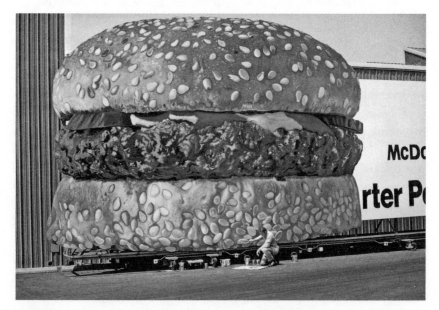

Figure 4.2 Even McDonald's advertisements are super-sized, as shown in this 1970 photo of a commercial artist working on a McDonald's billboard. Corbis Images.

This advertising influences children's food desires and choices, and creates customers for life. A study of young children aged three to five offered them identical combinations of foods and beverages, the only difference being that some of the foods were in McDonald's packaging. Children were significantly more likely to choose items perceived to be from McDonald's, showing the value of early imprinting of branding.[26]

All this advertising and other forms of marketing bring results. One 2009 national poll showed that a whopping 40 percent of parents reported that their child asked to go to McDonald's at least once a week, and 15 percent of pre-schoolers' parents said they fielded such a request every day. Most of the parents gave in: 84 percent reported bringing their two- to eleven-year-olds to a fast food restaurant within the previous week.[27]

Health authorities have criticized the McDonald's business model. According to a policy statement of the American Academy of Pediatrics, "Advertising directed toward children is inherently deceptive and exploits children under eight years of age."[28] David Ludwig, a professor of pediatrics at Harvard Medical School and a national authority on child obesity, has observed that "Fast-food consumption has been shown to increase calorie intake, promote weight gain and elevate risk for diabetes. Because African Americans and Hispanics are inherently at higher risk for obesity and diabetes, fast food will only fuel the problem."[29] An assessment of the nutritional quality of fast food carried out by researchers at the Rudd Center at Yale University found that only 10 percent of the 101 McDonald's food products they tested met three common nutritional standards. Of the 158 beverages served at McDonald's that Yale researchers tested, only a third met these standards.[30] Another study by investigators from U.C. Berkeley and Columbia University found that teenagers whose schools are within one-tenth of a mile of a fast food outlet are more likely to be obese than those whose schools are farther away.[31] In recent years, McDonald's has emphasized expansion in emerging markets such as Mexico, India, and China. By 2012, the company had more than 1,400 outlets in China, its third-largest market. In that year alone, McDonald's increased its investment in China by 50 percent.[32]

To respond to public and scientific criticism, McDonald's, like other corporations in the consumption complex, uses science and technology in a variety of ways. First, it hires its own specialists. Dr. Cynthia Goody, senior director of nutrition for McDonald's, has a doctorate and a master's in business administration from the University of Iowa. She is an active member of the American Dietetic Association and has served as a faculty member for the Culinary Institute of America and the Harvard School of Medicine Continuing Medical Education. Julia Braun, the company's director of global nutrition, is responsible for the integration of nutrition science into the development of new products. She's a registered and licensed dietitian and previously worked at the Center for Health Promotion and Disease Prevention in at the University of North Carolina in Chapel Hill.[33] Barbara Booth is the director of Sensory Science, Quality Systems, and U.S. Supply Chain Management. Among her jobs is to ensure that McDonald's french fries in Alabama and Australia taste the same.[34] These in-house experts oversee McDonald's laboratories and test kitchens and look to develop products that will make a profit. They also serve as liaisons with professional organizations and as "ambassadors" of health, challenging negative public perceptions of the company.

Second, McDonald's commissions outside researchers and companies to conduct studies. When the FDA ordered McDonald's to remove "trans fats" from its products by 2006, the company hired Cargill, Inc., the largest U.S. food and agricultural products company, to lead scientific blending and testing of oils. Cargill is also a principal supplier of beef and eggs to McDonald's. McDonalds settled on a blend of canola and soybean oils, which was then synthesized at Cargill solely for McDonald's use.[35] By turning to its giant corporate partner to solve a regulatory challenge, McDonald's was able not only to find a marketable solution but also to keep its fix proprietary, preventing its competitors and their consumers from benefiting.

Finally, McDonald's hires outside scientists to serve as public relations representatives. In 2003, McDonald's convened its Global Advisory Council on Balanced, Active Lifestyles, comprising independent experts in the areas of nutrition, public health, and fitness. The Council is charged with providing input and guidance to McDonald's on three questions: how to offer additional menu choices, how to promote physical activity, and how to provide accessible nutrition information. By bringing in researchers from universities and research institutes, McDonald's gains access to their expertise and networks and focuses public and scientific attention on questions that do not threaten McDonald's bottom line. For example, the Council was not asked to advise McDonald's on ending advertising to children or reformulating its unhealthy products, but simply to weigh in on adding a few healthier options.[36]

McDonald's claims that it offers its consumers choices, and that parents, not the company, have the responsibility to decide what their children should eat. And in recent years, in part in response to public pressure, "Mickey D's" (as the company is nicknamed) has made more choices available. It has added salads and fruit to its menus and recently made a half-order of apple slices and a half order of fries standard Happy Meal fare. However, according to market research, Happy Meals constitute only 10 percent of U.S. sales, and, as the economy worsened, many parents have ordered the higher fat, sodium, and sugar adult Value Meals to split between two of their young children, reducing the nutritional impact of the apples.[37]

Richard Adams, a former McDonald's executive who now works as a consultant for franchisees, says the average store sells roughly 50 salads a day and 50 to 60 premium chicken sandwiches, compared with 300 to 400 double cheeseburgers from the Dollar Menu.[38] In addition, one of the marketing triumphs of McDonald's and other fast food companies was to make breakfast into a fast food opportunity and to promote the need for a fourth meal in the wee hours of the night. By 2012, forty percent of McDonald's outlets were open 24 hours a day. In that year, McDonald's introduced a new advertising campaign, "Breakfast After Midnight," with the slogan, "The moon is full, you should be too."[39] A survey of male consumers had showed that 45 percent of the 18- to 29-year-olds and a third of the 30- to 39-years-old eat after seven in the evening every day.[40] McDonald's, by increasing the number of fast food visits, effectively negates the nutritional benefits of any marginal changes in product composition. Like Hardee's Monster Thickburgers, McDonald's Breakfast After Midnight puts young men, a population with high rates of heart disease in their future, at higher risk.

In a 2011 letter responding to critics of his company, McDonald's then-CEO James Skinner rejected the charge that his company contributed to diet-related diseases. He boasted of the company's "55-year track record of caring for kids, a core McDonald's value." "At McDonald's," he explained,

> we listen to what our customers tell us. For the past 30 years they have told us—again, overwhelmingly—that they approve of our Happy Meal program.... That's why we are confident that parents understand and appreciate that Happy Meals are a fun treat, with right-sized, quality food choices for their children. As Chief Executive Officer of McDonald's, I want you to know we will vigorously defend our brand, our reputation, our food and our people.[41]

However, Skinner misleads his readers when he emphasizes choice. The $2 billion his company spends annually on advertising is not a public service campaign on the benefits of choice; its intention is to direct consumers to the company's most profitable products: hamburgers, fries, and soda, the high fat, salt, and sugar products that contribute to diet-related chronic diseases.

To be fair, there have been some successes. McDonald's has vowed to make a 15 percent reduction in sodium across its American menu by 2015, and to cut sodium, added sugars, saturated fats, and calories in domestic meals by 2020, all good steps in the right direction. Overall, however, it is highly unlikely that McDonald's will abandon its reliance on its signature burgers and fries. As one former McDonald's executive observed, "(CEO) Jim (Skinner) is always the guy that takes us back to 'What difference is this going to make for the hamburger business? Is that going to help? If that's not going to help, forget it.' "[42]

On the business side, Skinner understood his company's profits depended on hamburgers, but on the public relations front, a different message was needed. "Ronald McDonald," he explained, "serves as an ambassador for children's well-being, promoting messages around physical activity and living a balanced, active lifestyle.... Children's well-being requires an ongoing effort and commitment to be a part of the solution. Going forward, we will continue to make more changes that are relevant to our customers and in their best interests, as we always have."[43]

Again, the message is misleading; McDonald's emphasizes the role of physical activity in obesity not because it cares about the "best interest" of its customers, but in part in order to distract attention from its products. Lori Dorfman of the Berkeley Media Studies Group, an organization that analyzes industry use of media, has observed that "promoting good works is a method used by many industry organizations across many different fields to deflect attention from their not-so-good works."[44] Through such distraction, the corporations that constitute the consumption complex create public images that mask their actual impact on health.

And the rewards for consumer corporate CEOs come from their success in promoting profit, not health. Skinner began his career flipping burgers as a McDonald's restaurant manager trainee in 1971 and rapidly worked his way up. Before he retired in 2012, several business groups named him one of the nation's best CEOs.[45] In 2009, his compensation package was about $17 million, of which $11.5 million was a performance bonus.[46]

To oversee its operations, McDonald's, like other corporations, has a board of directors. Its members, shown in Table 4.2, bring the experience of more than thirty other corporations and other institutions to help McDonald's plan strategy. Of note, six of its thirteen members bring experience in the financial sector, and four have experience in other companies targeting children and young people. Several serve companies that sell the type of goods or services that McDonald's uses. Boards of directors are the clubhouses and social networking sites of the corporate consumption complex, allowing leaders of the complex to exchange intelligence, plan strategies, make deals, and counter threats to the complex as a whole.

One of the lasting consequences of Lewis Powell's 1973 call for corporations to become more active politically is the growing corporate involvement in campaign financing and lobbying. McDonald's political activities show how big corporations engage energetically in the electoral, legislative, and legal arenas. They also demonstrate how the 2010 *Citizens United* Supreme Court decision has accelerated this involvement.

According to the Sunlight Foundation, a nonpartisan group that promotes government transparency, from 1989 through 2012, McDonald's has contributed $9,970,692 to candidates for public office, of which 52 percent has gone

Table 4.2 **McDonald's Current and Recent Board of Directors: Current and Recent Corporate Links for McDonald's Board of Directors (as of 2013)**

Board Member	Food and Agribusiness	Financial Services	Other Consumer Products	Retail	Services	Energy	Other
Andrew J. McKenna Non-Executive Chairman			Schwarz Supply Source (packaging and promotional materials)				
Susan E. Arnold			The Procter & Gamble Company		The Walt Disney Company		
Robert A. Eckert			Mattel, Inc. (toys) Levi Strauss & Co.				
Enrique Hernandez, Jr.		Wells Fargo & Company	Wells Fargo & Co.	Nordstrom, Inc.	Inter-Con Security Systems (security services)	Chevron Corporation	
Jeanne P. Jackson		MSP Capital (private investment company)	NIKE, Inc.				
Richard H. Lenny	The Hershey Company ConAgra Foods, Inc.	Friedman, Fleischer & Lowe (private equity firm) Discover Financial Services					
Walter E. Massey		Bank of America				BP Oil	Morehouse College School of the Art Institute of Chicago National Science Foundation
Carry D. McMillan	Sara Lee (and apparel)			American Eagle Outfitters	True Partners Consulting LLC (tax and other financial services)		

(continued)

Table 4.2 (Continued)

Board Member	Food and Agribusiness	Financial Services	Other Consumer Products	Retail	Services	Energy	Other
Sheila A. Penrose					Jones Lang LaSalle Incorporated (global real estate and money management) Penrose Group (strategic advisory services)		
John W. Rogers, Jr.		Ariel Investments (institutional money management)				Exelon Corporation (energy services)	
Roger W. Stone		Stone Tan China Holding Corporation (investment holding company) Stone Tan China Acquisition ("blank check" company created to acquire Chinese business)					
Donald Thompson President and CEO						Exelon Corporation	Caterpillar Inc.
Miles D. White			Abbott Laboratories (pharmaceuticals)				
Total	3	8	7	2	5	4	4

Note: McDonald's board members serve as senior managers or board members of listed companies, former affiliation in *italics*.

Source: McDonald's. Board of Directors Biographical Information. Available at: http://www.aboutmcdonalds.com/mcd/investors/corporate_governance/board_of_directors.html. Accessed on January 5, 2013.

to Republicans, 27 percent to Democrats, and 20 percent to other types of candidates. Its two largest overall recipients were Barack Obama and Arnold Schwarzenegger, showing its bipartisan approach to giving. In the 2010 election, after the *Citizens United* decision, the McDonald's Political Action Committee's contributions to congressional candidates jumped 360 percent from 2008, according to Open Secrets, another government watchdog group.[47] In 2012, McDonald's contributed more than $500,000 to candidates for the House and Senate, including contributions to 75 Republican and 61 Democratic House candidates, and 21 Republican and 14 Democratic Senate candidates.[48] These contributions assured that the "McDonald's" delegation to Congress could be a bipartisan force available to advance the company's interests. In the last six years, according to the Federal Elections Commission, former CEO Skinner has himself contributed more than $71,000 to political candidates, mostly Republicans.[49]

McDonald's also lobbies actively. Between 1989 and mid-2012, the company paid 10 lobbyists more than $8 million, a figure that does not include the salaries of its own paid lobbyists. Between 2007 and 2010, reported expenditures for lobbying almost tripled.[50] One of McDonald's own lobbyists is Chester C. "Bo" Bryant, Jr., the senior director of government relations for McDonald's Corporation. Prior to joining the company, he had served as the chief of staff for Georgia Republican congressman Mac Collins and as a legislative analyst at the White House,[51] illustrating how revolving-door employment helps companies get the expertise they use to gain access to, then influence, public officials.

Much of McDonald's lobbying explicitly seeks to thwart public health regulation. According to a 2012 special investigative report by Reuters, between 2009 and 2012, more than fifty leading food and beverage companies and trade associations, including McDonald's, spent $175 million to lobby the Obama Administration against the federal effort to write tougher—but still voluntary—nutritional standards for foods marketed to children.[52] This expenditure was more than double the $83 million spent in the previous three years, during the Bush Administration. The food and media companies hired Anita Dunn, Obama's former White House communications chief, to run their media strategy. In contrast, Reuters found, the Center for Science in the Public Interest, widely regarded as the leading public health advocacy organization lobbying against the food industry, spent about $70,000 lobbying last year—roughly what those opposing the stricter guidelines spent every thirteen hours.[53]

In 2009, Jon Leibowitz, chairman of the Federal Trade Commission, the agency proposing the new guidelines, told a congressional hearing, "We are calling on the food industry to tackle this threat and boldly reinvent the food marketplace." Three years later, after the industry onslaught, the Obama Administration conceded defeat and abandoned its effort to implement new voluntary standards for food advertising to children. The FTC's Leibowitz said the effort to write voluntary food standards was no longer an agency priority. "It's probably time to move on," he said.[54]

In addition to lobbying, McDonald's also influences the federal government by having its staff sit on six federal government advisory committees at the Departments of Agriculture, Commerce, and State.[55] Bo Bryant, for example, was appointed by the Secretary of Agriculture and the U.S. Trade Representative to sit on the Agricultural Technical Advisory Committees for Trade in Processed Food, along with representatives from Cargill, Coca-Cola, Hershey, Yum Restaurants, and Walmart.[56] This committee helps these companies learn about and influence trade agreements with other nations.

Another way that McDonald's uses its power to influence policy is through its membership in trade associations. The company is a member of the U.S. Chamber of Commerce, the National Council of Chain Restaurants, the National Restaurant Association, and the International Franchise Association, among others. Through these organizations, McDonald's amplifies its voice in Washington, coordinates strategies with other corporations, and gains access to additional lobbying and campaign contributions clout. For example, by the end of 2012, the National Restaurant Association had contributed almost $14 million to candidates since 1989 and spent just under $25 million on lobbying, far more than McDonald's alone. McDonald's is also a member of an industry-sponsored advocacy organization, Americans Against Food Taxes, which lobbies against taxes on unhealthy foods. These associations allow complex members to pool their assets to achieve their common policy goals.

For example, when the Food and Drug Administration proposed federal calorie-labeling rules as mandated by the 2010 Patient Protection and Affordable Care Act, McDonald's, the National Council of Chain Restaurants, the National Restaurant Association, the California Restaurant Association, and many other companies and trade groups submitted their objections to the proposed rules, which were subsequently modified in response.[57] McDonald's also helped create the Children's Food and Beverage Advertising Initiative (CFBAI), a group of food manufacturers that also includes Burger King, PepsiCo, and Kraft Foods. This initiative developed its own guidelines defining foods healthy enough to market to kids, using their standards as an alternative to standards proposed by the government or independent nutrition experts.[58]

McDonald's also seeks to influence federal and state legislation before it is written. Ed Conklin, senior director of governmental affairs for McDonald's, represented the company on the Executive Committee of the American Legislative Exchange Council's (ALEC's) Commerce, Insurance and Economic Development Task Force. ALEC claims that more than 1,000 of the bills its members draft are introduced by legislators every year, with one in every five of them enacted into law.[59] Conklin is also a member of the corporate-funded Council of State Governments and the State Government Affairs Council. These organizations provide McDonald's with an opportunity to draft proposed legislation and meet privately with state legislators to discuss policy issues.

Like other consumer corporations, McDonald's furthers its objectives through a skillful blend of marketing and public relations, often creating citizen marketers to advance its causes. Its Quality Correspondents program seeks to win over mothers by taking them on tours of its kitchens, highlighting food quality and healthful options. This cadre of volunteer moms helps enhance the company's image and overcome the single largest barrier to more McDonald's sales to children: mothers' health concerns.[60] In a message sent to "mother-oriented social networks and freebie product sites," McDonald's offered mothers a chance at "behind-the-scenes access to the farms [where] our fresh ingredients are grown." The winning mothers "are expected to participate in as many as three 'field trips' lasting two to three days, and receive payment for 'reasonable travel expenses.'" A McDonald's spokesperson said the company will then give these mothers "avenues to be able to share their findings."

When sweet talk from moms does not work to enhance its image, McDonald's also has a retinue of lawyers, who take a tougher line. In 1986, McDonald's sued two U.K. environmental activists—David Morris, a postman, and Helen Steel, a gardener—for distributing a pamphlet that charged, among other things, that McDonald's sells unhealthy, addictive junk food; alters its food with artificial chemistry, and exploits children with its advertising.[61] At the end of the two-and-a-half-year "McLibel" trial, the longest case in British history, McDonald's was finally awarded about $66,000, but its legal fees exceeded $16 million,[62] and the media attention the case generated hurt the company more than it helped. The case did, however, serve to deter critics who feared lengthy litigation. This type of suit, labeled a "strategic lawsuit against public participation" or "SLAPP," is intended to censor, intimidate, and silence critics by burdening them with the cost of a legal defense until they abandon their criticism or opposition.[63] A growing number of corporations use SLAPP suits to deter their critics.

In other legal actions, McDonald's lawyers have filed numerous trademark and defamation cases and actively defend the company's interest in consumer lawsuits. (An example: In 1996, McDonald's tried to force the Scottish sandwich shop owner Mary Blair of Fenny Stratford to drop "McMunchies" as her trading name).[64] To date, McDonald's has won court cases for damages brought by parents of obese children. But the fears of having to pay billions for the costs of the illnesses generated by its products, as in the case of the Tobacco Master Settlement Agreement, led McDonald's, other fast food companies, and their trade associations to sponsor what came to be known as Cheeseburger Bills. These laws prevent consumers from suing food outlets for making their customers obese or suffering from other diet-related diseases. By 2012, the National Restaurant Association reported that twenty states had passed some version of a cheeseburger bill.[65]

McDonald's is a global corporation, but that does not stop it from getting immersed in local politics when it perceives that its interests are threatened. In the fall of 2010, San Francisco passed an ordinance that set nutritional standards for restaurant food accompanied by toys or other youth-focused incentive items.[66] At every step, McDonald's, in partnership with Yum! Brands (a conglomerate of several national fast food chains) and the California Restaurant Association, made a determined effort to block the ordinance. When the bill finally passed, McDonald's found a way to get around it by asking parents to pay ten cents for the toys, thus escaping the ban on giveaways.[67]

This profile of McDonald's shows how the multinational corporations that constitute the corporate consumption complex have developed the capacity to think and act locally, nationally, and globally. They find friends and partners in high and low places and use their networks of business and political connections to advance their economic and policy objectives. While these impressive accomplishments have made McDonald's an international business success story, they have also left a deep footprint on the world's health, environment, and economy. By contributing to rising rates of diet-related diseases, unsustainable agricultural practices and environmental damage, lower wages, rising income inequality, and diminished democracy, McDonald's demonstrates that's what's good for business may be bad for human well-being.

PhRMA Urges Governments and Consumers to Just Say Yes to Prescription Drugs

In a speech in the House of Representatives in Congress in 2002, Independent Vermont congressman (later senator) Bernie Sanders told House Speaker Dennis Hastert, "Mr. Chairman, even the New York Yankees sometimes lose, and it has been known that, on occasion, the Los Angeles Lakers lose a ballgame. But, Mr. Chairman, one organization never loses, and that organization has hundreds of victories to its credit and zero defeats in the United States Congress, and that is the pharmaceutical industry."[68] A primary reason for Pharma's winning track record is the work of its trade association, the Pharmaceutical Research and Manufacturers of America, known as PhRMA. An examination of its history and accomplishments further illuminates the power of the corporate consumption complex.

PhRMA is a trade association that represents forty-eight of the world's leading pharmaceutical research and biotechnology companies. Its public mission is to invent "medicines that allow patients to live longer, healthier, and more productive lives...leading the way in the search for new cures."[69] In its media statements, PhRMA emphasizes its role in medical innovation, but behind closed doors, the organization works to create laws, court decisions, and regulations that enable its member drug companies to maximize profits and defeat any policy that might interfere with this goal.

Every industry has trade associations, and, as we have seen, individual corporations like McDonald's use these organizations to advance their case. PhRMA exemplifies how a powerful, savvy, well-resourced trade association can help the corporate consumption complex advance its goals in state capitals, Washington, and in countries around the world. Of note, PhRMA enables the world's largest drug companies to advance their common interests, rather than individual company objectives, replacing the rhetoric of competition with the reality of cooperation.

The Pharmaceutical Manufacturers Association was founded in 1958. The name was changed to the Pharmaceutical Research and Manufacturers of America (PhRMA) in 1994 to better publicize its commitment to research, the face it wants to show the public. PhRMA is headquartered in Washington, D.C., and also has offices in ten other U.S. cities, as well as Amman, Jordan; and Tokyo.[70] PhRMA's advance team is its lobbyists: about twenty on its own staff, plus others paid on a freelance basis. In 2012, PhRMA paid more than $29 million to forty-four outside lobbying firms to bring its messages to every level of government on issues from patents, Medicare, and taxes to rules for generic drugs. Among the lobbying firms PhRMA hired are Akin Gump, Arnold & Porter, Cassidy & Associates, Ogilvy Government Relations, and Williams & Jensen, a *Who's Who* of Washington influence peddlers. Between 1989 and mid-2012, PhRMA spent a staggering $225 million on lobbying.[71] Like the drug "detail men" and women who sell pharmaceutical products to doctors by wining, dining, and gifting them, PhRMA lobbyists sell policy change by dispensing information, access to campaign contributions, and gifts to politicians and federal agency staff.

At will, PhRMA can deploy this swarm of lobbyists, many of whom are highly qualified graduates of the revolving door between government and corporations. In 2012, 104 of PhRMA's lobbyists had previously held government jobs.[72] PhRMA's director of policy, Gregory Gierer, previously served as a legislative analyst for Connecticut senator Chris Dodd, and Alan Gilbert, former senior vice president and counsel for federal affairs at PhRMA, first did a stint at the White House as a special assistant to President George W. Bush. According to Open Secrets, PhRMA employed more revolvers than any other organization that was not a lobbying firm, except for the U.S. Chamber of Commerce.[73] And, of course, the revolving door spins both ways. In 2011, Representative Mary Bono Mack (R-California, and Sonny Bono's widow), chairwoman of the House

Subcommittee on Commerce, hired Ken Johnson, PhRMA's top spokesman for the past five years, as senior adviser for policy and communications.[74]

Like McDonald's, PhRMA also plays in the electoral arena. In the 2012 election cycle, it contributed $1,629,788 to PACs, parties, candidates, and outside spending groups; 56 percent of its campaign contributions went to Republicans and 43 percent to Democrats. Since 1994, these contributions totaled more than $13 million.[75] When an elected official friendly to PhRMA gets in electoral trouble, its deep pockets can save the day. In the 2012 election, Republican senator Orrin Hatch faced a primary challenge from more-conservative activists. According to the Center for Public Integrity, PhRMA gave $750,000 to Freedom Path, a nonprofit group that spent big to help Hatch win another term.[76] A leader of an opposing super PAC explained, "Orrin Hatch has always worked hard for the drug lobby. He has always been an advocate for their positions."

PhRMA is also active in state elections. In 2005, it contributed a whopping $86 million to support one California ballot initiative that would have created a new prescription drug discount program for low-income Californians and to oppose another initiative that would have subsidized more people and changed state law to make it illegal to engage in profiteering from the sale of prescription drugs.[77,78] Both failed to win passage, but the result was the maintenance of a status quo that benefited the pharmaceutical industry.

An examination of PhRMA's role in two major federal healthcare legislative outcomes, the Medicare Modernization Act of 2003 (MMA) and the Patient Protection and Affordable Care Act of 2010 (ACA, "Obamacare"), shows how the organization spends the political capital its lobbying and campaign contributions buy. (I am indebted to the research of my student William Cabin for this section). More broadly, these stories illustrate how the corporate consumption complex uses its carefully nurtured networks to achieve policy goals.

In the 2000 election, the drug industry as a whole spent $80 million to support Republicans to, as the *Wall Street Journal* put it, "ensure that any Medicare drug benefit would be administered by private insurers rather than the government."[79] The drug industry also wanted any plan to prohibit Medicare from negotiating drug prices directly. These contributions came from individual companies such as Bristol Myers, Squibb, and Pfizer, as well as the Chamber of Commerce and PhRMA itself.[80] Citizens for Better Medicare, a front group created by PhRMA and other industry groups, received $50 million to buy television, radio, newspaper, and direct mail ads to rally opposition to a federal role in the prescription drug program. The Chamber of Commerce spent another $10 million on ads. The Citizens for Better Medicare ads introduced Americans to "Flo," a skeptical senior often spotted with her friends at the bowling alley. She repeatedly tried to scare seniors with the specter of a "big government" program.[81]

Beginning in about 2000, PhRMA began to bankroll various organizations such as Citizens for Better Medicare, as well as United Seniors Association, the 60 Plus Association, and the Seniors Coalition.[82] According to a 2004 report by Public Citizen, PhRMA quietly channeled as much as $41 million to four "stealth PACs" in 2002 to help elect a Congress sympathetic to the pharmaceutical industry's interests.[83] These and other "astroturf" organizations looked like any other grassroots group but were in fact serving as fronts for industry, giving PhRMA a way to influence the public and Congress on drug issues.

With George W. Bush in the White House and the Republicans at least temporarily in control of Congress, the MMA was enacted to, among other things, create the Medicare Part D outpatient prescription drug benefit program. Part D is subsidized (and nominally run) by the government, in which people buy prescription drug insurance policies provided by private companies. Passing the MMA required overcoming the opposition of conservative Republicans and think tanks such as the Cato Institute, the American Enterprise Institute, and the Heritage Foundation, who objected to the expanded government role in healthcare. PhRMA's success in winning passage illustrates its capacity to split Republicans and build alliances, in this case with rural Democrats, to achieve priority goals.[84]

A key player in this close vote, which ended after the longest roll call in the history of the House of Representatives, was Representative Billy Tauzin, R-Louisiana, who as chair of the powerful House Committee on Energy and Commerce steered the MMA through the House. To those who objected to the unusual process, Tauzin explained, "It's just a messy process...the old adage about if you like sausage or laws, you should not watch either one of them being made is true. It's a messy process."[85]

To supporters of the MMA, it was a realistic compromise in which drug coverage was expanded but private companies stayed in control. To its opponents, however, it was an opening for privatization of the largest government health program. The Gray Panthers, an activist group of older Americans, denounced the legislation as "bait in an insidious strategy to undermine traditional Medicare and convert it into a private industry using taxpayers' subsidies to pay for it."[86]

In an assessment of the winners and losers of the MMA battles, a team of healthcare researchers noted that seniors had gained some additional coverage, although the so-called doughnut hole, which required recipients to spend $3,850 out of pocket before full benefits kicked in, imposed hardships on many beneficiaries. The biggest winner, the researchers concluded, was the pharmaceutical industry.[87] Drug companies could "now expect a higher demand from their best customers, and they prevailed on all three of their priority issues: no direct administration of benefits by the federal government, no explicit cost-control measures, and no legalization of drug reimportation."

The *Washington Post* observed that the decision to reject provisions that would have allowed Americans to legally import drugs from Canada and Europe, where medications retail for as much as 75 percent less than in the United States, was a striking political victory for the industry.[88] Polls showed that that an overwhelming majority of Americans supported the change, and the House approved the provision by 243 to 186. But the Bush Administration and pharmaceutical lobby said the move was dangerous and would cut into future research and development. The provision was dropped from the bill's final version.

In its support for the MMA, PhRMA showed its ability to change with the times. In contrast to prior legislative battles, by 1999, PhRMA was no longer unalterably opposed to prescription drug benefits under Medicare, perhaps because it realized that such legislation was inevitable and ought to be shaped to the industry's liking. One factor making such a policy more likely was the Republicans' realization that a drug benefit plan could be a potent issue for winning senior votes, long a Democratic constituency. According to conservative writer Robert Novak, the prescription drug benefit was "an audacious effort to co-opt the votes of seniors, reflecting (Republican adviser Karl) Rove's grand design of building on the electoral majority by adding constituency groups."[89] In this case, the interests of the Republican Party and the pharmaceutical industry intersected to create an alliance that succeeded in passing major federal health legislation, an accomplishment that had eluded the Clinton Administration in the previous eight years.

Six years later, PhRMA demonstrated its ability to win political victories under Democratic as well as Republican administrations. They applied the lessons they had learned from 2003: spend generously to achieve policy goals, limit government control of any future program by assigning major responsibility to the private sector, and keep a sharp eye on the industry bottom line.

In the debates on healthcare reform in 2010, the Center for Responsive Politics found that PhRMA spent $22 million and sent fifty-two representatives to make its case to Congress and the White House, more than any other organization.[90] Heading the organization until the end of 2010 was none other than Billy Tauzin, the Louisiana congressman who had twisted arms and rules to get the House to pass the MMA.

In the fifteen years before joining PhRMA, Tauzin had raised more than $218,000 in campaign contributions from pharmaceutical manufacturers. A star "revolver," he had switched from the Democratic to the Republican Party in 1995, then from Congress to PhRMA in 2004, after helping shepherd the MMA through Congress. According to a 2008 congressional report, in the first two years of MMA, one component crafted by Tauzin that switched 6.5 million low-income people from Medicaid, which did have the power to negotiate drug prices, to Medicare, which did not, produced "a windfall worth over $3.7

billion for drug manufacturers."[91] This windfall for the industry came out of the pockets of taxpayers and consumers covered by the new benefit. Tauzin told the *Washington Post* that he decided to take the PhRMA job after a successful battle against intestinal cancer. "When you become a patient, you get a sense of how incredibly valuable these medicines are," he said. "As I worked through my recovery, I realized that I wanted to work in an industry whose mission is no less than saving and enhancing lives."[92]

In 2009 and 2010, Tauzin was credited with brokering a deal with the Obama White House in which the drug industry agreed to forego $80 billion in revenues in an effort to win passage of the Affordable Care Act by lowering some prices in exchange for promises of increased business from the millions of additional insured Americans.[93] As in 2003, PhRMA again insisted on two provisions that undermined a government role in making prescription drugs more affordable: a continued ban on reimportation, and no federal negotiating on drug prices. PhRMA's deal was branded one of the top ten lobbying victories of 2010 by *The Hill*, a congressional insider media outlet.[94]

The photograph (Figure 4.3) of three senators and two congressional representatives meeting with President Bush to discuss Medicare and the

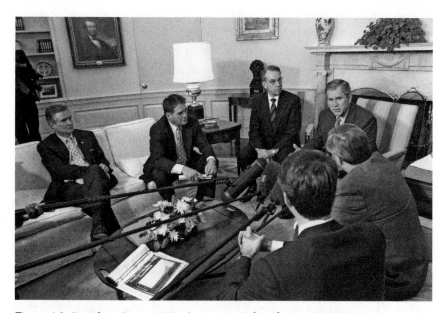

Figure 4.3 President George W. Bush meets with (*L–R*) senators John Breaux (D-Louisiana), Bill Frist (R-Tennessee), and Charles Grassley (R-Iowa), and Reps. W. J. Billy Tauzin (R-Louisiana) and Bill Thomas (R-California) to discuss Medicare and prescription drug benefits on March 5, 2001. Corbis Images.

prescription drug benefit in 2001 provides a snapshot of PhRMA's reach over the next decade. By 2010, Breaux's firm the Breaux Lott Leadership Group, a subsidiary of the Patton Boggs LLP law firm, was lobbying for PhRMA, as well as Citigroup, Goldman Sachs, General Electric, AT&T, and Tyson Foods.[95] In 2006, then–Senate Majority Leader Bill Frist (R-Tennessee) inserted text into the Department of Defense appropriations bill late on a Sunday night that added a sweeping liability provision that shields the pharmaceutical industry from law-suits over drugs used to treat pandemic illnesses, even in cases of gross negligence or gross recklessness, according to a report issued by Public Citizen.[96] The bill was strongly favored by PhRMA and other drug industry trade groups. Senator Chuck Grassley (R-Iowa) has been an outspoken critic of the drug industry and is the only Republican member of Congress who supports more stringent regu-lation in the health industries. He did, however, support the PhRMA-endorsed Medicare Modernization Act of 2003 and its Part D prescription drug benefit, and PhRMA has continued to provide Grassley with campaign donations.[97] Over his career, he has received more than $2.5 million in campaign contribu-tions from the insurance, pharmaceutical, and healthcare industries. Billy Tauzin, as described previously, went on to become the president of PhRMA in 2005. In 2000, before the photo was taken, Bill Thomas, the chairman of the House Ways and Means subcommittee on health, was accused of having an improper relationship with a drug industry lobbyist, a charge he denied, replying it was a personal matter, not a political one.[98] In 2007, Thomas joined the lobbying firm of Buchanan, Ingersoll & Rooney, which lobbies for pharmaceutical and healthcare companies on Medicare, Medicaid and other health issues.[99] These long-term relationships between elected officials, PhRMA, and the pharmaceu-tical industry illustrate the formal and informal ways by which the corporate consumption complex conducts its business.

In 2011, PhRMA hired Cassidy and Associates, a long-time Washington powerhouse lobbying firm, to ensure that new Medicare regulations to guide research on drug effectiveness would not enable Medicare and private health plans to refuse to cover certain treatments based on cost.[100] In other words, PhRMA advocated avoiding regulations that linked reimbursement too closely to effectiveness.

As in 2003, PhRMA was willing to broker political deals, even if they angered political allies. After PhRMA negotiated its deal with President Obama on healthcare reform, an enraged House Speaker John Boehner wrote to Tauzin, "When a bully asks for your lunch money, you may have no choice to fork it over. But cutting a deal with the bully is a different story, particularly if the 'deal' means helping him steal others' money as the price of protecting your own."[101]

Once it had won its political goals, PhRMA could afford to "make nice." According to The Hill, when PhRMA replaced CEO Tauzin with John Castellani in

2010, the group earned back some goodwill from the Republicans.[102] In one of his first statements after assuming PhRMA leadership, Castellani, the former president and CEO of the Business Roundtable, an organization of corporate executives, reinforced this message. "We're not in the business of picking sides," he said. "We're in the business of doing what is best for the patients we serve. Every day we strive to do just that and it is reflective in our outreach to members on both sides of the aisle."[103]

More broadly, PhRMA's wheeling and dealing shows that the corporate consumption complex is not aligned with one political party or another. True, its members contribute more often to Republicans than Democrats. But its ability to work with either party to achieve its goals demonstrates that the complex is the true bipartisan force in Washington. In the three election cycles between 2008 and 2012, the pharmaceutical and health products industries as a whole contributed almost $50 million to the campaigns of Republican federal candidates and almost $46 million to the campaigns of Democrats, ensuring ready access to the ears of policy makers on both sides of the aisle.[104]

For the most part, as the lobbying campaigns of 2003 and 2010 show, PhRMA has had no hesitation about lobbying Congress directly. It knows that its deep pockets enable it to stand out in the crowd and that its generous campaign contributions get the attention of lawmakers. But in the last decade or so, public opinion has turned against the drug industry, with fewer people viewing it as the representative of high science and medical innovation and more as just another money-making business.

A 2005 public opinion poll by the Kaiser Family Foundation showed that 70 percent of Americans believe that drug companies put profits ahead of people, compared with about a quarter who say drug companies are most concerned with developing new drugs that save lives and improve quality of life. People also blame drug companies for rising healthcare costs. Nearly six in ten say prescription drugs increase overall medical costs because they are so expensive—compared with fewer than one in four who say drugs lower medical costs by reducing the need for expensive medical procedures and hospitalizations.

"Rightly or wrongly, drug companies are now the number one villain in the public's eye when it comes to rising health-care costs," said Kaiser Foundation president Dr. Drew E. Altman. In the 2005 survey, overall, half of Americans said they had an unfavorable view of drug companies, while 44 percent said they had a favorable opinion. Drug companies were viewed more favorably than oil companies (36 percent favorable) and tobacco companies (17 percent), but less than doctors (82 percent favorable), hospitals (78 percent) and banks (75 percent).[105] PhRMA's use of astroturf groups in 2003 and 2010 illustrates the capacity of the corporate consumption complex to operate simultaneously on several levels and to use its resources to overwhelm the more limited capacity of its opponents.

Preempting government regulations that could jeopardize profits is a key goal of all trade associations. Lobbying is the main strategy used to achieve this goal, but even more efficient is to preempt regulation by developing voluntary standards for industry behavior. In 2002, in response to growing media attention on conflicts of interest between drug makers and health professionals, PhRMA developed its Code on Interactions with Health Care Professionals. Another motivation to act was that more aggressive government enforcement of even the weak existing rules on marketing had resulted in $1.2 billion in fines against drug companies.[106]

The PhRMA code defined appropriate and inappropriate activities (e.g., drug companies can offer physicians occasional modest meals but not meals with entertainment). While the code acknowledges the problems that critics had identified, an expert on industry ethics observed that it serves industry purposes by accepting its premise that drug companies' primary goal in interacting with health professionals is to educate them rather than to promote its products. The code thus seeks to manage, not end, this conflict of interest. It encourages member companies to adopt procedures to "assure adherence" but has no force of law and no formal organizational structure to support it.[107]

PhRMA has developed similar codes on the conduct of clinical trials and on communicating results of such trials to the public, both also efforts to avoid stricter regulation. PhRMA is a participant in the International Conference on Harmonisation of Technical Requirements for Registration of Pharmaceuticals for Human Use (ICH), a global body that seeks to harmonize different nation's drug regulatory process. According to John Abraham of the Centre for Research in Health and Medicine at the University of Sussex in the United Kingdom, "the ICH process has permitted scientists from industry to renegotiate extensively the scientific standards that the regulatory agencies are supposed to be using to protect public health."[108]

Still another way to influence the regulatory process is to "capture" a regulatory agency—that is, to gain enough influence to shape its decisions. In part, the legislative changes PhRMA advocated redesigned the FDA to make it more business-friendly. Once these new rules were in effect, the industry then looked for ways to make the FDA more dependent. In 1992, drug companies and the FDA made a deal in which, in exchange for the companies' agreeing to pay user fees, the FDA would review new drugs in twelve months or less. In fiscal year 1993, the industry's $8.9 million in user-fee money accounted for just 7 percent of the FDA's drug-review budget, but by 2004 it represented 53 percent of the total drug-review budget. Over the years, PhRMA and the Biotechnology Industry Organization have negotiated ever more comprehensive agreements. In exchange for higher fees, drug companies got expedited reviews and informal pre-approval meetings with FDA staff.[109]

However, it turned out that expedited review had health consequences. In a 2008 article in the *British Medical Journal*, University of Colorado researcher Dr. David Kao found that the faster a drug is approved, the more likely it is to be withdrawn or have safety warnings added later. In addition, the rapid rollout of mass marketing increases the risk that large numbers of patients will be quickly exposed to unknown risks, as was illustrated by the case of Vioxx.[110]

Recognizing the threat from this viewpoint, PhRMA reacted sharply, telling CBS News, "Unfortunately, the paper published today by the *British Medical Journal* suffers from a number of flawed assumptions, among the most glaring that Food and Drug Administration (FDA) deadlines for approving drugs have shifted the Agency's focus away from patient safety."[111] PhRMA further complained that, "It is erroneous to conclude that marketing plays a dominant influence on which medicines physicians prescribe. Marketing is only one of many factors that impact which remedies are prescribed to patients."[112] Merck's experience with Vioxx, GlaxoSmithKline's with Avandia, and Eli Lilly's with Darvon, each heavily marketed drugs that reached millions of people before being withdrawn or restricted in its use, as described in Chapter 2, show the harm that mass-marketing of inadequately tested drugs can create.

Although PhRMA is a U.S.-based organization, its member companies operate around the world, and PhRMA supports their global business by playing a key role in bilateral and multilateral trade agreements. In pursuing its goals of protecting the patents of its members and resisting any provisions that could reduce their profits, PhRMA often takes stands that prevent other nations from providing affordable medicines to their citizens. For example, in 2007, when Thailand decided to authorize the production of generic versions of two AIDS drugs that are still under U.S. company patents, as well as one cardiovascular drug, PhRMA threatened to ask the U.S. government to eliminate trade preferences that allowed some Thai imports to enter the country duty-free. Its concern was that other big market countries such as Brazil and India could emulate Thailand's decision. PhRMA CEO Billy Tauzin warned that, in the long term, this move could cost American jobs and cause the entire system of protecting intellectual property "to crumble."[113] He threatened that U.S. customers would be forced to pick up the tab for drug companies' research and development costs. He did not mention that at the time, drug makers were enjoying record profits and continued to rely on National Institutes of Health funding, not the industry, for most basic drug-development research.[114]

The UN High Level Meeting on Non-Communicable Diseases highlighted the critical importance of the pharmaceutical industry in combating chronic diseases around the world. The industry could meet these threats in two ways. On one hand, drug companies could balance their quest to make higher profits with a desire to find new ways to make the existing drugs that are effective in treating or managing chronic diseases more affordable and more available. They could develop new, affordable drugs that promise prevention or earlier intervention for major chronic diseases. They could pledge not to use their economic and political clout to manipulate democratic decisions about health.

Or they can choose a second path, the one PhRMA has followed for the last two decades: business as usual. According to the Organization for Economic Co-operation and Development, annual spending on pharmaceuticals is $947 per person in the United States, nearly twice the average of $487 for other developed nations.[115] Thanks in part to the success of PhRMA and the companies it represents, Americans spend more on drugs than any other nation, but experience worse outcomes, including in the treatment of chronic diseases that drug companies say is a main concern. By insisting on the priority of its patent protections, the need to make windfall profits, and the right to decide which drugs to develop and which to abandon based on market principles, not health needs, PhRMA has consistently put the industry goal of promoting consumption of prescription drugs ahead of patient health.

Any corporation or industry would welcome a friend like PhRMA, a powerful, effective friend who could advance its interests in the larger world. But for society as a whole, single-minded trade associations like PhRMA make it much easier for companies to choose the path that puts profits before health.

When fifty leading food and beverage companies and trade associations worked to derail the Obama Administration's plan to write tougher but still voluntary nutritional standards for foods marketed to children, they demonstrated the power of the corporate consumption complex to veto policies it opposes. When PhRMA and its drug industry partners successfully lobbied for modifications to the Medicare Modernization Act and the Affordable Care Act to benefit the industry's bottom line at the expense of making safe, affordable, and effective drugs available to more Americans, they showed the complex's capacity to safeguard corporations' bottom line. Both examples also illustrate its ability to override public opinion and undermine democracy.

Despite its accomplishments, the corporate consumption complex has significant vulnerabilities. McDonald's has to be intensely worried that caring parents, policymakers, and health professionals might decide that promoting products that put children at risk of illness is unacceptable. PhRMA fears that declining respect for an industry that puts its profits ahead of patient needs may risk losing the government protection that has enabled them to enjoy windfall rewards. More broadly, corporate leaders fear that their damage to health, the environment and democracy may again provoke a backlash, as has happened before in American history.

In his speech warning Americans about the military industrial complex, President Eisenhower suggested a remedy. "Only an alert and knowledgeable citizenry," he said, "can compel the meshing" of the complex with the American values of peace and democracy.[116] And Lewis Powell, in his confidential memo to his friend at the U.S. Chamber of Commerce, claimed that just such an informed and active citizenry was threatening the continued dominance of corporate control. To counter these threats, the corporate consumption complex mobilized to acquire unprecedented political and economic clout. But this power may not be sufficient to protect the complex's vulnerabilities. What is also needed is a softer but perhaps more insidious approach: to get inside people's heads. In the next chapter, we turn to the complex's efforts to create an ideology that makes people want what it has to offer.

5

The Corporate Ideology
of Consumption

How is it that the few men and women who control the world's major multinational consumer corporations have accumulated the power to shape patterns of health and disease among the world's billions of people? One answer, as we have seen, lies in a system that gives them the resources, rule-making authority, and skills to control the environments in which people decide what to buy and consume.

Another equally important explanation is the success of the corporate consumption complex in getting inside the minds of ordinary people. For more than a century, and especially since the 1970s, corporate leaders have created, then enlisted support for, an ideology that they incessantly broadcast around the world. These ideas are carefully rooted in the longstanding American values of individualism, self-reliance, and distrust of government. At times, social movements and economic events have challenged free market ideology—after the Depression, for example, or in the 1960s—but its tenets have long dominated what people think and how they act.

Today the beliefs that markets are the best shapers of public policy and that the products of consumer corporations are the surest road to prosperity and economic growth are accepted by most of the world's business and political elites. For many ordinary people, these views have become as natural as the air we breathe. In 1980, British prime minister Margaret Thatcher famously observed, "There is no alternative" to free market capitalism. To shake the belief that the status quo is inevitable and to pose credible alternatives will require challenging this ideological power of the corporate consumption complex.

Core Beliefs on Individualism, Markets, and Government

The corporate consumption ideology has several key tenets that constitute the foundation of its public messages. I summarize these in Box 5.1. Let's consider each to understand its origin and rationale.

LIFESTYLE IS THE MAIN INFLUENCE ON AN INDIVIDUAL'S HEALTH, AND INDIVIDUALS, NOT COMPANIES OR GOVERNMENT, ARE RESPONSIBLE FOR THEIR OWN LIFESTYLE AND BEHAVIOR

In this view, lifestyle is the major determinant of health. Since individuals decide what to eat, smoke, and drink, they have the personal responsibility to make healthy choices. As John Mackey, co-founder and CEO of the supermarket chain Whole Foods put it, "Rather than increase government spending and control, we need to address the root causes of poor health. This begins with the realization that every American adult is responsible for his or her own health."[1] And former British Prime Minister Tony Blair noted that most health problems were "not, strictly speaking public health problems at all...(but) questions of individual

---

Box 5.1 Core Beliefs of the Corporate Consumption Complex

1. Lifestyle is the main influence on health. Individuals, not companies or government, are responsible for their own lifestyle and behavior.
2. Companies produce what customers want. If people didn't demand these products, companies would not produce them.
3. Education is the best solution for helping consumers to make better choices. Advertising provides consumers with the information they need to choose wisely.
4. Government shouldn't tell people what to do. Government is the problem, not the solution.
5. Government shouldn't tell companies what to do or say; market forces and self-regulation work better and more efficiently to discourage dangerous business practices.
6. Free trade is good for everyone and is inherently fair trade.
7. Criticizing big business is un-American.
8. Promoting consumption is essential for economic growth and prosperity.

lifestyle—obesity, smoking, alcohol abuse, diabetes, sexually transmitted disease. These are not epidemics in the epidemiological sense—they are the result of millions of individual decisions at millions of points in time."[2]

If poor health is the result of individuals' bad choices, then corporations are not the problem; indeed corporations have only a constructive role to play, that of encouraging healthier choices. "I think the most important thing a food and beverage company should be doing is looking in at changing lifestyles," observed PepsiCo CEO Indra Nooyi.[3] The goal is to offer options to consumers who want healthier products, while those who prefer unhealthy products can, at their own peril, continue to enjoy their less responsible choices. "The key is choice," Nooyi said. "By expanding our portfolio, we are making sure our consumers can treat themselves when they want with 'Fun For You' products, but are able to buy a range of appetizing and healthy 'Good For You' snacks when they are being health-conscious."[4]

Burger King explains this core tenet of consumption ideology more simply in its corporate slogan, "Have It Your Way." In this view, corporations have no responsibility for the consequences of encouraging poor health. They fulfill any social responsibility they may have by offering choice. If irresponsible consumers choose their less healthy, fun-for-you products, the consequences are the fault of the consumer, not the company.

For children, according to corporate ideology, it is parents, not society, who have the responsibility to make healthy choices. In a 1996 speech, J. H. Fish, the vice-president of external relations for the tobacco company RJ Reynolds, explained:

> As the father of young children, I talk regularly with them about the pressures they face in today's world. It is the responsibility of every parent to encourage their children to make proper choices about lifestyle decisions. It is not the role of the federal government to mandate how children ought to behave. No matter how many rules and regulations bureaucrats put on the books, they are destined to fail without the reinforcement and commitment of family to act responsibly. It is time for all of us to take responsibility for ourselves and our children. It is time for us to stop inviting the government into our homes to fix the problems that we have failed to fix ourselves.[5]

By emphasizing individual and family responsibility, corporate leaders can blame the health problems associated with their products on the irresponsible individuals and parents who fail to make informed choices, not on their marketing or product design. Carlos Brito, the chief executive officer of Anheuser-Busch InBev, the world's largest beer maker, put it simply:

We don't need irresponsible drinking to have a great business.... Unfortunately, there is always that 0.5, 1 percent, 0.1 percent of the population that use our product in the wrong way, like they could use a car in the wrong way, right? And they are on the front page of the paper. So I think this whole thing about irresponsible drinking is something that we fight very hard with governments, parents, NGOs, to curb it. It's bad for our industry, bad for our business, we don't need it.[6]

COMPANIES PRODUCE WHAT CUSTOMERS WANT. IF PEOPLE DIDN'T DEMAND THESE PRODUCTS, COMPANIES WOULD NOT PRODUCE THEM

Corporations simply provide Americans with wanted *choices* in products and lifestyles. When a journalist asked Ford CEO Alan Mulalley how Ford lives up to its reputation as a green company when it sells gas guzzlers like the Expedition SUV and Mustang, he replied, "We're a consumer company, and we're market-driven. We're making the vehicles people want and value."[7]

Advertising provides customers with information to make the choices that define American freedom. In defending his company against charges it targeted children for advertising, McDonald's former CEO James Skinner asserted that Ronald McDonald

does not advertise unhealthy food to children. We provide many choices that fit with the balanced, active lifestyle. It is up to them to choose and their parents to choose, and it is their responsibility to do so. This is about choice, this is about personal, individual right to choose in the society we live in. That's where we play, that's where you play, and we have every right to do so.[8]

The assertion that corporations are simply responding to consumer demands also has the effect of making consumers complicit in the hyperconsumption status quo. According to this belief, if we didn't love our Marlboros, Big Macs, Budweiser, Hummers, and Prozac so much and demand that our need for them be fulfilled, we wouldn't be facing the health problems that these products cause.

EDUCATION IS THE BEST SOLUTION FOR HELPING CONSUMERS TO MAKE BETTER CHOICES

If the diagnosis of our health problems is that individuals and families are making poor lifestyle and behavioral choices, then a logical prescription is to educate them to make better choices.

According to Dawn Sweeney, president and CEO of the National Restaurant Association, the group's 380,000 restaurant members who serve 130 million meals a day are key nutrition educators. "As more and more nutritional information becomes available in restaurants, consumers should have the education they need to make the choices that are ideal for their individual health needs and lifestyle."[9]

Similarly, Coca-Cola asserts on its website: "Education is the essential link that enables people to select healthful diets and become more physically fit. We are committed to supporting educational programs designed to expand consumer knowledge and understanding about the benefits of a healthy lifestyle."[10] And the main rationale for direct-to-consumer advertising of prescription drugs is that it helps individuals make more informed decisions. Sydney Taurel, former chairman, president, and CEO of the drug maker Eli Lilly, put it this way:

> I think direct-to-consumer advertising has some very important public health benefits. One is you can see for the majority of the products which are advertised that they deal with conditions which, according to medical experts and the data available, are under-treated—diseases such as depression, such as diabetes, such as hypertension, such as high cholesterol. All of these areas are today under-treated, and direct-to-consumer advertising helps educate patients and bring them to the doctor's office. The most expensive disease is the one which is not diagnosed or treated.[11]

GOVERNMENT SHOULDN'T TELL PEOPLE WHAT TO DO. GOVERNMENT IS THE PROBLEM, NOT THE SOLUTION

In his first inaugural address in 1980, President Ronald Reagan told the nation, "In this present crisis, government is not the solution to our problem; government is the problem."[12] This view, now widely echoed by political and business leaders, serves to delegitimize and discredit government efforts to correct the problems that corporations cause.

More recently, corporate leaders and their conservative supporters have created a potent bogey man: the so-called Nanny State, defined as excessive meddling by the state in areas that some consider matters of personal responsibility. For example, in opposing the New York City Department of Health's proposal to ban trans fats, a food additive associated with increased prevalence and premature deaths from diabetes and heart disease, food industry lobbyist Richard Berman cautioned, "if they can declare New York City a trans fat-free nanny state by bureaucratic fiat, what can't (New York City Health) Commissioner

Thomas Frieden and his minions ban? Throwing out all the ice cream in the city might lengthen a few people's lives, too. But New Yorkers probably wouldn't appreciate it."[13]

Corporate spokespersons warn that Americans face a new threat to their cherished freedoms—the Nanny State that wants to deprive us of french fries and burgers, stop us from enjoying a cigarette or martini, and prevent us from benefiting from new medicines. By shining a spotlight on the government response to the health problems their products cause, corporations are able to deflect attention from their own practices. Moreover, by portraying government as the problem, corporations tap into the deep distrust of the public sector that has been a persistent theme in American society.

GOVERNMENT SHOULDN'T TELL COMPANIES WHAT TO DO. REGULATIONS KILL JOBS AND INDUSTRY. SELF-REGULATION WORKS BETTER AND MORE EFFICIENTLY

Distrust of government informs another element of corporate ideology: when government tells companies what to do, only bad things happen. Government regulations are alleged to kill jobs, impose unnecessary costs on business, and offer less effective solutions to the problem at hand than voluntary industry self-regulation. In a sweeping indictment of government presented at the Washington Press Club in 1998, Steven F. Goldstone, then chairman and CEO of the food and tobacco company RJR Nabisco, outlined his company's public relations message:

> We're also going to talk...about the intrusion of government into the free enterprise system and the censorship and coercion of individual liberty. We're going to talk about protecting our constitutional right to advertise, market and communicate with adults, and protecting the rights of adults in a free society to hear us and make their own personal judgments, free from government coercion. We're going to see if adults want their federal government to censor the images they are permitted to see, like that dangerous camel that has been on the front of our package for 85 years.[14]

Another example comes from Kenneth Frazier, CEO of the drug company Merck, who wrote in the *Wall Street Journal* that federal proposals to lower the costs of prescription drugs will "dampen incentives for innovation and job-creation, ultimately reducing access to life-saving and cost-saving treatments... (and) could kill 130,000 or more U.S. jobs in and around the pharmaceutical industry."[15]

Dawn Sweeney from the National Restaurant Association explains her organization's opposition to regulating the sodium content of restaurant and processed food, the source of 75 percent of the salt in the American diet:

> In an industry that incorporates a broad array of concepts and ethnic cuisines, tastes and expectations of food choices differ across the country and among cultures…we are opposed to one-size-fits-all federal, state, or local mandates around sodium content. Because of this variety, a flexible, voluntary, incremental approach is needed, and bears a greater likelihood for success. Many within the industry have been working for some time to reduce sodium in menu items—or at least to offer a number of selections that are lower in sodium. This is also an area where we have been partnering with our supply chain as restaurants cannot reduce the sodium level of products or ingredients that we purchase.[16]

The American Medical Association estimates that cutting the amount of salt in processed foods by half could save 150,000 lives in the U.S. every year.[17]

Corporate ideologies also hold that the First Amendment protects the commercial and political speech of corporations in addition to individuals. In 1996, when the Food and Drug Administration first proposed new rules to protect young people from tobacco advertising, Steven Parrish, senior vice-president at Philip Morris, objected to:

> the irrational and unconstitutional nature of the proposed regulations themselves.…FDA's proposals go far beyond measures to prevent youth access to cigarettes. FDA wants to ban practices that are legitimate tools for marketing a legal product to adults. Brand-sponsored racing, ashtrays with cigarette logos, and any non-tobacco item that bears a tobacco brand trademark will be wiped out by fiat of FDA. FDA would also effectively deny us the right to use common methods, such as direct mail, billboards, and point of sale materials, used to market many other legal products to adults.[18]

A softer version of anti-regulatory rhetoric is the call for government–industry partnerships to decide on health rules. PepsiCo's Indra Nooyi articulated this perspective: "Today's problems of the world cannot be solved by governments alone, cannot be solved by people alone. It has to be solved in partnership between companies and governments. Public–private partnerships are the only way things can work."[19] By insisting on their right to a place at the table, corporations can ensure that their interests are taken into account, even if such participation results in compromises on public health goals.

Despite its dour view of the public sector, corporate ideology has a more optimistic vision of what government could be: a protector of big business. Carlos Ghosn, CEO of Renault and Nissan, a global auto manufacturing conglomerate, explained, "The government's responsibility is to create the condition for the market to perform—to initiate technology, or to offer the basic conditions for this technology to flourish, or to serve as a catalyst for something to happen. That's where I see government cannot be replaced. But then after this, the faster you move to market forces, the better it is."[20] In this common corporate perspective, government is good when it provides services and advantages to corporations, but bad when it seeks to level the playing field by providing safeguards for consumers against the power of corporations.

FREE TRADE IS GOOD FOR EVERYONE

Promoting free trade is a core tenet of corporate ideology. In this view, free trade brings more, better, and cheaper goods to consumers everywhere. It promotes market efficiencies and stimulates economic growth. Free marketeers concede that some people get hurt by the expansion of free trade—namely, the employees and owners of small businesses who can't compete with big multinational companies like Walmart or McDonald's. Additionally, these big companies have more political clout than small producers, and can thus set the terms of trade to their benefit. In their judgement, however, these costs of free trade's collateral damage are far outweighed by its benefits.

In theory, free trade would eliminate all barriers to economic exchanges between countries. But in reality, free trade agreements include thousands of pages of exceptions, designed to protect intellectual property, local producers or, in a few cases, public health. In practice, the question is not free trade versus not-free trade, but rather, who sets the terms for trade, and to what purpose? In corporate consumption ideology, free trade is defined as agreements in which corporations and global markets set the rules and objectors are labeled as protectionists, seeking to block progress and economic growth for their selfish interests.

In order to satisfy investors' desire for growing profits, most American and European multinational corporations that produce consumer goods need to expand their markets in other countries, especially as wealthy countries impose restrictions on consumer products in order to protect public health or the environment in their own nations. To allow multinationals to penetrate these markets, importing countries are encouraged—or required—to reduce or remove tariffs or other rules that block free trade.

It is not surprising, therefore, that these companies should vigorously defend free trade. When Philip Morris International feared that the Uruguayan, Filipino, and Indonesian national governments might launch more aggressive anti-tobacco campaigns, thereby limiting these important markets, the company filed protests with the World Trade Organization. It argued that these countries were interfering with their ability to conduct legitimate business. In its complaint about Uruguay, Philip Morris lawyers wrote, "We have supported and will continue to support effective and sensible tobacco regulations, but the...measures challenged are neither. They are extreme, have not been proven effective, have seriously harmed the company's investments in Uruguay and have deprived the company of its ability to use legally protected trademarks and brands."[21]

A common rhetorical strategy of free traders, illustrated by the Philip Morris lawyers, is to acknowledge the right of governments to regulate trade in theory but to object to any actual rules that jeopardize profits or market share.

CRITICIZING BIG BUSINESS IS UN-AMERICAN

Borrowing a lesson from the Cold War, corporate ideology also seeks to paint criticism of business practices as misguided, unpatriotic, and, ultimately, un-American. In a television interview, 2012 Republican Senate candidate Rand Paul observed that President Obama's complaints about the energy company BP's inadequate clean-up of its Gulf Coast oil spill "sounds really un-American in his criticism of business."[22] New York City billionaire Mayor Michael Bloomberg, a strong defender of public health but not of critics of the free market system, described Occupy Wall Street protestors as "trying to destroy the jobs of working people in this city," even while defending the right of people to protest.[23]

When 2004 Democratic vice-presidential candidate John Edwards urged Americans to give up their SUVs to reduce pollution and the nation's dependence on foreign oil, Jason Vines, Chrysler Group's vice-president of communications fired back, "Last time I checked, America is about choice.... This kind of reminds me of book burnings of the past. Shouldn't a president try to preserve freedoms? So let's lay off any suggestions of vehicle choice by government committee."[24]

By painting their critics as unpatriotic or misguided radicals who want to restrict the freedom of ordinary citizens, corporations hope to tap into Americans' fears of disruption and political conflict.

PROMOTING CONSUMPTION IS ESSENTIAL FOR ECONOMIC GROWTH AND PROSPERITY

In the depth of the economic crisis of 2008, Thomas J. Donahue, the president and CEO of the U.S. Chamber of Commerce, described its "Campaign for Free Enterprise" to a *Business Week* reporter:

> We are going to remind, promote, educate and encourage in every way we can so that people remember, or learn, what made the greatest

economy in the history of the world—[*what*] created more jobs, created more wealth, created more innovation, created more opportunity—was a free-enterprise economy with free and open trade with open capital markets, with the right to fail and fall right on your face and get up and try it over again, the right to make money, and the right to make it in a system with moderate regulation and taxes.[25]

These words from Donahue, a leader of business's most powerful lobbying organization, illustrate the celebratory view of free market capitalism, even in the throes of the world's most serious crisis since the Great Depression. Echoing Thatcher's "there is no alternative," its supporters describe free market capitalism as "the only system that increases both growth and freedom."[26] Thomas Friedman, the *New York Times* columnist and champion of free markets, compares market-driven globalization to the reality of the sun rising every morning:

Generally speaking, I think it's a good thing that the sun comes up every morning. It does more good than harm.... But even if I didn't much care for the dawn there isn't much I could do about it. I didn't start globalization, I can't stop it—except at a huge cost to human development—and I'm not going to waste time trying. All I want to think about is how *I* can get the best out of this new system, and cushion the worst, for the most people.[27]

For those who don't believe they are benefitting from the status quo, the consequence of these beliefs is skepticism or despair that another world is possible, a very potent obstacle to change.

At times, corporate leaders suggest an orchestrated crusade against their rights. In 2003, the CEO and chair of the pharmaceutical company Eli Lilly warned of a "worldwide campaign against pharmaceutical innovation" by governments and healthcare systems that failed to protect "the two most important preconditions for innovation in my industry...market-based pricing and intellectual property protection."[28] By painting themselves as the beleaguered victims of misguided policies that jeopardize economic growth, corporations and their allies hope to win sympathy from policymakers and the public.

Consumption ideology is not the only belief system in the church of free markets. Other variants focus on military security, relations with workers, or the primacy of shareholder value. But consumption ideology is the mass religion of corporations—the set of beliefs used to manufacture consent from consumers, to win their support for a political and economic system that offers the masses ready access to products in exchange for acquiescence in a world where corporations increasingly make the decisions that shape our lives.

While the proponents of the corporate consumption ideology don't agree on everything, and the nuances of the beliefs change somewhat over time, it has been a remarkably powerful and consistent set of ideas for the last several decades. To remain relevant, even corporate critics are forced to engage with beliefs that may have little basis in fact (e.g., that free trade benefits all). The corporate consumption complex uses this ideology to enlist support from both business and political élites and ordinary people for its economic and political agenda of promoting consumption as the only feasible path for economic prosperity. What may strike readers is how reasonable and self-evident the ideology's tenets seem to be, even to those who know its grounding in truth is limited. To reduce the influence of the complex in causing premature death and preventable illness will require tackling the foundations of its ideology.

Taking on Corporate Consumption Ideology

The power of corporate consumption ideology lies in its capacity to engage people and to disarm threats to the status quo. To identify possible vulnerabilities in this world view, let's first review the extent to which corporations' practices follow the ideology they promulgate, then examine public support for its various beliefs. Finally, I explore counter-ideologies that could effectively compete with the corporate consumption ideology.

As we have seen in previous chapters, the practice of corporations does not always match their ideology. PepsiCo and other food and beverage companies promote their unhealthy fun-for-you products much more heavily than their healthier alternatives because fun-for-you foods are more profitable. Choice is the smokescreen that enables these companies to promote ready access to their most profitable—and often unhealthy—products. Despite claims by alcohol maker CEOs that their companies do not need to promote irresponsible drinking to make a profit, independent studies show that alcohol companies target youth and problem drinkers with their advertising, relying heavily on these populations for current and future market share.[29] Tobacco, alcohol, and food companies say they want parents to make decisions about their children's consumption habits but use every advertising strategy at their disposal to reach children directly, thereby bypassing parental involvement. And all the industries I have described extol the benefits of education but spend billions on marketing approaches that are explicitly designed to bypass cognitive processes and appeal directly to deeper, more primitive urges, the antithesis of education. In the political arena, they consistently oppose accurate, effective independent health education.

By exposing how corporations exploit the value of freedom to choose so they can promote choices that benefit their profit at the expense of well-being, advocates of healthier patterns of consumption can disarm a powerful ideological weapon. In his book *Development as Freedom,* the philosopher Amartya Sen asks whether choice nourishes or deprives us, builds or undermines self-respect, encourages or diminishes participation in democratic society.[30] Using these criteria to judge corporate promises of choice can help to separate the dross from the gold.

Another corporate claim is that governments have too much power, an assertion that enables corporate America to find common cause with traditional conservatives who believe that more government authority means less individual freedom. But as David Rothkopf observes in *Power, Inc.,* "history demonstrates that when the power of states is reduced, with alarming regularity, it does not benefit average citizens as much as it does big private actors well positioned to swoop in and take best advantage of the opening." [31] What corporations fear from government is not loss of individual freedom but of their right to set the agenda, to design, market and distribute their products with as little interference as possible, irrespective of the health, environmental, or social consequences.

Corporations also use the demand for their products and the lifestyle of hyperconsumption they promote to further their attack on government. Juliet Schor, an economist at Boston College, has observed that as private consumption crowds out public use of resources for education, healthcare, and recreation. Since people "need" to buy more things and to borrow to buy, they want to pay lower taxes.[32] Quick to realize an opportunity, corporate promoters of starving the beast of government use their muscle to advocate leaving more money in the pockets of consumers. With this extra cash—and the expanded credit that the financial sector has made available as another source of profit—consumers can buy more of the goods and services corporate America offers. In effect, lower taxes and easy credit subsidize hyperconsumption at the expense of clean air, better education and health care.

In summary, the assertions of the corporate consumption complex need to be taken with a grain—or perhaps a shaker—of salt. They are often based on dubious or nonexistent evidence, they contradict the practices of corporations in the real world, and they are self-serving. Does this matter? In the short run, no. The corporate system has the power to define its own reality. Karl Rove, adviser to President George W. Bush, once said, "When we act, we create our own reality. And while you're studying that reality—judiciously, as you will—we'll act again, creating other new realities, which you can study too, and that's how things will sort out. We're history's actors...and you, all of you, will be left to just study what we do."[33] Similarly, the corporate consumption complex uses all the tools as its disposal to create its own reality, expecting critics to lament but not change its practices.

In the longer run, however, other American traditions—valuing equality, truth, fairness, justice, community, and democracy—challenge the domination of corporate ideology. Exposing the contradictions of this ideology, revealing the false claims it makes, and documenting its undermining of core values creates the opportunity to engage the American people—and those of other nations—in a search for alternatives.

Public Opinions on Corporate Core Beliefs

Proponents of the corporate consumption ideology would have us believe that not only corporate leaders but also the masses support these beliefs. A review of national and international public opinion polls suggests that the reality is more complex. In a 2009 BBC poll in 27 countries, only 11 percent of those questioned thought free-market capitalism was working well. Almost a quarter (23 percent) thought capitalism was fatally flawed, including 43 percent of the French sample, 38 percent of Mexican respondents, and 35 percent of Brazilians. In 26 of 27 countries (Turkey was the exception), a majority of respondents wanted government to be more active in regulating business.[34] The 2008 economic crisis no doubt contributed to these dark views of market forces.

Several polls suggest that American people don't trust corporations very much. A 2011 Gallup poll found that 67 percent of respondents thought corporations had too much power.[35] A 2010 Gallup Poll found that while 19 percent of respondents had a great deal or quite a lot of confidence in big business, 38 percent reported very little or no confidence, almost the same rates making these judgements as in 1981.[36] A separate poll showed that more than a quarter of respondents thought that Big Business was a greater threat to the country than Big Government or Big Labor.[37] Another series of Gallup polls found that the proportion of Americans who wanted major corporations to have less influence in this nation grew from 52 percent in 2001 to 62 percent in 2011, an increase of almost 20 percent.[38]

These findings suggest that many Americans, including substantial portions of those who have benefited least from the post–World War II prosperity, have doubts about corporations and the economic and social arrangements that the corporate consumption complex has celebrated. By themselves, these doubts do not constitute a counter-ideology, much less a program for action, but they may provide an opening for a different national conversation on consumption, well-being, democracy, and health.

On the question of the role of government in regulation, polls also show that Americans are divided—and that the corporate campaign against regulation seems to be succeeding. In 1993, according to a Gallup Poll, 37 percent of respondents thought government regulated too much and 28 percent too little. By 2011, Gallup found that 50 percent thought the government regulated too much and 23 percent too little.[39] Annual Pew Research Center polls showed that between 1987 and 2012, support for government regulation increased among Democrats but fell among Republicans and Independents, suggesting further polarization on this issue. Overall, in 2102, 63% of the population agreed that "a free market economy needs government regulation in order to best serve the public interest."[40] However, another series of polls by Pew suggest that when it comes to public health, support for stronger regulation has not declined much since 1995. In a 2012 survey, more than half the respondents support stronger federal regulation of food production and packaging and environmental protection, and about two in five support stronger regulation of car safety, workplace health and safety, and prescription drugs.[41] Protecting public health might constitute a useful starting point for public discussion on the costs and benefits of regulation.

Polling data provide only limited snapshots into the minds of people; translating such findings into the deeper knowledge needed to understand the values and beliefs that guide behavior is more challenging. Finding the language, issues, and political strategies that can exploit these openings in public opinion to construct alternatives to the corporate consumption ideology will require new approaches to health education, community organizing and political strategizing.

Constructing Alternatives to Consumption Ideology

Constructing an alternative to consumption ideology requires taking on several intellectual and political tasks. First, the myths and misinformation on which corporate ideology rests need to be debunked. Challenging the tenuous "facts" that corporations use to justify their health-damaging practices will not be sufficient to bring about change, but it is a necessary step in contesting business's credibility. The high proportion of people who mistrust corporations suggests many people are ready to hear such messages. Second, alternative beliefs, lifestyles, and patterns of behavior that appeal to human needs and desires—other than those tapped by corporate interests—need to be identified, promoted, and forged into an attractive and credible counter-ideology. Third, and perhaps most difficult, the institutions and governance systems that the corporate consumption complex uses to advance its ideology and maintain the status quo need to be confronted and ultimately transformed.

Already, many movements and organizations around the world are immersed in these daunting tasks—an analysis of their successes and failures, which I present in the following chapters, provides the foundation for moving forward. In this chapter, I focus more narrowly on the role that scientists and health professionals have played both in supporting corporate consumption ideology and in developing alternatives.

Debunking Myths and Misinformation

Capitalism has always depended on science and technology for innovation. In the past few decades, the corporate consumption complex has expanded this use by employing ever more scientists to design more profitable products; convince people that hyperconsumption makes them safer, happier, and healthier; and thwart regulation by creating doubt and confusion about the scientific evidence. In each of these tasks, scientists and health professionals have played an important role.

In designing products, scientists provide both material support, e.g., creating hyperpalatable products that blend fat, sugar and salt; and ideological cover—how can anything devised by highly educated researchers in white coats be bad for health? In their marketing, companies borrow the legitimacy of science to make their claims more credible and to cloak their real goals—selling more products—in the mantle of the modern era's religion of science.

Corporate slogans like those from DuPont, "The Miracles of Science" (which replaced "Better Things for Better Living...Through Chemistry") and Bayer USA's "Science for a Better Life," illustrate how companies embrace and even flaunt science. Consider a few advertising campaigns that have made health claims: L&M Cigarettes: "Just what the doctor ordered,"[42] SUV ads claiming that these vehicles are safer because they are bigger and more powerful,[43] and Merck's direct-to-consumer ads for Vioxx promoting its use "for everyday victories" for arthritis sufferers who wanted to overcome their disabilities.[44] In each of these cases, misleading scientific claims have contributed to preventable deaths.

In the political arena, corporations and their allies use science to create confusion and doubt in order to thwart regulation and convince policymakers not to act and the public not to worry.[45,46] Public health policies to reduce the toll from tobacco, alcohol, firearms, automobiles, pharmaceutical products, and food have consistently been opposed by industry-paid scientists whose goals were to cast doubt on the evidence that justified public oversight. "Doubt is our product," a cigarette executive once observed, "since it is the best means of competing with the 'body of fact' that exists in the mind of the general public. It is also the means of establishing a controversy."[47]

While corporations have used science and scientists as a weapon to advance their business and political interests, it is also true that scientists and health researchers have been in the forefront of efforts to protect the public against corporate misinformation and harm. Researchers first documented the appalling toll of tobacco, and then an army of health advocates and professionals led the successful campaigns to reduce tobacco use, first in the United States and later in other developed nations and around the world. The work of scientists like Rachel Carson on pesticides, Barry Commoner on petrochemical products, Irving Selikoff on asbestos, and organizations like the Environmental Defense Fund and the committees for occupational safety and health helped to create the environmental and occupational health movements and to spur the spate of new regulations that were passed in the United States in the 1960s and 1970s. Today researchers, public interest science groups and health professionals are actively engaged in confronting the pharmaceutical, firearms, automobile, and food industries.

Scientists and health professionals play an important role in constructing an alternative to the edifice of corporate consumption ideology because they have the capacity to challenge several of its pillars. Corporate ideology depends on four science-based claims:

(1)   that genetic (or cultural) factors best explain disease causation and that controlling disease can best happen on an individual basis,
(2)   that its views of human nature, health and disease are the only objective scientifically valid ones,
(3)   that its prescriptions for the marriage of corporate power and modern science and technology is the key to better living and good health, and
(4)   that the future it has created for us will benefit, not harm, our children and grandchildren.

Independent scientists are challenging each of these claims. Just as churches depend on divine authority for their continuing hold, industry depends on science to provide the moral stature needed to justify these claims. By withdrawing their support for corporations' misappropriation of science, researchers can deprive corporations of one of their ideological bulwarks. By demonstrating in practice the alternative of using science to benefit humanity rather than corporate profits, they can contribute to a healthier future.

Several strands of cutting-edge scientific research challenge the scientific claims of corporate ideology. New epigenetic research questions the twentieth-century view that the DNA we are born with determines our health over our lifetimes. It suggests instead that environments and genes interact in complex ways and that changing environments to prevent the expression of genetic diseases may be a more feasible ways to reduce disease than engineering the genes of individuals.[48] For example, modifying the obesity-producing food environments that seem to trigger manifestation of type 2 diabetes is a far more efficient strategy for reducing the growing burden of diabetes than treating its metabolic consequences one person at a time. Hence, restricting the relentless promotion and ubiquitous availability of sugary beverages, fast food, and processed snacks may do more to prevent future cases of diabetes than any drug or gene therapy.

Public health research on asthma, obesity, heart disease, and cancer also suggest that clinical interventions and behavioral strategies may be less fruitful paths for improving the health of populations than changing environments, policies and social structures.[49,50] As the evidence for these new approaches grows and moves into the scientific mainstream, it will be more difficult for corporate ideologues to insist that biomedical and individual approaches are the best or only ways to solve the world's health problems. In 2020, according to the National Institutes of Health, Americans will spend at least $158 billion on treating cancer. Today many cancer patients pay more than $100,000 for a single course of drug therapy.[51] Ending the global promotion of tobacco to young people, on the other hand, can prevent more cases of cancer than all these drugs combined and at a fraction of the cost.

As scientists document and expose the role of corporate practices and products in producing the world's most serious health problems, industry will find it more difficult to claim that its use of science is what brings the world progress. The clearest illustration of how serial misinformation can discredit an industry comes from tobacco, where researchers have documented the systematic corporate misrepresentations of scientific evidence on the impact of tobacco on health and the industry's long history of deceiving its customers and policymakers.[52] As a result, the tobacco industry today is a much less credible participant in public policy discussions than it was fifty years ago.

Another claim of consumption ideology is that corporate use of science and technology to maximize profits is inevitable—that there is no alternative. This inevitability rests on two claims. First, corporations assert they "own" the science—it is their intellectual property to do with as they please rather than the collective product of generations of humanity. Second, since only corporations have the infrastructure to deploy the science to market, critics can object to their practices but as Karl Rove said about the Bush Administration's foreign policy, only corporations have the power to make their own reality. Examples include the food industry's decision to make cheap obesogenic food and beverages more available than healthier alternatives; the pharmaceutical industry's focus on "me-too" copycat drugs rather than new products to cure major diseases; and the auto industry's decision to make building individual passenger cars a higher priority than producing buses, trains, or other forms of mass transit.

By providing policymakers, consumers, and advocates with the specific knowledge and tools to contest these claims, scientists can arm the public with the evidence needed to propose alternatives. These can be as simple as discovering ways to produce food without using disease-inducing trans fats or making airbags or trigger locks standard features of automobiles and guns, to more complex proposals such as designing local food systems to rely less on industrial agriculture. When the industry monopoly on applying science and technology to solving human problems is broken, then policy makers and the public can debate which proposals best advance human well-being. Today, too often the corporate solution, which always puts profits first, is accepted without question.

A third science-based claim is that the corporate solutions to human problems are sustainable, at least in the short run. As the contrary evidence grows, corporate supporters initiate frantic campaigns to defend their beliefs, making themselves vulnerable to more rational voices. This is well illustrated by the determined corporate assault on climate science that shows that human-induced global warming threatens health, prosperity, and ultimately human survival. As the author and activist Naomi Klein explains:

> Climate change detonates the ideological scaffolding on which contemporary conservatism rests. There is simply no way to square a belief system that vilifies collective action and venerates total market freedom with a problem that demands collective action on an unprecedented scale and a dramatic reining in of the market forces that created and are deepening the crisis.[53]

In recent years, corporations and conservative think tanks have spent hundreds of millions of dollars to support climate deniers to discredit what most scientists believe is true.[54] Public opinions polls demonstrate that this disinformation campaign has had some success.[55] But as Klein argues, the willingness of the energy industry and its supporters to continue spending to defend increasingly indefensible science shows their understanding of a new reality. If public support for policies to act against global warming grows, fears the industry, several of the core beliefs of corporate ideology would be subject to challenge. That understanding makes the investment in climate denial a rational, albeit a socially destructive, act for the energy industry.

Might critics of hyperconsumption exploit corporate vulnerabilities by extending this argument? What if health advocates could convince parents and concerned citizens that current policies allowing food, tobacco, and alcohol companies to promote their products to children and young people with only minimal restrictions effectively doom our children and grandchildren to premature death and horrible suffering from diabetes, cancer, and heart disease? Could we then undermine support for laissez-faire regulation of marketing to children? If the governments and people of China, India, Brazil, and Mexico understand that if their countries follow Western patterns of automobile and energy use millions of preventable injuries, illnesses, and deaths will ensue, will their publics demand another direction?

While scientists and health professionals lack the resources that the energy industry has poured into its campaign for climate change denial, they do have the knowledge, skills, and credibility to make these arguments to a wider public. Their success in engaging the public on these issues will make it much harder for corporate claims to be accepted without question.

More broadly, if concerned scientists and health professionals, professional organizations and universities could launch a sustained campaign to insist that scientific knowledge belongs to all humanity, not only to the corporations with the resources to deploy it, they could contribute to a climate more hospitable to evidence-based policy.

Equally important, they could set the stage for more rationale use of science in the future. Today several emerging technologies may be creating the health hazards of the next century: assisted reproductive technologies, genetically modified organisms, electromagnetic radiation, and widespread commercial use of endocrine disruptors, to name a few. Industry scientists insist these technologies are safe; critics are portrayed as Luddite radicals. Without ideological support for independent science, these debates are more likely to be settled by post-marketing body counts, as we have seen for the consumer products contributing to today's epidemics of chronic diseases and injuries.

What makes the hope for a campaign for independent science more than a naïve pipe dream is the on-the-ground work of organizations like the Union of Concerned Scientists, the Center for Science in the Public Interest, Physicians for Social Responsibility and many others. By extending and amplifying this work, scientists and health professionals can help to create a body of knowledge and a practice that can provide a concrete alternative to the ideology of corporate science.

Appealing to Human Desires and Needs

Corporations successfully resist challenges to their political and economic dominance in part because they have persuaded people that Big Business gives people what they want. This success rests not so much on rational arguments but on appeals to our deepest wants, needs and fears. Let's again look at a few corporate slogans, shown in Box 5.2, and advertising messages that illustrate this appeal to human desires.

By associating their brands with feelings and sensations, corporations build a bond between products and their customers that transcends cognitive processes or rational analysis. The experience of consuming can become a way of relieving stress, fighting off insecurity and loneliness, establishing connections to others, and asserting one's masculinity or femininity—some of the emotional demands precipitated by an unfettered market economy. Figure 5.1, for example, shows the Dodge Ram pickup truck, designed to look as big and menacing as a Mack truck and to appeal to customers' "reptilian instincts." Its popularity led other automakers to supersize their SUVs and pickups and to launch advertisements that prescribed these vehicles as the antidote to suburban fears about crime and urban disorder.[56] With such potentially rewarding and often subconscious pay-offs, it is hardly surprising that many people choose to consume, even in ways that can cause illness, death, pain, and suffering. To interrupt the cycle of emotional reward that consumption (and especially hyperconsumption) offer, those who claim another world is possible will need to offer alternative benefits that are equally or more attractive.

What might such an alternative ethic of consumption look like? To succeed, it cannot rely on abstention and moralism. People eat, drink, and consume in part for pleasure, and asking people to give up these pleasures is unlikely to offer a viable alternative to corporate consumption. Instead, we need to find ways to create patterns of consumption that bring pleasure, create community, and support health. In the 1960s, some parts of the youth counterculture offered such rewards and offered an alternative to the corporate-dominated culture and patterns of

---

Box 5.2 Corporate Slogans That Tap Human Desires

Dreaming—Honda—The power of dreams; Jaguar—Don't dream it, drive it

Adventure—Marlboro—Come to Marlboro Country; Taco Bell—Head for the border; Dodge Ram—Grab life by the horns; Butterfinger Candy Bar—Break out of the ordinary

Youth—Pepsi, the taste of a new generation

Love—McDonald's "I'm Lovin' It"; Volkswagen: *Aus Liebezum Automobile*, translated as, "Out of love to automobiles"

Feeling and pleasure—BMW—Sheer driving pleasure; Toyota, Oh what a feeling

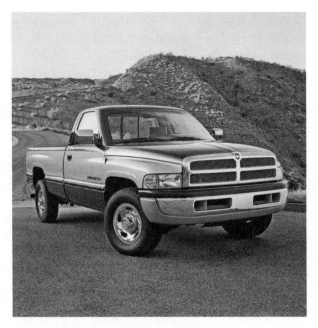

Figure 5.1　The 1994 Dodge Ram pickup. Corbis Images.

consumption of the 1950s. It celebrated, among other things, personal freedom, expansion of consciousness, freedom from traditional gender roles, and participatory democracy. Corporate marketers soon realized they could co-opt these desires, using youth culture to sell products, thus tarnishing the idealism that had been one part of youth counterculture. Today, new forces—such as the food justice movement, ethical consumption groups, and environmental sustainability advocates, are striving to create contemporary alternatives to corporate consumption. They will also need to find ways to resist the inevitable cooptation that corporations will attempt. The growing involvement of global multinational food companies in the organic food market illustrates one such effort.

Dismantling the Corporate Consumption Complex

In practice, the American people have made significant changes in their patterns of consumption. Sometimes these changes are motivated by health, other times by economic forces or changing values. As we have seen, the prevalence of cigarette smoking in the United States fell from 42 percent in 1965 to 19 percent in 2011.[57] Per capita consumption of ethanol, the active ingredient in alcohol beverages, fell by 13 percent from 1977 to 2009.[58] In 1998, Americans on average drank 54 gallons of soda a year. But by the end of 2012, the total stood at just 44 gallons, a decline of 18.5 percent.[59] And, to the consternation of the auto industry, young people are driving less and buying fewer cars. If current trends continue, predicts one study, driving could remain below its 2007 peak through 2040, even though the population is expected to grow by 21 percent.[60]

In a sensible society, these declines in unhealthy and unsustainable consumption would be celebrated and all sectors would work together to accelerate these changes. For the corporate consumption complex, however, declines in hyperconsumption translate into falling profits. And so when consumption falls, the tobacco, alcohol, soda, automobile and other industries go all out to find replacement consumers or re-engage former customers by offering price deals, super-sizing products, or making unsubstantiated health claims.

Ultimately the success of creating new approaches to consumption will require more than weaving together the evidence, ideas and emotions that will constitute an alternative ideology. It will also require confronting, then dismantling the power of the corporate consumption complex. Big business succeeds in shaping patterns of health and disease not because it has better evidence or ideas, or a deeper understanding of human needs, but because it has more power to get inside people's heads and into the rooms where policy decisions are made. Through their advertising, public relations, lobbying, campaign contributions, and their influence on media coverage, philanthropy, and scientific research, corporations and their allies have a dominant voice in most of our society's channels of communication.

Offering an alternative to corporate ideology, therefore, is not simply a question of framing a better message or communicating more effectively. It also requires creating movements, organizations and institutions that can challenge corporate control in many sectors of life, including those that influence health at all levels from the household to the global. This will require a jiu-jitsu political strategy, which, like the Japanese martial art, uses the agility and deftness of health advocates to convert the size and power of its corporate opponents from an asset into a handicap.

One important function of the corporate consumption ideology is to pre-empt criticism of the health and social consequences of corporate domination. To disarm this function, proponents of an alternative perspective need to expose the vulnerabilities of the corporate consumption complex. One such weakness is that the economic costs of products that cause premature deaths and preventable illnesses are often externalized to consumers and taxpayers, who then suffer this burden for generations. Another is the extensive use of deception and manipulation in advertising, lobbying, and public relations. A third is systematic efforts to undermine democracy and public health protection through lobbying and campaign contributions. Finally, all evidence suggests that current patterns of consumption are economically and environmentally unsustainable, enabling today's generations to consume at the expense of the well-being of future generations. These political and moral vulnerabilities create windows of opportunity for public discussion and community mobilization.

Today, many sectors of society grapple with weaving these vulnerabilities into a narrative that can offer a compelling alternative to corporate consumption ideology. Some are listed in Box 5.3. Together these and other groups are weaving these disparate strands into a counter-ideology that can, over time, provide a comprehensive and appealing moral belief system. What role does health play in its construction?

Box 5.3 **Social Groups Acting to Create Ideological Alternatives to Corporate Consumption**

Types of Groups	*Ideological Contribution*	*Source*
Ethical consumer groups	What people consume shapes their moral identity	a
Slow and local food groups	Maintain local food traditions and practices, link gastronomic pleasure and environmental responsibility, and resist corporatization of food	b
Fair trade groups	Trade practices should not jeopardize workers, nations or the global environment. All nations should have the right and opportunity to benefit from global trade.	c
Environmental justice groups	The environmental consequences of business practices and economic development should not unduly burden any group; all people have the right to a clean and healthy environment.	d
Faith-based social action groups	Moral and religious values can motivate believers to take action to protect the environment, promote justice, or defend the vulnerable.	e
Farmer and peasant movements	Food systems need to support workers and consumers and create sustainable patterns of agriculture and food marketing.	f

(continued)

Box 5.3 (**Continued**)

Other labor groups	Workers and consumers can benefit from production and regulation systems that protect both.	g
Patient advocacy groups	By challenging corporate practices that contribute to their illnesses, people with these conditions can improve their own health and contribute to a healthier society	h
Cultural jamming groups	By subverting corporate messages, one can expose corporate domination and foster democratic change.	i
Global justice groups	Corporate controlled globalization damages health, democracy and the environment while globalization from the bottom promotes more equal distribution of the world's resources	j

References for Box 5.3:

a. Lewis T, Potter E. *Ethical Consumption: A Critical Introduction*. London: Rutledge, 2011.
b. Andrews G. *The Slow Food Story*. Montreal: McGill-Queen's University Press, 2008.
c. Bowes J. *The Fair Trade Revolution*. London: Pluto Press, 2011.
d. Bullard RD, ed. *The Quest for Environmental Justice: Human Rights and the Politics of Pollution*. San Francisco, CA: Sierra Club Books, 2005.
e. Wallis J. *Rediscovering Values: A Guide for Economic and Moral Recovery*. Brentwood, TN: Howard Books, 2011.
f. La Via Campesina. *Sustainable Peasant and Family Farm Agriculture Can Feed the World Via Campesina Views*. Jakarta, Indonesia: Via Campesina, 2010.
g. Frank D. Where are the workers in consumer-worker alliances? Class dynamics and the history of consumer-labor campaigns. *Politics & Society*, 2003;31(3):363–379.
h. Brown P, Morello-Frosch R, Zavestoski S, eds. *Contested Illnesses: Citizens, Science, and Health Social Movements*. Berkeley: University of California Press, 2011.
i. Lasn K. *Culture Jam: How to Reverse America's Suicidal Consumer Binge—And Why We Must*. New York: William Morrow, 2000.
j. Della Porta D, ed. *The Global Justice Movement: Cross-National and Transnational Perspectives*. Boulder, CO: Paradigm Publishers, 2007.

First, advocates of a counter ideology have begun to create a language that allows them to communicate with the public. Corporations have appropriated what some have called America's first language of individualism, personal responsibility, limited government, and individual freedom. Those proposing an alternative seek to become fluent in America's "second language" of common good, collective action, fairness, and using government to achieve common purposes.[61,62] One way to do this is follow the advice of the sociologist C. Wright Mills, who said that activists ought to "turn personal troubles and concerns into social issues and problems."[63]

In matters of health, they can do this by helping people to understand that the diabetes, cancer, and asthma that they or their family experience are in part the result of a political and economic system in which companies put profit ahead of health. Advocacy groups of people with AIDS, breast cancer survivors, and parents of children with asthma have shown how to link illness experiences with political analysis in order to mobilize communities.[64] By transforming personal troubles into a social problem, as Mills advocated, these activists create an identity that makes collective action an essential part of their response to illness.

In ideology, as in so many things, one size does not fit all. As I wrote in the Preface, those who lived though the social movements of the 1960s or younger participants in successor movements might find it easy to summon the optimism and hope that ordinary people can change history. For those exposed only to the individualism and consumerism of the 1970s and beyond, however, other approaches may be necessary. Perhaps focusing this latter group's skepticism on bogus corporate claims may be a starting point. The anti-tobacco industry Truth Campaign, which in the late 1990s and early 2000s encouraged rebellious teenagers to reject the tobacco industry's effort to profit at their expense, succeeded in changing attitudes towards the tobacco industry and smoking behavior. These campaigns showed that those exposed to the counter-advertising had more negative perceptions of tobacco industry practices and were less likely to smoke,[65] illustrating the potential of such an approach to reach skeptical young people.

A second element of a counter ideology is to ground consumption in human needs that transcend the infantilization and appeals to insecurities that now motivate commercial promotion of consumption and hyperconsumption. The Super Bowl television ads provide a window into Madison Avenue's views of the typical consumer. Eight of the top ten Super Bowl advertisers are automobile or food and beverage makers, and these corporations pay on average more than $3.5 million for a thirty-second ad.[66] These commercials present images of babies, dogs, and women in bikinis, usually presented at a level that would seemingly appeal to immature eight-year-olds rather than adult Super Bowl viewers. In a Coca-Cola ad shown for the 2012 Super Bowl, for example, an animated polar bear urges its companion to drink a bottle of Coke (65 grams of high fructose corn syrup and 57 mg of caffeine) to allay its fears about who might win the Super Bowl. The closing message: "Coca-Cola: Open Happiness." [67] The social critic Benjamin Barber describes contemporary commercialism as "induced childishness: an infantilization that is closely tied to the demands of consumer capitalism in a global market economy."[68]

Alternative approaches to consumerism might appeal to feelings of happiness, solidarity, sense of community, or fairness. The "slow food movement," which seeks pleasure from the preparation and consumption of locally grown food; alternative transportation groups that promote biking, walking and mass transit; fair trade activism, which seeks to ensure that the workers producing goods are not subject to corporate abuses; and climate activism, which seeks individual, collective and municipal action to reduce global warming, are all examples of alternatives to corporate consumption. To date, these efforts have been modest and often more attractive to middle-class people, but their continuing appeal demonstrates the potential for engaging communities, organizations, and activists in forging alternatives to corporate consumption. The success of the environmental and food justice movements in mobilizing low-income communities and people of color show that by speaking to their concerns it is possible to broaden movements that challenge current patterns of consumption.[69,70]

One attraction of these alternatives is their practicality: anyone can find some way to change what they eat, drink, buy, or how they get around. The many entry points to transformed consumption mean it can accommodate individual differences and preferences. In addition, politicized consumers can choose the pace and trajectory of transformation—from avoiding fast food outlets to becoming a vegan. Moving back and forth between individual change and political change highlights the possibility and the necessity of working at multiple levels. This flexibility opens the door for wide cross sections of the population to explore such alternatives, including the substantial portions who distrust corporations. On the other hand, a counter ideology that has a thousand variants, each with its own adherents and practices makes the creation of a clear, unified political agenda for transformation more difficult, a challenge I will take up in the last chapter.

A third element of a counter ideology is respect for democracy. Across the political spectrum, Americans lament the erosion of core democratic principles of fairness, such as one person-one vote and the ability to participate in decisions that affect one's well being. A 2012 Rasmussen public opinion poll showed that 57 percent of a sample of U.S. likely voters believed that it is not possible to seek the presidency without ties to lobbyists and special interest groups.[71] Addressing the public's dissatisfaction with the growing tilt of the political playing field towards corporations and their allies will require the many groups now exploring alternative forms of democracy and governance to develop a coherent political program that offers people concrete ways to participate in the political process. It will also require bringing together the mostly-separate efforts to change laws on campaign finance, lobbying, voter registration, and revolving door rules, to name a few.

Finally, any alternative ideology must address the issue of sustainability. For those able to think beyond their own generation, the unsustainability of hyperconsumption is the Achilles heel of corporate America. Already some religious groups have made faith-based arguments that corporate promotion of hyperconsumption shows disrespect for children and families, an abandonment of our responsibility to be stewards of the earth, and a challenge to traditional religious values of humility and living simply.[72] "What would Jesus drive?" asked an evangelical environmental group in their campaign against SUVs.[73]

At its starkest, carbon fuel-based consumption contributes to human-induced climate change. As Bill McKibben points out in his book *Eaarth*, humans already live on a different planet than the one we inherited. The last century's patterns of production and consumption have led to persistent droughts, desertification, melting ice caps, flooding, shortages of drinking water, the emergence and spread of new infectious diseases, more frequent extreme weather, rising acidity in our oceans, and disruptions of food production.[74] Continuing this type of consumption for another century and extending it to China, India, Brazil, Russia, and other emerging nations will dramatically reduce the prospects for humanity's survival and life as we know it.

In sum, multiple streams of social and cultural activism and scientific inquiry can inform the creation of a system of beliefs and values that provides a coherent alternative to the ideology of consumption and the practice of hyperconsumption. Health constitutes a central theme in this alternative, as shown in Box 5.4, an effort to create a consistent response to the core beliefs of the corporate consumption complex shown in Box 5.1. By consistently using these core messages in advocacy and educational campaigns and by encouraging their public discussion, advocates for healthier more sustainable consumption can nurture a belief system that can contribute to building a movement for change.

For some, the threats to the survival of our children and grandchildren as well as to human civilization and the environment that supports life may be too distant or dire to motivate action. For those, the more immediate consequences of continuing our current patterns of corporate consumption—high rates of diabetes, heart disease, and cancer, as well as automobile and firearms injuries and deaths—may be what inspire action.

Already rising health care costs jeopardize economic growth, most acutely in the United States but also in other developed nations. In 2009 a bipartisan panel on Social Security appointed by the president and Congress concluded in its report *The Unsustainable Cost of Health Care* that "we believe that the rising cost

---

Box 5.4 **Core Beliefs and Values of Advocates for Healthy, Sustainable Consumption**

1. Making a profit by sickening others is wrong.
2. Parents, families, teachers, and health professionals, not corporations, should educate people about health, nutrition, and moral values.
3. Nanny corporations that seek to exploit children's vulnerability and immaturity, not nanny states, are the real threats to health and freedom.
4. The goal of social policy should be to make healthy choices easy choices.
5. In a globalized world, economic activity anywhere affects people everywhere; shifting the harms of such activity to another region or country in order to protect one group is wrong.
6. Every generation has a responsibility to leave the world a better place for future generations. Knowingly bequeathing our children and grandchildren a burden of disease, damaged environments, or corrupted democracy violates most of the world's moral codes.
7. Science belongs to all humanity; appropriating it to profit at the expense of health or the environment is wrong.

---

of health care represents perhaps the most significant threat to the long-term economic security of workers and retirees."[75] Turning off the faucets of tobacco, unhealthy food, alcohol, and polluting automobiles—the primary causes of the flood of people with expensive chronic illnesses into our health care system—is one of the most straightforward ways to lower these costs.

By itself, a coherent and compelling alternative to the corporate consumption ideology may not be sufficient to reverse the trends that jeopardize health in the United States and around the world. But without this necessary component of transformation, the forces now challenging corporate control will have difficulty weaving together the disparate strands that constitute an emerging movement for a healthier world. For some, this task may seem like one more example of "there is no alternative," a hopeless tilting at windmills. For others, however, consumption ideology was created by humans to achieve a goal and therefore other people can now offer healthier and more sustainable ways to meet human needs.

6

The Health Impact of Corporate
Managed Globalization

In the next decade or so, the people and governments of China, India, Indonesia, Brazil, Mexico, and other emerging nations will need to make a momentous decision: whether to follow the Western developed nations down the road of hyperconsumption that leads to premature deaths, preventable illnesses, and injuries, or to chart a different path of healthier, more sustainable consumption. Their choices will shape global health and the environment for the next century and beyond.

Since the first humans trekked north from sub-Saharan Africa more than 70,000 years ago, globalization has influenced public health. People, goods and services, money, and ideas traveled around the world, carrying prevalent diseases with them. What's different today is the magnitude and speed of these global interchanges of health and illness. Money that once took months to move is now wired around the world in milliseconds. Diseases that once took weeks or years to cross national borders can now spread globally in hours or days. HIV became a global pandemic within a few years after spreading slowly for a few decades in Africa. Avian flu and H1N1 spread around the world within a few weeks.

What is also different is the growing power of multinational corporations to make the decisions that shape global trade. Companies that used to produce for local or national markets now send their products around the world, creating the potential for global outbreaks of acute illnesses or chronic diseases. Baby formula produced in China in 2008 was contaminated with melamine, a byproduct of plastic manufacturing illicitly added to formula to mimic high-protein additives. As a result, infants in dozens of nations suffered from kidney problems, and some died.[1] Aggressive and sophisticated marketing of tobacco, alcohol and unhealthy food, once confined to advanced industrial nations, has now spread around the world, contributing to premature deaths and preventable illnesses in Africa, Asia, and Latin America as well as in North America and Europe.

The corporate consumption complex and its ideology, born in the United States and Europe, has become a global force. If an alternative political or economic agenda is to lead to improvements in world health, it, too, must operate globally. The success of the tobacco control movement in curtailing tobacco use in advanced industrial nations but not in developing and emerging markets provides a grim reminder of the peril of ignoring the global dimensions of lethal but legal products and practices. As tobacco use grows in Africa, Asia, and Latin America, tobacco mortality is predicted to increase tenfold compared to the last century. Already, hyperconsumption has established a beachhead in the growing middle classes of emerging nations. Allowing these trends to continue will accelerate the global rise in chronic diseases and injuries and the growing health gap between the better-off and the poor.

Exporting Obesity and Diabetes: NAFTA and the Health of Mexico

Constructing an alternative to hyperconsumption and its disease burden will require an understanding of the strategies that multinational corporations use to distribute their unhealthy products around the world. To begin this task, let us examine the impact of the North American Free Trade Agreement (NAFTA) on the health of the people of Mexico, a story that illustrates how free trade can harm health. The United States, Mexico, and Canada signed NAFTA in 1994 to create the world's largest trading bloc.[2, 3]

In the late 1980s, these three nations began to negotiate a new treaty designed to eliminate barriers to trade and investment. The political battle to pass NAFTA pitted industries in these countries that were big enough to prosper from expanded markets—tobacco, processed food, and automobiles—against smaller ones that preferred the continued protections that tariffs and subsidies offered. NAFTA opponents included industries like textiles, apparel, rubber, and plastics, as well as labor unions and environmental groups, who feared that the agreement would hurt their interests.[4] The industries that had saturated the domestic U.S. market with unhealthy products and were now attracting greater regulatory scrutiny favored NAFTA and its successor treaties as a way to reach new customers in markets with less stringent public health and environmental standards. In testimony at a Senate hearing on the Central America–Dominican Republic Free Trade Agreement, a NAFTA spinoff treaty approved in 2005, Kraft's executive vice-president for global corporate affairs, Mark Berlind, explained:

> The 50 U.S. states are currently Kraft's largest market. Given U.S. demographic realities, however, future growth for Kraft—as well as for the

entire U.S. food and agriculture complex—is inextricably tied to our ability to access export markets. Mr. Chairman, as you and most other farm state Members know, 95 percent of the world's consumers live outside the U.S. That is where future growth will take place.[5]

For the U.S. food and agricultural sectors, the quest for new international markets was the consequence of the subsidy, trade, and land policies that Secretary of Agriculture and former Ralston Purina director Earl Butz had implemented during the Nixon Administration, as described in Chapter 3. These policies, approved at the behest of the agribusiness interests Butz represented, had led to overproduction of cheap, processed food and the need for new customers to sustain profits.

President Bill Clinton, who became a champion of NAFTA when he took office in 1993, responded to critics by saying that he supported the treaty because it would create jobs in the United States:

> NAFTA will generate these jobs by fostering an export boom to Mexico; by tearing down tariff walls....Already Mexican consumers buy more per capita from the United States than other consumers in other nations....The average Mexican citizen...is now spending $450 per year per person to buy American goods. That is more than the average Japanese, the average German, or the average Canadian buys....So when people say that this trade agreement is just about how to move jobs to Mexico so nobody can make a living, how do they explain the fact that Mexicans keep buying more products made in America every year? Go out and tell the American people that....And there will be more if they have more money to spend. That is what expanding trade is all about.[6]

Although the United States had long had trade agreements with other countries, NAFTA was the first proposed agreement among countries of such unequal size and levels of development in which governments chose to ignore these differences.[7] It was also the largest trade agreement to be negotiated since the emergence of the Washington Consensus, the U.S.-driven push to elevate free trade, deregulation, and privatization to paramount political and economic priorities. For these reasons, NAFTA was important both in its own right and for setting precedents that guided the creation of the World Trade Organization (WTO) in 1995 and subsequent bilateral and multilateral trade agreements.

The NAFTA treaty called for a variety of changes, some to be implemented immediately, and others to be phased in over fifteen years. These included reductions in tariffs between the three countries, increased protection for corporate intellectual property rights, and the relaxation of restrictions on foreign direct investment. On the whole, it opened wide the doors that enabled U.S.-based corporations to export many products, including those that harmed health.

In the years after NAFTA, the pattern of food exchanges between Mexico and the United States changed significantly, as did the diet of Mexicans. American exports of sugar, high-fructose corn syrup, snack food, dairy products, and breakfast cereals to Mexico increased dramatically. In 1994, the United States exported about 50,000 metric tons of sugar and other sweeteners to Mexico; by 2007, this had climbed to almost 950,000 metric tons, a nineteen-fold increase. U.S. exports of corn and soybeans, the foundation of industrial processed food for both American and Mexican producers, also increased significantly. In this same period, exports of livestock and other meat products more than tripled. In the decade after NAFTA passed, sales of processed food in Mexico increased by 5 to 10 percent annually.[8]

U.S. foreign direct investment in Mexico also spiked after NAFTA. In just five years, from 1994 to 1998, U.S. direct investment in the Mexican food and beverage industries almost quadrupled, from $2.3 billion to $8.8 billion.[9] Between 2002 and 2007, U.S. foreign direct investment in Mexican beverage companies increased by 35 percent to almost $6 billion. In 2012, grains, oils, and meat—products associated with obesity, diabetes, and other diet-related diseases—accounted for 75 percent of the U.S. agricultural exports to Mexico.[10]

NAFTA also changed food retailing in Mexico. With tariff barriers lowered, large multinational supermarket chains began to move into Mexico and rapidly came to dominate the market. Between 1997 and 2006, market share of the five largest retail chains doubled from 24 percent to 48 percent.[11] Walmart was a leading player: between 1993 and 2001, the number of its stores grew from 114 to 561, and by 2005, Walmart controlled about 20 percent of the Mexican food retail market.[12]

In 2012, an investigation by the *New York Times* revealed that Walmart facilitated this expansion by bribing local and national officials to overlook a variety of rules, and that an internal inquiry into the matter had been suppressed at corporate headquarters in Arkansas. Challenging Walmart's defense that it was the victim of a corrupt culture, the *Times* investigation concluded:

> Walmart de Mexico was an aggressive and creative corrupter, offering large payoffs to get what the law otherwise prohibited. It used bribes to subvert democratic governance—public votes, open debates, transparent procedures. It used bribes to circumvent regulatory safeguards that protect Mexican citizens from unsafe construction. It used bribes to outflank rivals.[13]

The *Times* reported that deciding how to manage the bribery charges provoked "a prolonged struggle at the highest levels of Walmart, a struggle that pitted the company's much publicized commitment to the highest moral and ethical standards against its relentless pursuit of growth." The Mexican government and the United States Department of Justice and the Securities and Exchange Commission began investigating the bribery and cover-up. In a regulatory filing shortly after the story broke, Walmart warned investors that its reputation could be affected by the bribery scandal, with inquiries from the media and law enforcement authorities adversely affecting the "perception among certain audiences of its role as a corporate citizen."[14] In 2012, Walmart spent $157 million on its probe of alleged bribery allegations in Mexico, Brazil, China and India, and on improvements to its compliance programs. Walmart also boosted the pay of its CEO Mike Duke by 14 percent to $20.7 million for the year.[15]

In the short run, Walmart's business model makes cheap food more available, but in the longer run it puts pressure on local growers to lower their prices, often to the point of driving them out of business. Walmart can always find other suppliers in another part of the world, but for Mexico, such practices diminish the supply of locally grown food and increase unemployment among small farmers and local store owners.[16] The bribery also contributed to weakening the rule of law in Mexico, further diminishing its government's capacity to protect its citizens rather than special interests.

U.S.-based multinational fast food outlets also grew in the post-NAFTA era. The first McDonald's restaurant opened in Mexico City in 1985; by 2012, there were more than 500 McDonald's outlets in eighty-three cities in thirty-one states in Mexico.[17] Yum! Brands, the owner of Kentucky Fried Chicken (KFC), Pizza Hut, Taco Bell, and Long John Silver's, and other U.S.-based fast food corporations, also expanded their presence in Mexico.

By the time NAFTA was fully implemented, the Mexican diet had been transformed. Between 1992 and 2000, for example, calories from carbonated soft drinks increased by almost 40 percent, from 44 to 61 calories per capita per day. By 2002, the average Mexican was drinking 487 servings of Coca-Cola per year, more than the 436 8-ounce servings U.S. residents downed annually.[18] Between 1992 and 2000, in part as a result of economic changes precipitated by NAFTA, the cost in pesos per calorie of food tripled, making the low-cost, low-nutrient foods that NAFTA brought in more attractive, especially to families with low incomes.[19]

Aggressive marketing of soft drinks and other high-calorie, low-nutrient snack foods by global and national beverage makers further encouraged consumption.[20] Companies like Coke, Pepsi, McDonald's, and Kraft hired global advertising companies to use their U.S.-tested skills in winning over young customers by targeting advertising to urban children and young adults. These were the fastest growing segment of the Mexican population and the multinational companies' best hope for long-term increased market share.[21] One study of a large sample of Mexican children aged five to eleven found that, between 1999 and 2006, the number of calories consumed annually from sugary beverages more than doubled.[22] The growing exports of snack foods from the United States to Mexico increased competition between local and U.S. manufacturers. This in turn led to more aggressive advertising and price competition, further increasing consumption of these high fat, salt, and sugar products.[23]

Not surprisingly, the changes in food consumption, availability, and prices that NAFTA had triggered led to changes in the health of Mexican eaters. Between 1988 and 1999, the national prevalence of overweight and obesity almost doubled, rising from 33 percent to a shocking 59 percent.[24] Among some groups, the rise was even more striking. Among female adolescents in Mexico, obesity and overweight more than tripled between 1988 and 2006.[25] By 2006, 26.3 percent of Mexican children aged two to eighteen were overweight or obese. In the 1990s, the overall prevalence of diabetes in Mexico increased by 30 percent.[26] Another study found significant increases in deaths due to diabetes, hypertension, and acute myocardial infarctions in Mexico in this period, which the authors attributed to increases in the prevalence of obesity.[27]

So Bill Clinton was right to predict an export boom to Mexico as a result of NAFTA. Unfortunately, some of the boom was the result of products that significantly worsened Mexico's health profile and raised its health care costs. Did NAFTA cause Mexico's obesity and diabetes epidemics? Of course not. Obesity is too complex a problem to have a single cause, and weight and body mass have been expanding around the world, not just in Mexico. Nevertheless, the evidence is clear that NAFTA, a trade agreement shaped by multinational food, agriculture, and other industries to increase their profits, transformed Mexico's food environment and diet. These NAFTA-induced changes increased the availability, promotion, and consumption of the processed foods, sugar-sweetened beverages, and fast food most associated with obesity, diabetes, and other diet-related chronic diseases. In Mexico, NAFTA provided the platform from which multinational food companies could launch their program of hyperconsumption.

And Mexico is not the only country to suffer the consequences. China, India, South Africa, and Indonesia, among others, are witnessing similar transformations of their diet and health.[28,29,30] Moreover, as we shall see, the food industry is not the only sector to use trade agreements and foreign investments to pursue profits at the expense of health. Tobacco, automobile, firearms, and other global industries have also used trade agreements to increase exports of their side products of premature death and preventable illnesses and injuries.

Drivers of Corporate Practices that Harm Health

NAFTA's role in the rise of obesity and diabetes in Mexico illustrates the health impact of what Laura Wallach of Public Citizen's Global Trade Watch calls "corporate managed trade."[31] By 2013, 159 nations had joined the World Trade Organization, making it the leading global influence on trade. An additional approximately 500 bilateral and regional trade agreements further guided commercial relationships among nations. To understand how new forms of trade privilege business over public interest requires an examination of the procedures and rules used to develop and implement these agreements.

The NAFTA and WTO treaties were negotiated in closed sessions where health and environmental representatives were excluded, but hundreds of security-cleared representatives from industry and trade associations acted as formal, appointed advisors to the U.S. government, reducing the likelihood that health concerns were addressed in public or in private.[32] While treaties have always included private negotiations, in the new trade discussions, only some voices were welcome. In addition, the WTO created new rules for resolving trade disputes that allow companies to bring conflicts to an independent body that often favors corporations over national governments or health or environmental groups. As a result, explains Wallach, these agreements have created a platform in which business can advance its agenda of privatization, deregulation, and added protections for corporate intellectual property rights, with fewer opportunities for national governments or public health organizations to safeguard health.[33]

What had in the past been settled by diplomatic negotiations between nations was now decided in a business-dominated international forum. This dispute resolution process lacks the procedural safeguards found in the American judicial system, or in other world forums such as the United Nations.[34] Cases are decided by tribunals of trade experts who are not required to disclose actual or potential conflicts of interest, nor to follow other due process standards. The dispute resolution process in NAFTA and the WTO is secretive: documents are confidential; oral arguments are closed to observation or participation by any entities except national government representatives; and no outside appeal is available, nor can nongovernmental entities submit amicus briefs. Federal, state, or local laws and regulations judged to be out of compliance with NAFTA or the WTO must be eliminated or changed, or the "winning" country can place economic sanctions on the country whose law is ruled to be outside the NAFTA or WTO agreements.[35] Such penalties encourage governments to reach business-friendly agreements. A WTO staff person told the *Financial Times* that the WTO "is the place where governments collude in private against their domestic pressure groups."[36]

Another way that United States trade agreements circumvent normal demo-cratic procedures is by granting the president the power to "fast-track" trade trea-ties. Under fast track, the president can negotiate trade agreements with foreign countries without consulting Congress or state legislators. After the Executive Branch makes a trade deal, Congress is permitted only a yes or no vote, while states are virtually left out of the process. Thus, state and congressional officials elected to represent the public interest have no role in the process but to approve or disapprove the whole package.[37]

While the original fast-track authorization expired in 2007, in the previous decade, the United States Trade Representative has used fast track to push con-troversial pacts through Congress, including the Central America Free Trade Agreement (CAFTA) as well as dozens of bilateral trade agreements with coun-tries such as Chile, Singapore, Morocco, Australia, Bahrain, and Oman. Trade negotiations have been accelerated, denying American legislators and the public the time to consider the health, environmental or economic consequences of these agreements. In other countries, pro-business governments often approve trade agreements with minimal public consideration of the health or environ-mental consequences.

In 2013, the Obama Administration pressed Congress to approve a revised fast-track plan, labeled the Trade Promotion Authority, in time to allow another major trade agreement, the Trans Pacific Partnership (TPP), to win fast-track approval. The TPP includes 12 Pacific Rim nations that represent 40 percent of the world's gross domestic product.[38] It proposes new trade rules for tobacco, pharmaceuticals, and other products that influence public health.

Business has also gained an influential voice in writing the specific rules that govern trade. In the food industry, for example, trade agreements, includ-ing both NAFTA and the WTO, rely on the *Codex Alimentarius,* standards for food safety and quality developed by an international body in Rome. A study showed that more than four-fifths of the nongovernmental participants in *Codex* committees represented industry, while only one percent represented public interest organizations.[39] Companies like Nestlé, Hershey Foods, Kraft, General Foods, Coca-Cola, and PepsiCo, along with trade groups such as the Grocery Manufacturers of America and the National Food Processors Association, often have far more staff people at these standards-setting ses-sions than do governments from low-income countries. In short, industry and its trade associations are often the judges, juries, and expert witnesses in making decisions about trade agreements, leaving little space for health considerations.

Another important goal of international trade organizations is to "harmo-nize" individual national regulations with larger NAFTA and WTO mandates, a process that often leads to the weakening of national standards to meet the more business-friendly trade rules. Under NAFTA and the WTO, international standards influenced by business often serve as a ceiling that countries cannot exceed, rather than as a floor that all countries must meet.[40]

COMPONENTS OF GLOBAL TRADE

Trade agreements establish rules for several categories of commercial exchanges, each of which influences health.

Foreign Direct Investment. Free-trade proponents claim that entrepreneurs from wealthier nations contribute to economic growth when they invest in companies in poorer countries and also bring technical expertise and better access to foreign markets. They point to countries like Singapore, Malaysia, and more recently, China, that have benefited from such foreign direct investments.[41] Beginning in the 1980s, free traders have argued that trade, not aid, contributes to real development. By 1992, foreign direct investment overtook aid for the first time since World War II, making investment a more important influence on development than international assistance programs.[42] By 2008, annual global foreign direct investments totaled $1.7 trillion dollars, about three times the gross domestic product of the world's forty-eight poorest nations.[43] Recently, China has been the largest recipient of foreign direct investment, with an estimated $260 billion in investments in 2012.[44]

How do these investments affect health? First, as we saw in Mexico, many of the companies making investments in emerging economies are producers of unhealthy products. Between 1990 and 2002, for example, the foreign assets of the world's twelve largest food companies, based mostly in the United States and Western Europe, increased in value from $34 billion to $258 billion.[45] These investments significantly increased the capacity of these companies to bring highly processed foods high in fat, sugar, and salt to the world's fastest growing consumer markets. In the case of supermarket chains like Walmart, their expansion through investments in emerging economies like Mexico and China favors products with long shelf lives and the potential for economies of scale, such as snack foods and sweetened beverages, the same packaged products associated with diet-related chronic diseases.[46]

In alcohol and tobacco, as well as food, foreign direct investment leads to more competition with domestic producers, forcing prices down and increasing aggressive marketing. In free-market ideology, increased competition is good for consumers. But when it leads to lower prices, increased availability, and more marketing for unhealthy products, the consequence is wider exposure to pathogenic agents and higher rates of associated diseases. One study in the former Soviet republics found that in the countries that received direct foreign investment from multinational tobacco companies between 1991 and 2001, tobacco consumption increased by 51 percent. This contrasted with a 3-percent *decline* in countries that did not receive direct investment.[47]

Liberalization of foreign direct investment has other health consequences. Increased competition among nations for such investment contributes to a race to the bottom in occupational health, environmental regulation, and other standards. It can also force local companies to go out of business, reducing employment opportunities and diminishing local self-sufficiency. The mobility of foreign investment, and its susceptibility to economic crises, also means that today's investment can be tomorrow's disinvestment. This economic churning can undermine social stability, and therefore health, especially in the poorest nations.[48] In addition, investors with capital to spare and rules that allow them to invest anywhere often turn to speculation—taking high risks in new business areas in the hopes of greater return. In the last decade, investors have bought up commodities such as food and fuel in the hopes that higher prices would yield windfall profits, a hope that was often realized at the expense of growing hunger and food insecurity.[49]

Tariffs and Subsidies. National governments impose tariffs on imported goods in order to protect domestic industries. These governments also offer subsidies to locally produced products in order to spur national economic development. An overriding goal of the current quest to liberalize trade is to remove such tariffs and subsidies in order to encourage expanded trade. Free traders argue that even if reductions in tariffs and subsidies cause some short-term harm to local producers or consumers, in the long run they benefit everyone, because they increase trade and therefore grow the economy. Thus, with only a few exceptions that I will describe, the WTO forbids countries to impose tariffs or offer subsidies that treat imports differently from domestically produced goods.

For some nations, however, especially poor ones, tariffs and subsidies provide governments with health benefits. Tariffs on unhealthy products can keep them out of the country, or at least make them more expensive. In 2004, three years after joining the WTO, China cut its tariffs on imported cigarettes from 65 percent to 25 percent, making the popular imported brands much more affordable.[50] Today, 54 percent of Chinese men aged fifteen to sixty-nine smoke tobacco; one of the highest rates in the world.[51] In the early 1970s, average annual use in China was 730 cigarettes; today, it is 1,711.[52] Chinese smokers consume one-third of the world's cigarettes each year, and 100 million Chinese under the age of eighteen smoke.[53] These lowered tariffs presented Philip Morris International and other global tobacco companies with a business opportunity to win new customers in China, dooming millions more Chinese to tobacco-related death and disease.

Similarly, when the WTO forced South Korea, Japan, Thailand, and Taiwan to eliminate their tobacco import tariffs, cigarette consumption skyrocketed.[54]

After new European Union trade rules required Finland to lower taxes on imported alcohol, a study found that alcohol-related health problems increased, especially among heavy drinkers.[55] Tariffs also provide government revenues, which in poor nations can be an important source of funding for health care and other services. Few developing nations have been able to replace the revenues lost from tariff reductions with other forms of taxation, weakening their capacity to protect public health.[56]

Subsidies can also benefit health, encouraging production of healthier products, promoting national food self-sufficiency, and keeping healthy products more affordable. In some developing nations, WTO-mandated reductions in subsidies to farmers encouraged agricultural production for export, diminishing the availability of local staple produce and increasing reliance on imported, processed food. In Mexico, NAFTA's termination of corn subsidies and tariffs on imported food has led to a collapse of its corn economy, triggering large increases in corn prices, and food riots.[57] In this case, Mexican corn could not compete on price with the still-highly subsidized corn from the United States, which is also the basic ingredient in much of the processed food the United States sent to Mexico.

Some critics have charged that the WTO's positions on tariffs and subsidies unfairly serve the interests of wealthy nations. In the twentieth century, developed nations used these now-forbidden policies to protect their domestic industries, but they now want to deprive emerging nations of these same tools that helped fuel their growth.[58]

Intellectual Property Rights. Another goal of trade liberalization is to strengthen protection of patents and other intellectual property rights. In the negotiations that led to the creation of the WTO in 1995, the United States and others developed nations insisted that their companies needed stronger protection of these property rights than most developing nations then offered. Drug companies wanted to be able to sell their drugs without fear of competition from generics that violated their patents. Multinationals branded companies like Coca-Cola and McDonald's wanted better protection for their registered trademarks, which American manufacturers claimed were losing them $24 billion a year in unpaid royalties.[59]

The 1995 Agreement on Trade-Related Intellectual Property Rights (TRIPS) committed all current and future WTO members to provide protections of patents, trademarks, and copyrights comparable to those available in the developed world. After a transitional period, TRIPS specifies a minimum of twenty years of protection from the date of application.[60]

A few stories illustrate how the application of TRIPS can harm health. In 1983, Guatemala passed a law requiring infant-formula companies to adhere to the World Health Organization's International Code on Marketing of

Breast-Milk Substitutes, which bans direct-to-consumer marketing of infant formula and various misleading claims. A substantial body of evidence shows that early termination of breastfeeding increases the risk of premature infant death and a variety of chronic diseases for both infants and mothers.[61]

When the U.S.-based multinational baby food company Gerber (now owned by Nestlé) refused to stop advertising to women; to remove its trademark picture of a chubby, smiling baby from its product labels; or to add a phrase to its advertisements saying breast milk was superior to infant formula, Guatemala took Gerber to court. The government believed the ad images and text wrongly implied that infant formula contributed to healthy babies. Ten years later, after the company lost its final appeal, Gerber opened a new line of attack on Guatemala, arguing that the Guatemalan law was illegal under international statutes because the law was, in Gerber's view, an "expropriation of Gerber's trademark." In 1995, when the WTO came into being, Gerber dropped this claim about illegal expropriation of its trademark and instead threatened to bring Guatemala before a WTO tribunal. Acknowledging that it was unlikely to win in this business-friendly arena, the Guatemalan government changed its law to allow Gerber to continue to use its trademark baby, illustrating how multinational companies can use just the threat of invoking TRIPS to force poor countries to open their markets.[62] Gerber's victory allowed it to continue promoting infant formula in Guatemala in ways that had been outlawed by the 1981 WHO code.

Agricultural producers have used intellectual property rights to justify applying for patents for seeds. In 1997, for example, Ricetec, a Texas rice company, patented the seeds for Basmati rice, claiming that such protection gave it the right to take the 250,000 farmers in India and Pakistan who had traditionally grown this type of rice to court for allegedly violating its patent rights. The Indian scholar and food activist Vandana Shiva has called this practice "biopiracy."[63] She writes, "This perverse intellectual property rights system that treats plants and seeds as corporate inventions is transforming farmer's highest duties—to save seeds and exchange seeds with neighbors—into crimes."[64] In the Basmati rice conflict, more than 50,000 people demonstrated in front of the United Sates Embassy against the patent. The Indian government protested the patent at the Seattle meeting of the World Trade Organization and challenged the U.S patent in court. Ultimately, five years later, the Indian government and the U.S. Patent Office reached an agreement that narrowed but did not withdraw patent protection for Ricetec's products.[65]

This story is characteristic of the corporatization of the worldwide seed market. Between 1985 and 2008, market share of the top ten global seed companies increased from 20 percent to 50 percent. One company, Monsanto, controlled 35 percent of the world's seed market in 2008. When big companies use their market power to gain a monopoly on seed patents, they diminish the diversity of the world's food supply, increase vulnerability to global crop failures, drive farmers who can no longer afford their seeds off the land, and contribute to rising food prices that put affordable food out of reach of the poor.[66] For Monsanto, its domination of the global seed market also provides a platform to advance its efforts to introduce its patented (and profitable) genetically modified seeds to new markets.[67]

Pharmaceutical companies use TRIPS to extend and globalize patent protections on their most profitable products. They argue that extended patent protection rewards the high costs on developing new drugs and encourages innovation. Critics counter that many drug development costs are subsidized by national research institutes in the United States, the United Kingdom, and other developed nations, not by drug companies themselves.[68]

In 2001, the WTO Fourth Ministerial Conference in Doha, Qatar, modified TRIPS to expand the rights of national governments. The Doha Declaration recognized the importance of implementation and interpretation of the TRIPS Agreement "in a manner supportive of public health, by promoting both access to existing medicines and research and development into new medicines."[69]

The Doha Declaration also reaffirmed and slightly expanded the TRIPS rules for compulsory licensing, a process by which governments can allow a national company to produce for domestic consumption the patented product or process without the consent of the patent owner.[70] As I will describe, Brazil, Thailand, and South Africa have all used compulsory licensing to allow production of generic antiretroviral drugs to make these life-saving medications affordable to people with HIV in their countries. [71]

While the Doha Declaration in theory put the WTO on record as supporting the "right to medicine for all," the multinational pharmaceutical industry has found new ways to protect its patents, thus limiting wider availability of essential medicines. By creating a "TRIPS Plus" option in bilateral trade agreements, Big Pharma has extended patent protections by narrowing the types of products that can be excluded from patentability. These new rules allow genetic sequences to be patented, guarantee patentability if health authorities issue patents promptly, and limit experimental studies on generic drugs while the patent is still valid.[72] Currently, these "TRIPS Plus" provisions are incorporated in bilateral agreements with Australia, Morocco, Jordan, Bahrain, Singapore, Peru, and Colombia, overriding TRIPS protections. In these and other nations, TRIPS Plus places strict limits on the ability of governments to encourage generic entry or issue compulsory licenses for pharmaceutical products, the protections offered by the Doha Declaration.[73] Since 2006, applications for compulsory licenses have declined, suggesting that the stricter TRIPS Plus agreements are discouraging their use.[74]

The ostensible business rationale for TRIPS was to allow pharmaceutical companies in developing *and* developed nations to expand trade. But an investigation of this claim by researchers at the London School of Hygiene and Tropical Medicine found that "TRIPS has not generated substantial gains for developing countries, but has further increased pharmaceutical trade in developed countries."[75] The authors concluded that TRIPS and TRIPS Plus provisions had worsened access to life-saving drugs in developing nations.

In sum, growing foreign direct investment, declining use of tariffs and subsidies, and increased protection of intellectual property rights—the three primary goals of the new regime of corporate-managed trade inaugurated by the WTO—have harmed health in two ways. First, they have increased exposure to the products and practices that encourage hyperconsumption and the burden of chronic disease and injuries that follow. Second, they have limited the authority of national governments to protect public health, transferring decisions on trade from public health authorities to business-dominated international organizations. In combination with the lax regulatory approaches advocated by the World Bank and the International Monetary Fund, this latter development has led to a serious weakening of the public health capacity of national governments.[76]

PRIVATIZATION OF INTERNATIONAL HEALTH ORGANIZATIONS

Another contributor to weaker public control of harmful multinational corporate practices has been the increased influence of private interests on international organizations such as the World Health Organization and the parallel rise of corporate-funded global health philanthropy.

In recent years, WHO has been unable to raise the money it needs to achieve its goals from the national governments that created it, a trend worsened by the 2008 economic crisis. As a result, it has turned to private partners to make up the shortfall. In 2008, the Bill and Melinda Gates Foundation was the WHO's second biggest contributor after the United States government. The Gates contribution of $338.8 million constituted 10 percent of the organization's budget. Why isn't this generosity simply a win for all? The fear is that private donations will influence WHO's priorities. As one journalist asked, "Will the WHO continue to be in charge of the world's health policy, or will its role be reduced to that of a mere coordinator?"[77]

An investigation of conflicts of interests of global health philanthropy found grounds for concern.[78] The Gates Foundation, for example, is heavily invested in food and pharmaceutical companies, including McDonald's, Coca-Cola, Walmart, Schering Plough, and Merck. Its leaders are current or former board members or senior managers of companies such as Coca-Cola, Kraft, Unilever, Merck, and Novartis. Among the questions such relationships raise is whether major donors to the WHO seek to influence policy to benefit the corporations whose directors guide their work and whose profits fund it. Certainly, the willingness of WHO to allow corporations to shape the content and wording of its policy statements on NCDs, as described in Chapter 2, show the extent to which private interests have infiltrated its deliberative processes.

WHO is an indispensable player in global health. Its constitution grants the agency extraordinary rule-making powers, but in more than sixty years, the agency has promulgated only two major treaties, one being the Tobacco Convention. To achieve its potential to confront the most serious global health problems of the twenty-first century, WHO will need to find new ways to ensure that private interest are not distorting its public mission.

Responses to Globalization

To counteract the public health threats posed by corporate-driven globalization, several types of organizations have created new global forms of resistance. In the following examples, I will examine the successes and limitations of these strategies and assess their potential for creating healthier, more sustainable alternatives to corporate-managed trade.

TREATIES

Framework Convention on Tobacco Control. If the trade agreements of World Trade Organization show the power of multinational corporations to set trade terms that protect profits, then the Framework Convention on Tobacco Control (FCTC), described briefly in Chapter 1, demonstrates the potential of national governments and non-governmental organizations to forge international measures to protect health. Adopted by the World Health Assembly in 2003 and ratified in 2005, the Framework Convention has been signed by 175 nations. By 2013, 168 of these governments had formally approved the treaty, making it one of the most widely and rapidly accepted of UN treaties.[79] The United States signed the FCTC in 2004, but Congress has not yet ratified it. The World Health Organization's Commission on the Social Determinants of Health hailed the FCTC as "an excellent (if rare) example of coherent, global action to restrain market availability of a lethal commodity" [80] and suggested it could serve as a model for treaties to control other health-damaging commodities like alcohol and processed food.[81]

The FCTC process was initiated by the WHO, the one international body with an explicit mandate to propose global health treaties. During the FCTC negotiations, nations that profited from tobacco (United States, Great Britain, Germany, Japan, and China), influenced by their powerful tobacco lobbies, worked to water down the treaty. In this case, the determination of WHO and health officials from many other nations hard hit by tobacco deaths thwarted at least some of these efforts, making the FCTC's ratification a partial victory for the developing world.[82]

The FCTC requires participating nations to fulfill seven tasks:

1. Exclude the tobacco industry and other commercial interests from setting public health policies on tobacco control.
2. Protect people from exposure to tobacco smoke.
3. Regulate the contents of tobacco products and tobacco product disclosures.
4. Package and label tobacco products so that "every person should be informed of the health consequences, addictive nature and mortal threat posed by tobacco consumption and exposure to tobacco smoke."[83]
5. Provide education, communication, training, and public awareness on tobacco and its harms to all relevant constituencies.
6. Limit tobacco advertising, promotion, and sponsorship.
7. Take effective measures to promote cessation of tobacco use and adequate treatment for tobacco dependence.[84]

Every two years, nations are required to submit and make public reports documenting their activities and progress in these seven areas. In addition, the FCTC enables non-governmental organizations not linked to the tobacco industry to participate in its implementation and the reviews of progress. This has provided an opportunity for health advocates to influence the negotiation and implementation process, an effort accelerated by the formation in 1999 of the Framework Convention Alliance, a group that now includes more than 350 like-minded NGOs from more than 100 countries, working to ensure the full enactment of the treaty.[85] This contrasts with the exclusion of these types of groups from the NAFTA and WTO processes. A participant in the Alliance explained that it became "one of the most important factors driving in support of stronger treaty" in which the group's interactions

> served as a sort of global university for the 500 or so national delegates. And over time...you could feel the level of knowledge and understanding of these issues increased among the body of delegates...the more you learn about the science and evidence, the more willing you become to support stronger policies because the science supports stronger policies.[86]

In creating a platform for national governments and non-governmental organizations from around the world to exchange information, learn from their successes and failures, and develop more effective tobacco control strategies, the WHO's FCTC shows a bottom-up response to globalization that serves as a morally and politically powerful alternative to the top-down corporate globalization that promotes hyperconsumption.

Despite these accomplishments, public health critics have noted the FCTC's limitations. Professor Jeff Collin at the Centre for International Public Health Policy at the University of Edinburgh, Scotland, noted the agreement "focuses overwhelmingly on seeking to reduce demand for tobacco products rather than curtail their supply."[87] By accepting that a world awash in tobacco is the unchangeable reality, the FCTC missed opportunities to limit access.

Collin observed that the relationship between tobacco control and the World Trade Organization was "perhaps the dominant issue during FCTC negotiations, and a clear majority of countries favored the inclusion within the Convention of language that would give precedence to health over trade."[88] However, the FCTC does not clarify this relationship. This failure has allowed the tobacco industry to use the WTO and other trade agreements to limit the impact of the FCTC and protect its right to promote its products in emerging markets. Collin concluded that by giving up the chance to establish the importance of public health over free trade, "the FCTC can be seen as having preserved prospects for the future growth of transnational tobacco companies."[89]

The persistent and determined efforts by the tobacco industry to undermine and subvert the FCTC show that ratifications of global health treaties are at best a first step in controlling harmful corporate practices. From the start, companies like Philip Morris acted aggressively to limit the treaty's threats to profitability. In the late 1990s, it hired the public relations firm Mongoven, Biscoe & Duchin to limit the impact of the treaty.[90] The company advised Philip Morris to focus its efforts on weakening the language of treaty protocols rather than frontal opposition:

> The history of framework conventions shows that successful weakening of the language of an article in the framework convention can be easily undermined by the protocol process. The potential protocols are more important to the company in the long-term than the framework convention itself.... It would be in the company's best interest to have the treaty focus entirely on protecting children and leaving adult choice protected.[91]

In 2012, the WHO chose "tobacco industry interference" as the theme for its recognition of World 'No Tobacco' Day. In a speech in Singapore that year, WHO director-general Dr. Margaret Chan, shown in Figure 6.1, first recounted the many successes of the FCTC, including national smoking bans, tobacco

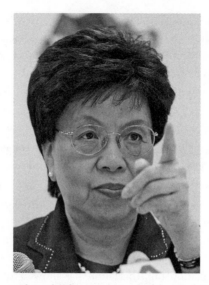

Figure 6.1 Dr. Margaret Chan, the director-general of the World Health Organization, and an outspoken critic of the tobacco industry. Corbis Images.

tax increases, and hard-hitting educational campaigns, each contributing to reductions in tobacco use. She then described the changing face of the tobacco industry:

> Unfortunately, this is where the balance no longer tips so strongly in our favour. The enemy, the tobacco industry, has changed its face and its tactics. The wolf is no longer in sheep's clothing, and its teeth are bared. Tactics aimed at undermining anti-tobacco campaigns, and subverting the Framework Convention, are no longer covert or cloaked by an image of corporate social responsibility. They are out in the open and they are extremely aggressive.[92]

Then, in language unusual for an international conference, she spoke directly to the tobacco industry:

> We've come a long way, bullies. We will not be fazed by your harassment. Your products kill nearly 6 million people each year. You run a killing and intimidating industry, but not in a crush-proof box. Tobacco industry: the number and fortitude of your public health enemies will damage your health.[93]

Advocates for public health can take two views of industry opposition to treaties like the FCTC. On one hand, they can say this is what free market democracy looks like: corporate interests use their money and clout to advance their agenda in every way possible. In these asymmetrical battles, opponents do their best to use their resources to thwart health-damaging policies and practices.

Those who, like Dr. Chan, assert that another world is possible make a different case. They argue that political rules that allow special interests to undermine duly ratified international health treaties need to be changed. The experience of the FCTC demonstrates both the possibility of this approach and the obstacles it inevitably encounters.

With the partial success of the FCTC, national governments, public health officials, and non-governmental organizations have called for other global treaties to limit the rights of corporations to engage in practices that harm health.

Small Arms Treaty. In 1996, the World Health Organization declared that violence was a leading public health problem worldwide and urged nations to assess its extent. In a 2001 report prepared for the first UN Conference on Illicit Trade in Small Arms and Light Weapons, WHO stated that "violence is . . . an important health problem—and one that is largely preventable. Public health approaches have much to contribute to solving it."[94] Such public health approaches include health-oriented regulations, anti-violence programs, and conflict resolution.[95] A year later, WHO made securing treaties to control the trade in small arms one of its priority recommendations, calling on the UN "to seek practical, internationally agreed responses to the global drugs trade and the global arms trade."[96]

Premature death and serious injuries from gunshots are a major health and financial problem in many developing nations, especially for males and young adults. One study on injuries from violence in hospitals in five African countries found that the probability of death due to gunshot injuries was forty-six times greater than death from other types of interpersonal violence, underscoring the lethality of firearms.[97] Military governments, insurgent movements, and criminal organizations import small arms to arm their combatants. With time, these weapons find their way into the retail market where they contribute to further crime, family violence, and accidental injuries and deaths.[98]

In July 2012, after three years of preliminary meetings, officials gathered at the United Nations in New York to negotiate the terms of a treaty covering the trade in international arms. Ultimately, however, delegates from the 170 nations who attended the meeting failed to reach agreement. Arms-control activists blamed the United States and Russia, two of the world's largest arms exporters, for the inability to reach a decision, as both countries said there was not enough time left for them to clarify and resolve issues they had with the draft treaty.[99] Part of the reason for the defeat was strong opposition from the U.S. gun lobby, which falsely charged that the treaty would restrict the U.S. government's right to set gun policy within the United States. Richard Patterson, the managing director of

the Sporting Arms and Ammunition Manufacturers' Institute, the trade association of U.S. gun makers, testified "that hundreds of millions of citizens regularly
use firearms for the greater good," and that a "treaty that does not support the
positive use of firearms is doomed to cause more harm than good."[100]

As with the FCTC, non-governmental organizations have also played an
important role in advocating for the Smalls Arms Treaty. The International
Action Network on Small Arms, a global network that includes policy organizations, national gun control groups, women's groups, research institutes, aid
agencies, faith groups, gun violence survivors, and human rights and community action organizations, advocates passage of the Small Arms Treaty and campaigns for "policies that will protect human security."[101]

Although the Obama Administration supported the Small Arms Treaty, it has
also proposed to relax restrictions on the export of small arms in order to increase
market share for U.S. gun manufacturers. Two federal agencies, the departments
of Justice and Homeland Security, voiced concerns about these proposals, fearing they would make it easier for terrorists and criminals to get guns.[102] In a rare
example of shared interest, the senior vice-president of the National Shooting
Sports Foundation endorsed the White House proposal. "Our industry totally
supports the White House efforts on this," the official said. "The U.S. loses out to
European and Israeli competitors who aren't forced to deal with these delays."[103]

As with tobacco, an alliance between gun makers and governments of countries with big gun makers has used the goal of promoting trade to delay and
weaken a treaty that has the potential to save lives. On the day the UN treaty
failed to win approval in 2012, Anna MacDonald, head of arms control at Oxfam,
observed, "Today was the day for political courage—not delays and dithering.
Some 50,000 people lost their lives through armed violence during the course
of these month-long negotiations. The out-of-control arms trade must—and
will—be stopped."[104] In April 2013, the United Nation's General Assembly
finally approved a modified treaty; within five months, more than eighty nations
had endorsed the treaty.[105]

Food Marketing to Children. In 2007, an International Obesity Taskforce
(IOTF) Working Group met in Sydney, Australia, to develop recommendations
for action on changing food and beverage marketing practices that target children. The group proposed that global and national measures to reduce marketing to children should: "(i) Support the rights of children; (ii) afford substantial
protection to children; (iii) be statutory in nature; (iv) take a wide definition of
commercial promotions; (v) guarantee commercial-free childhood settings; (vi)
include cross-border media; and (vii) be evaluated, monitored and enforced."[106]
Industry groups opposed the call for statutory guidelines, calling instead for voluntary industry-developed standards, the road now being pursued in the United
States and the United Kingdom.

The Working Group advocated a rights-based approach that invoked the United Nations Declaration on the Rights of Children to justify elevating the rights of children to a level that supersedes potentially conflicting rights claimed by food marketers. However, as Shiriki Kumanyika, an expert on child obesity at the University of Pennsylvania, observed, "The concept that the rights of children will take precedence over the rights of others may be more idealistic than practical.... The question of power is inevitable. That is, operationally, having rights may be less important than having the power (collective and individual agency) to exercise one's rights or obtain one's entitled protections."[107]

More recently, as part of its effort to reduce non-communicable diseases, the WHO has also developed and endorsed a set of recommendations on the marketing of food to children, and its member states are encouraged to adopt these recommendations. In 2011, an editorial in the British medical journal *Lancet* argued that "one immensely important next step in the fight against non-communicable diseases could be the agreement on a framework convention on obesity control." This recommendation was based on the assessment that all indications so far are that the voluntary standards proposed by the food and beverage industry are ineffective.[108] Moreover, the global reach of major food companies makes uniform international rules imperative. As yet, no action has been taken to negotiate a framework convention on food marketing.

NATIONAL GOVERNMENTS

Some national governments have also resisted corporate-managed free trade. As I described previously, the Doha Declaration affirmed WTO rules permitting countries to issue compulsory licenses for essential medicines, even if such licenses bypass the patent rights of pharmaceutical companies in developed nations. Let's examine how Brazil has used this power to develop an internationally recognized model for reducing the burden of HIV infection and AIDS.

Brazil. In 1996, the Brazilian president signed a law establishing free distribution of drugs to people living with HIV/AIDS, the first nation to make such treatment a universal right.[109] Pushed by a large and energetic AIDS movement, the Brazilian government made human rights, public health, and economic arguments for maintaining and strengthening the free distribution program. A 2002 report by Brazil's Ministry of Health concluded that the cost savings of the free distribution program were almost $1.1 billion, all due to its prevention of opportunistic infections and averted hospitalizations.[110]

Brazil used both threats and action to get the changes it wanted from multinational pharmaceutical companies. In 2001, Brazil announced it was considering breaking patents for two antiretrovirals: nelfinavir, produced by Roche, and efavirenz, produced by Merck, if the companies did not reduce their prices. Merck agreed to lower the price of efavirenz by 60 percent, but when Roche offered a smaller reduction for nelfinavir, the Brazilian government said it intended to break Roche's patent and to produce nelfinavir domestically at a government laboratory. A few weeks later, Roche agreed to further reduce the price of the drug, and Brazil dropped its plans to break the patent.[111]

Earlier that year, the United States asked the WTO to examine the compatibility of Brazilian patent laws on compulsory licensing with TRIPS requirements— in essence calling for an investigation of Brazil's price reduction on life-saving medications. A spate of protest from international AIDS organizations and the UN Human Rights Commission led the United States government to withdraw that request a few months later.

Six years later, after it was revealed that Merck was still charging Brazil $1.59 per pill, while charging Thailand only 65 cents, Brazil did issue a compulsory license for efavirenz.[112] The country began manufacturing its own generic version, saving $30 million in 2007 and providing the medication to nearly 65,000 of the 170,000 people in Brazil receiving free HIV treatment.

Predictably, Brazil's decision elicited a variety of responses. Merck said it was "profoundly disappointed" by the decision and warned that the "expropriation of intellectual property sends a chilling signal to research-based companies."[113] Merck contended that it "cannot sustain a situation in which the developed countries alone are expected to bear the cost for essential drugs." Pedro Chequer, the former head of Brazil's AIDS program, said, "I am really proud of this wonderful political decision." James Love, an economist who runs Knowledge Ecology International, a think tank in Washington, D.C., that supports access to essential medicines, observed that the actions of Brazil, Thailand, and other countries threaten Big Pharma, who worry that this movement could go beyond AIDS to heart disease and other ailments. "There's a big push in Thailand to do it for everything."[114]

India. In 2012, the patent authority of the Indian government issued a compulsory license for sorafenib, a patented anti-cancer drug used to treat of advanced-stage kidney and liver cancer. Bayer, the German-based manufacturer of the patented version, Nexavar, said it was "disappointed" with India's decision to issue a compulsory license and later decided to appeal to a higher court.[115] The new license India issued requires the domestic company producing the generic version to sell sorafenib at a 97 percent discount to Bayer's existing product, making the drug available to thousands more people. In its approval of the compulsory license, the patent authority noted that Bayer's branded drug Nexavar sells for $5,181 for a month's supply while the generics competitor which brought the case planned to sell its version for $160 a month.[116]

WHO estimates that 1.7 billion people in the world have little or no access to essential medicines, a clear indication that the market has failed to meet this human need.[117] Compulsory licensing offers governments an opportunity to shrink this population at the expense of revenues for multinational drug companies. As the demand for drugs to treat the burgeoning epidemics of NCDs in China, India, Brazil, and other emerging nations rises, the stakes of compulsory licensing will grow both for governments and pharmaceutical companies.

GLOBAL CORPORATE CAMPAIGNS

In Brazil, Thailand, India, and elsewhere, AIDS became a driving force for rethinking the connections between trade and health. Two researchers on the influence of non-governmental organizations (NGOs) on the drug industry concluded that "there would not have been a good case for trade policy activism without the HIV/AIDS crisis."[118] This activism made demands on both governments and directly on drug companies.

Treatment Action Campaign (TAC). TAC was created in South Africa in 1998 to ensure that every person living with HIV has access to quality comprehensive prevention and treatment services to live a healthy life. With more than 16,000 members, 267 branches, and 72 full-time staff members, TAC has become the leading civil society force behind comprehensive healthcare services for people living with HIV and AIDS in South Africa.[119] Zachi Achmat, one of TAC's founders, explained the source of its activists' passions: "Mostly our anger was directed at the pharmaceutical companies, and their excessive profiteering on medicines, particularly HIV medicines."[120] In its campaigns to lower the price of AIDS drugs, TAC demonstrates the power of grassroots organizations to channel this anger into challenges to corporate-managed trade.

The foundation for TAC's actions, explained TAC activist Mark Heywood was the human rights guaranteed by the post-apartheid South African constitution. The organization believed that that excessive pricing of essential medicines by multinational drug companies violated constitutionally protected rights to life, equality, dignity, autonomy, and access to healthcare services.[121] In TAC's view, intellectual property was not an inviolable human right, but a device granted by the state for a public purpose, one that could be modified if needed.[122] Based on this analysis, TAC carried out campaigns to enforce these rights, using a combination of negotiation, litigation, and mobilization to get the South African government and multinational drug companies to fulfill their obligations. In the course of their history, they have developed alliances with global NGOs, faith organizations, and philanthropies. Many of TAC's founders were also members of the African National Congress, the party that led South Africa's struggles against apartheid, giving them deep roots in the nation's history of resistance and struggle.

TAC's concerns about drug prices were precipitated in part by a success-ful effort by the Pharmaceutical Research and Manufacturers of America (PhRMA), the U.S. drug trade group profiled in Chapter 4, to persuade the U.S. government to pressure South Africa to repeal legislation that gave it added power to set drug prices and override patent protections. In addition, forty-one multinational pharmaceutical companies called on South Africa to change its law.[123] James Joseph, then U.S. Ambassador to South Africa, wrote a letter to rep-resentatives of the South African Government, strongly urging South Africa to alter its patent law. In 1998 and 1999, the U.S. Trade Representative put South Africa on a special watch list based on a determination that South Africa failed to provide adequate intellectual property protection, a step that set the stage for the United States to impose unilateral trade sanctions on South Africa.[124] In response, TAC called for international protests against what it called "drug profi-teering" that would cost lives.

The co-chairman of the United States/South Africa Binational Commission, a group created to improve communication and cooperation between the two countries, was U.S. Vice-President Al Gore. At PhRMA's request, Gore had become actively involved in pressuring South Africa to give in to industry demands to change its laws. In an important example of global solidarity, TAC asked American AIDS groups, including the combative ACT UP, to use Gore's presidential campaign to raise the issue in the U.S. national media. Chanting "Gore's Greed Kills: Africa Needs AIDS Drugs," the group disrupted a number of his campaign events, including the announcement of his run for the presi-dency. In addition, the U.S. Congressional Black Caucus sent Gore a letter urg-ing him to support more affordable HIV medicines in South Africa.[125]

In response to this pressure, a few months later, the U.S. and the South African governments announced that the controversy was resolved and that the U.S. government would no longer pressure South Africa. In return, South Africa promised to adhere to its obligations under TRIPS.[126]

Despite this agreement, drug companies continued to charge prices that put anti-retrovirals out of reach of the tens of thousands of HIV-infected South Africans who needed them. On at least five occasions, TAC has undertaken constitutional litigation to challenge the pricing structures of GlaxoSmithKline, Boehringer Ingelheim, and other drug companies.[127] As in Brazil, in some cases the mere threat of legal action by TAC or other groups was enough to bring about a reduction in the price of several essential medicines for HIV-related opportu-nistic infections.[128] When TAC was founded in late 1998, the price of the tradi-tional first-line regimen of anti-retroviral medicines was approximately R4500 per month. By 2007, the first-line regimen cost less than R300 per month.[129]

Infant Formula Action Coalition (INFACT). Global activist campaigns against corporations have achieved other important victories. In one of the first corporate campaigns to focus on public health, the U.S.-based INFACT launched a boycott of Nestlé's products in 1977 that sought to persuade the multinational food company to stop promoting its infant formula. Researchers had shown that bottle-fed babies were much more likely to die or get sick in their first year of life, and that the advertising campaigns of Nestlé and other infant formula companies were designed to give the false impression that infant formula was a healthy alternative to breast feeding.[130,131] The boycott soon spread to Australia, Canada, New Zealand, and Europe. Nestlé hired the public relations firm Mongoven, Biscoe & Duchin, the same company Philip Morris International later hired to assist in weakening the FCTC, to help it counter the boycott.[132]

In 1981, despite industry opposition, 118 national governments voted to approve the WHO/UNICEF International Code on Marketing of Breast-Milk Substitutes,[133] the code that Guatemala had used in the previously described litigation to force Gerber to change its infant formula advertising. The Code calls upon the baby formula industry to stop giving free formula samples to new mothers and hospitals; eliminate "Milk Nurses," salespeople disguised as health professionals; halt direct promotion to mothers; and restrict promotion to the health professions. In 1984, after Nestlé signed an agreement pledging to abide by the Code, INFACT suspended the seven-year boycott against the Swiss food giant. While the United States initially voted against the Code, in 1994, the Clinton Administration in effect endorsed the Code, giving it the support of every WHO member state.[134]

Thirty-five years later, the campaign against Nestlé illustrates both the strengths and weaknesses of a campaign approach. On the positive side, activists played a key role in pushing WHO and UNICEF to pass a global code of marketing—a tool that, like the FCTC, continues to be used by international organizations, governments, and advocacy groups to monitor industry practices and push for compliance. The Code contains clear, direct language that reflects the perspectives of medical and public health experts, not the industry's. This contrasts with the voluntary codes of conduct that the global food and alcohol industries have created, which strongly reflect their self-interests. The campaign against Nestlé also helped create an ongoing activist organization, now called Corporate Accountability International, which serves as a catalyst on other global health issues, including tobacco and fast food, and as a training ground for future activists.[135]

On the negative side, Nestlé and other infant formula companies still routinely violate the Code. A recent report by the International Baby Food Action Network (IBFAN) titled *Breaking the Rules, Stretching the Rules* found that, while 77 percent of signing countries have taken some action to implement the Code, monitoring and enforcement are still inadequate, particularly when laws and legal systems are weak.[136] IBFAN concluded that "only effective national legislation, properly enforced and monitored—independently from the companies—can protect child health."[137]

One conclusion from both the TAC and INFACT campaigns is that getting multinational corporations to agree to change their harmful practices is only a first step. Monitoring implementation of these commitments, taking action when guidelines or laws are not followed, and persuading reluctant governments to make companies uphold their pledges are continuing challenges.

We have seen that international treaties, public health regulation by national governments, and global activist campaigns can each claim victories in the battles for trade practices that support rather than undermine health. These stories show that often these three approaches combine to have a synergistic impact. They also show that local, national, and global alliances can create moral and political pressure that has at time forced the world's largest corporations to change their practices. In this way, they foreshadow an alternative approach to global trade that puts human need ahead of profits; provides a platform for the voices of concerned citizens, advocates, health officials, and national governments; and uses the powerful channels of globalization to expand rather than contract the common cultural and natural resources that bind humans everywhere together.

But these alternatives to corporate managed trade are fragile and do not yet constitute a consistently powerful alternative to the corporate consumption complex. As yet, few global organizations have the capacity to weave the disparate strands of people-managed globalization into a coherent and effective global force. In the next chapter, I describe some of the building blocks for a more sustainable and powerful movement against hyperconsumption and its health consequences.

Part Two

CREATING SOLUTIONS

7

Optimism Past, Present, and Future

The Building Blocks for a Movement

Some readers may be discouraged by the evidence of the immense power of corporations to shape health, or perhaps pessimistic about realistic solutions that can better protect well-being. But there are grounds for optimism in our past and present, and in our prospects for the future.

In the late nineteenth and early twentieth centuries, U.S. corporate power had reached new heights and corporate practices in the workplace, environment, and market threatened the living conditions and health of millions of Americans. Yet, in the following decades, mortality dropped precipitously. In the twentieth century, the average lifespan of people in the United States lengthened by more than thirty years; researchers attribute twenty-five years of this gain to advances in public health.[1] Living conditions improved significantly, and in the years between World War II and the early 1970s, income inequality declined. How did this happen? What can we learn from these successes in improving the quality of life and reducing mortality by mitigating the harm from corporate practices?

Today, thousands of organizations throughout the United States and many more around the world are organizing to protect people's health from corporations that put profit over well-being. They work at the local, regional, national, and global levels. They include governments, professional organizations, international non-governmental organizations, community organizations, researchers, advocates, and many more. They use tactics from legislation, litigation, and ballot initiatives, to demonstrations, boycotts, and civil disobedience. And together they have forced companies to label ingredients, improve working conditions, take products off the market, compensate victims of dangerous products, and reduce pollution.

And from our critical analysis of these experiences comes our hope for optimism about the world's future. What can we learn from the successes and limitations of these organizations and their campaigns? What lessons do they offer to those who seek to build a movement for healthy more sustainable consumption?

In this chapter, I analyze past successes in improving public health and survey the panoply of current activism and movements that are challenging the corporate role in health. My goal is to identify the building blocks for an alternative to the corporate consumption complex and its brand of hyperconsumption.

Optimism Past

FOOD AND DRUG SAFETY

> All day long the blazing midsummer sun beat down upon that square mile of abominations: upon tens of thousands of cattle crowded into pens whose wooden floors stank and steamed contagion; upon bare, blistering, cinder-strewn railroad tracks and huge blocks of dingy meat factories, whose labyrinthine passages defied a breath of fresh air to penetrate them; and there were not merely rivers of hot blood and car-loads of moist flesh, and rendering-vats and soap caldrons, glue-facto-ries and fertilizer tanks, that smelt like the craters of hell—there were also tons of garbage festering in the sun, and the greasy laundry of the workers hung out to dry, and dining rooms littered with food and black with flies, and toilet rooms that were open sewers.[2]

These words, from Upton Sinclair's 1906 exposé of the meat industry, *The Jungle*, played a critical role in persuading Congress to pass and President Teddy Roosevelt to sign two new laws: the Meat Inspection Act, which significantly expanded the U.S. Department of Agriculture's inspection of the slaughtering and packing of meats, and the Food and Drug Act of 1906, which created a national agency to protect the public from unsafe food and drugs.

Sinclair's descriptions—meat workers sick with tuberculosis spitting on the floor, then dragging butchered meat across it; sausages that included rat drop-pings; the selling of rotten meat and moldy sausages that had been rejected for sale in Europe; spoiled meat dyed with borax or rubbed with soda to remove the smell—sickened readers and led many to act. Within weeks of the publication of *The Jungle*, sales of meat fell by half. Horrified readers sent President Roosevelt a hundred letters a day asking him to act.[3] The American Medical Association also supported the creation of a new agency. Its leaders warned Republicans that if the Senate did not pass a bill, its 135,000 members would urge their patients to lobby the Senate.[4] Reluctantly, Roosevelt invited Sinclair to the White House to discuss conditions in Chicago's meat industry.[5] Sinclair, a socialist activist as well as a journalist, had hoped that *The Jungle* would improve working conditions for the exploited meat packers as well as food safety. He later wrote, "I aimed at the public's heart and by accident, I hit it in the stomach."[6]

Other exposés in popular magazines educated consumers about the risks of patent medicines, heavily advertised but often ineffective remedies sold over the counter. In *Collier's* magazine, the muckraking journalist Samuel Hopkins Adams informed readers of the limited effectiveness, side effects, and addictive properties of patent medicines. "Gullible America," he wrote in 1905,

> will spend this year some seventy-five millions of dollars in the pur-
> chase of patent medicines. In consideration of this sum it will swallow
> huge quantities of alcohol, an appalling amount of opiates and narcot-
> ics, a wide assortment of varied drugs ranging from powerful and dan-
> gerous heart depressants to insidious liver stimulants; and, far in excess
> of other ingredients, undiluted fraud. For fraud, exploited by the skilful-
> est [sic] of advertising bunco men, is the basis of the trade.[7]

Adams explained the benefits of regulation, encouraging consumers to lobby for new food and drug protections. The industry, of course, actively opposed the legislation. A representative of the Proprietary Association, the trade organizations of patent-medicine makers, said that a law requiring labeling "would practically destroy the sale of proprietary remedies in the United States," not because of the expense, but because the requirement "to disclose that fanciful products were actually as plain as the bottles of powder in any apothecary would be catastrophic."[8]

Congress was inundated with petitions from members of the General Federation of Women's Clubs and the Women's Christian Temperance Union, leaders of the home economics movement, and public health officials, all demanding regulation of patent medicines.[9] Another series of exposés showed how patent-medicine manufacturers were using their power over the press to defeat state regulation, highlighting the importance of strengthening democratic safeguards.

During the late nineteenth and early twentieth centuries, the practices of both the food and pharmaceutical industries threatened health. Contaminated meat, milk, and water caused many food-borne infections, including typhoid fever, tuberculosis, botulism, and scarlet fever.[10] Patent medicines, which in the early twentieth century accounted for nearly half of newspapers' advertising revenue, threatened health with the ingredients they did and did not include. Many contained alcohol, opium, cocaine, morphine, or chloroform, putting users at risk of addiction.[11] Coca-Cola was introduced in 1885 as a patent medicine that at first included both alcohol and cocaine. Its inventor, John Pemberton, claimed that the drink was an effective treatment for various conditions, including dyspepsia, headaches, impotence, and morphine addiction. In 1893, one William Radam sold Microbe Killer, another nostrum, about which he claimed, "No disease in the world will not yield to the Microbe Killer."[12]

Reformers made several efforts to pass new federal legislation during the late nineteenth century but failed due to industry opposition and lack of popular support. While several states passed laws regulating food safety or patent medicines, they were generally weakly enforced. Moreover, as both the food and pharmaceutical industries produced and distributed for national markets, state laws became inadequate to protect consumers. Some big companies decided to support national rather than state rules to enable economies of scale in production and as a competitive edge against smaller producers, who had more difficulty meeting national standards.[13]

As policymakers and health officials came to recognize that deceptive advertising often left consumers without the knowledge or skills to make informed decisions about complex and multi-ingredient products, support for stricter regulation increased. At the same time, science was developing the tools to help consumers make informed judgements. In 1902, a government scientist, Dr. Harvey Wiley (who later became the director of the newly established Food and Drug Administration), began human experiments with volunteers that tested the health effects of increasing doses of frequently used food preservatives. He found that several common preservatives, including borax and formaldehyde, caused gastric distress, headaches, and bowel troubles.[14]

Did the new federal regulations of the early twentieth century make a difference? In the case of food-borne infections, the answer was a clear yes. Once the sources and characteristics of food-borne diseases were identified, they could be mitigated through handwashing, sanitation, refrigeration, pasteurization, and pesticide application. Healthier animal care, feeding, and processing also improved food supply safety. In 1900, the incidence of one food-borne illness, typhoid fever, was approximately 100 per 100,000 population; by 1920, it had decreased to 33.8, and by 1950, to 1.7.[15] For consumer drugs, additional legislation was needed to adequately protect consumers. In 1938, Congress passed a law requiring that drugs be proven safe before they could be sold; in 1962, another law required they be proven effective.[16]

In addition to protecting public health, these regulations established important political precedents. As Philip Hilts wrote in his history of the FDA, "In creating a regime of food and drug regulation, Roosevelt and Congress were establishing the principle that it was now the job of government not just to champion commerce but to intervene when it got out of hand."[17] Teddy Roosevelt put it a different way: "Every new social relation begets a new type of wrongdoing—of sin, to use an old-fashioned word—and many years always elapse before society is able to turn this sin into a crime which can be effectively punished by law."[18]

WORKER SAFETY AND HEALTH

At the start of the twentieth century, as the United States was rapidly industrializing, worker diseases such as coal workers' pneumoconiosis (black lung disease) and silicosis were common. Workplace injuries and deaths in mining, construction, and other sectors were an especially important problem. As one observer noted in 1907,

> To unprecedented prosperity...there is a seamy side of which little is said. Thousands of wage earners, men, women and children, [are] caught in the machinery of our record-breaking production and turned out cripples. Other thousands [are] killed outright...How many there [are] none can say exactly for we are too busy making the record production to count the dead.[19]

During the Progressive Era of 1890 to 1920, reformers, labor unions, health professionals, public officials, and some business leaders came together to demand stronger government protection for worker safety and more rights for workers to participate in setting public policy.[20] Over the ensuing decades, their efforts paid off, with new state and federal laws regulating workplace health and safety, plus new agencies charged with enforcing the regulations. Labor unions were often at the forefront of persuading states and Congress to pass these types of standards for corporate behavior. These measures included workers' compensation laws and the formation of the Mine Safety and Health Administration (MSHA), the Occupational Safety and Health Administration (OSHA), and the National Institute for Occupational Safety and Health (NIOSH). The results were physical changes in the workplace, such as improved ventilation and dust suppression in mines; safer equipment; development and introduction of safer work practices; and improved training of health and safety professionals and of workers.[21]

Not surprisingly, these developments resulted in improved health for workers. According to the National Safety Council, deaths from work-related injuries declined 90 percent between 1933 and 1997—from 37 per 100,000 workers to 4 per 100,000.[22] If today's workforce had the same risk of dying from injuries as it did in 1933, then an additional 40,000 workers would have died in 1997.[23]

Remarkably, these health gains have not plateaued. Between 1980 and 2000, the rate of fatal occupational injuries declined an additional 40 percent.[24] Since the estimated cost of workplace injuries from medical care, lost wages, and lost productivity equals $146.6 billion annually, these reductions in deaths saved hundreds of billions of dollars. Although many workplace hazards persist and new ones related to the twenty-first–century workforce are emerging, the dramatic decline in workplace deaths and injuries led the U.S. Centers for Disease Control and Prevention to declare that improvements in workplace safety were one of the greatest triumphs of twentieth-century public health.[25]

CHILD LABOR

Another advance in workplace health was the mostly successful effort to end child labor in America. In 1910, more than 2 million children under the age of fifteen were employed in the United States, working in canneries, textile mills (see Figure 7.1), tobacco factories, and agriculture.[26] While some states had laws limiting children's work hours, these rules were generally weak and poorly enforced. In 1910, Edward Klopper, the Secretary of the Ohio Valley National Child Labor Committee, told members of the American Public Health Association,

> The standard child labor law may be a thing of beauty as it reposes tranquilly on the pages of an admiring commonwealth's statute books, but it can never become a joy forever until it is completely and impartially enforced. The preservation of the health, and therefore the future efficiency, of working children depend in large measure upon strict enforcement.[27]

A movement led by Florence Kelly, Jane Addams, and other reformers, aided by church groups, women's clubs, and civic organizations, persuaded Congress to pass federal legislation in 1916 to limit the age at which children could work without restrictions and parental consent.[28] However, the U.S. Supreme Court declared the law unconstitutional, saying it unduly interfered with interstate commerce. Only in 1941 did the Supreme Court reverse this decision, forcing businesses to abide by the rule and allowing children to work only outside of school hours and forbidding children under eighteen to hold jobs hazardous to their health.[29] By the 1950s, child labor in America had declined significantly, and with it the threats it posed to children's well-being.[30] However, as the movement to protect children dissipated after the 1960s, child labor re-emerged in new ways—in the fast food industry and in new types of agricultural work, again posing threats to the well-being of the nation's children.[31] Globally, it is estimated that 215 million children are still involved in child labor.[32]

In the last several decades, new threats to food safety, occupational health, and child welfare have emerged as businesses devise new strategies to overcome and thwart public oversight. But the early successes on food safety, worker

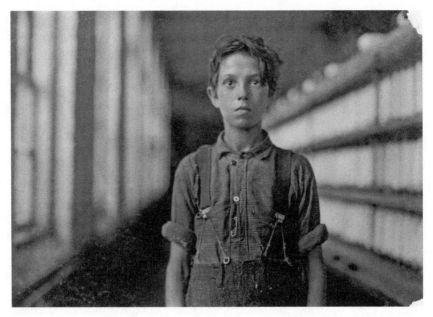

Figure 7.1 A boy inside the cotton mill where he worked in the late nineteenth century. Corbis Images.

health, and child labor demonstrate that it is possible for popular mobilizations to bring about changes in the practices of powerful corporations, and in so doing to create a healthier and more democratic society. These changes in corporate practices prevented premature deaths, extended the lifespan of the average American, and reduced injuries and disease. They also improved living and working conditions for millions of people. For the most part, these reforms have persisted into the twenty-first century, showing that public health protections that enjoy popular support can endure, even as corporations seek new profitable ways to cut corners.

Optimism Present

If past successes demonstrate that diverse sectors of society have successfully mobilized to change harmful corporate practices, current activities show that every sector of society has the potential to take action to change how corporations do business. In this section, I briefly describe six examples of recent efforts by a variety of individuals and organizations to modify corporate practices that contribute to premature death or preventable illness or injury. These vignettes, one from each of the six industries I have considered, demonstrate some of the accomplishments of recent campaigns to protect public health against risky corporate practices. Analyzing their successes to identify promising strategies and tactics can help synthesize these experiences into lessons that can guide organizers for a comprehensive movement to transform current patterns of illness and health. Equally important, probing the limitations of current activism can suggest new approaches to overcoming these failures.

NEW YORK CITY FOOD JUSTICE MOVEMENT: BLENDING ALTERNATIVE FOOD ACTIVISTS AND CRITICS OF CORPORATE FOOD

In New York City, a "food justice movement" is growing that, in its diversity of participants, issues, and strategies, illustrates the potential for a national food movement that can challenge the dominant industrial food system. New York City's emerging movement includes a wide cross-section of constituencies, listed in Table 7.1 below. These disparate individuals and organizations constitute a new force that is determined to change the choices the city's food environments now offer. Examining the accomplishments and limitations of this emerging movement provides insights into the dynamic tensions between those who seek to create personal alternatives to corporate consumption and those who want to reduce the influence of profit-seeking corporations on American society.

In the last five years, the movement has contributed to numerous changes in policy and public attitude. Some changes target corporations directly: New York City's food movement contributed to a requirement for calorie labeling in all restaurant and fast food chains, subsidies for supermarkets that operate in low-income neighborhoods, and a ban on trans fats in restaurant food. Others have begun to create alternative food systems, ones not so dependent on big corporations. Farmers' markets are now common throughout the city's five boroughs, with upstate farmers selling fresh, local food and accepting food stamps to encourage low-income customers. A farm-to-school program brings fresh food to some of the city's public schools. And Green Carts— mostly immigrant street vendors whose carts may have previously sold hot dogs and soft drinks—now sell fresh fruits and vegetables on city streets in low-income neighborhoods. In some cases, the food movement has supported initiatives of New York City's mayor, billionaire Michael Bloomberg, a public health champion. In other cases it has opposed mayoral policies, such as the requirement that food stamp recipients be fingerprinted prior to getting benefits, or his unwillingness to support a living wage for the city's low-income workers, many in the food sector.

Table 7.1 **Constituencies in New York City's Emerging Food Justice Movement**

Constituencies	Who want:
Parents	Healthier school food for their children and protection against the intrusions of marketers of unhealthy foods
Food workers	Living wages and safer working conditions
Chefs	Healthier, tastier, and more local foods on their menus
Churchgoers	Opportunities to manifest faith in food pantries, soup kitchens, and food justice activism and to reduce poverty and inequality
Immigrants	Familiar and healthy sustenance for their families and alternatives to ubiquitous fast food and soda
Residents of low-income neighborhoods	Healthier and more affordable food choices in their neighborhood
Staff and volunteers at New York's 1,200 food pantries and soup kitchens	Reductions in hunger, food insecurity, poverty, and inequality in the city
Health professionals and researchers	Reductions in city's epidemics of obesity and diet-related diseases and in health inequalities
People with diabetes and other diet-related diseases	Better food choices that help them manage disease and prevent complications
Elected officials, agency staff, and policymakers	Improvements in food policies and credit for change that will help them win votes

One of the largest and most diverse of New York City's food justice organizations is the Brooklyn Food Coalition (BFC), a grassroots organization with three overriding goals: making healthy, affordable food available for all; creating a sustainable food system; and seeking justice for food workers.[33] BFC was founded in March 2009, and its first conference drew 3,000 people of all ages and backgrounds. It has launched projects in school food, living wages for food workers, and establishing alliances with upstate farmers. In 2012, BFC offered education and advocacy to Brooklyn residents on the federal Farm and Food Bill, the legislation that authorizes farm support and food assistance. BFC made the case that the renewal provided an opportunity to take money away from big agribusiness corporations and redirect it to more local producers. Nancy

Romer, a founder of the Brooklyn Food Coalition, explained her view of the role of corporations:

> The biggest problem in the food system is the control of local, regional, state, and national governments by multinational corporations. If we could wrest control over our food choices back from the corporations, the opportunities for sustainable food systems are endless. The city of New York provides around 1 million meals every day; if city agencies could determine where they sourced the food for those meals, and could choose regional small- or medium-scale farmers as their go-to source, that alone would make a huge difference in strengthening the local food system, as well as the local economy. The same goes for processed and cooked foods—if local suppliers of these foods were given preference over multinational suppliers, New York's economy would be given a huge boost.[34]

The BFC's 2012 conference drew almost 6,000 people, some first-time participants and others experienced activists. They came from neighborhoods throughout Brooklyn and New York City and attended more than 160 workshops on such topics as "Corporations: Creating Impact Through the Food Chain," "Faith and Feeding the Hungry," "Organizing for Farmworker Justice," and "Free Trade vs. Safe, Just, and Sustainable Food." An important goal of the meeting, explained Romer, was to bring "all these activists out of their 'silos,' or the specific areas in which they are working. We need to work as a movement, not as factions with independent goals, because we are all working toward a healthier, fairer, and more sustainable global food system."[35] By enabling its participants to weave together the concerns that motivate food activists—problems such as child obesity and diet-related chronic diseases, hunger and food insecurity, climate change and loss of agricultural land, income inequality and unsafe working conditions for food workers—BFC seeks to create a stronger fabric that unites its members.

In 2013, in anticipation of the city's mayoral election, BFC joined with 10 other New York City food and hunger organizations to sponsor the city's first Mayoral Candidates Forum on food policy. Almost 2,000 people participated in the forum, and candidates answered a variety of questions on their positions on food policy. Several candidates proposed new policies to require food corporations to offer healthier fare to city residents. Marion Nestle, the NYU nutrition professor who moderated the forum, concluded that the New York City "food movement is strong enough to make candidates for office stand up, listen and take food issues seriously."[36]

Some BFC members are connected to regional, statewide, national, and international efforts to change food policies. Others rarely leave their neighborhoods.

One of the BFC's strengths is the multiple formal and informal networks of its members who belong to church, environmental, and labor rights groups. In its work on school food, BFC conducted aggressive outreach and education in black and Latino schools, enabling parents to become activists in their own schools and to join and influence citywide and national coalitions to support a federal bill that would provide more funding and higher nutritional standards for school food programs. When it was revealed that many school food programs still served "pink slime," the product made from leftover meat remnants and then treated with a puff of ammonium hydroxide to kill bacteria, BFC encouraged New York City schools to drop the product from its menus.[37]

BFC is also skilled in linking personal concerns with political concerns. As Romer put it:

> Our community gardens, our farmers markets, our food coops, our food pantries, our school food committees, our unions all bring us into human-scale communities that create real relationships and solve real problems on the ground. We grow, sell and cook local food. We feed the hungry. We protect the green spaces and the local farmland. We celebrate and educate ourselves through these communities and relationships. And for that we are a strong and vibrant movement.[38]

By creating an organization that can accommodate all these goals, BFC has helped bring thousands of people into food activism, and in doing so, deepen the New York City food justice movement. At the close of the 2012 Brooklyn Food Conference, Romer summed up the challenges facing the food justice movement:

> We need to link arms with others who share our concerns, who believe in the right of all people to healthy food, who want to see an end to corporate domination of our food system. We need to change the policies that shovel our hard-earned tax money to the richest corporations that...harm our people and our planet—Monsanto, Cargill, Nestlé, Unilever, General Mills. We need to regulate the largest farms that use the most dangerous techniques—chemical fertilizers and pesticides for plants and hormones and antibiotics for animals, long-distance distribution eating up outrageous amounts of oil and gas, all destroying our planet and giving unhealthy food. We need to regulate the largest food processors and fast food corporations to stop saturating our food with sugar, salt and fat and to stop preying on our children with media advertisements of cheap, fast foods promising happiness and delivering misery. The U.S. low-wage structure keeps us dependent on these

unhealthy foods because they are cheap at the checkout aisle but costly at the doctor's office.[39]

In her book *Change Comes to Dinner*, food writer and activist Katherine Gustafson observes that the United States has designed a food system perfectly designed for the purposes it serves, "creating low-quality, low-priced food and large profits for a handful of big corporations."[40] The task, she says is to "shrink all aspects of this system back down to a size that fits all our lives." In its work with parents, schools, churches, food retailers, farmers, and city officials, BFC shows one road to doing this in a city whose diversity and needs are the same as those facing urban Americans everywhere. BFC has not overcome the many tensions between "alternative foodies" and food justice activists, but by embracing these differences, it has shown the possibility of finding the common ground that nurtures activism.

BLACK COMMUNITIES CHALLENGE TARGETING BY THE ALCOHOL INDUSTRY

Like other industries, the alcohol industry targets blacks with marketing for profitable but risky products such as malt beer and distilled spirits. To promote its products, alcohol makers have hired black entertainers like Billy Dee Williams, who claimed that Colt 45 "works every time." The rapper Ice Cube promised that St. Ides would "get your woman in the mood quicker and make your jimmy thicker."[41] Malt liquors were so attractive to some young people that ministers labeled them "liquid crack."[42] Images on malt liquor ads included— and still use—guns and near-naked women, projecting images of danger and sexuality.

Although alcohol has always been available in poor communities, the proliferation of convenience stores, bars, chain restaurants, and other outlets made it even more available. As one activist from Raleigh, North Carolina, observed, "The sheer amount of alcohol sold in our neighborhood is a problem.... The fact that more alcohol is sold than any other legal product...that's a real problem because it encourages alcoholism, domestic abuse, trash, filthiness around the neighborhood."[43] Research studies confirmed that neighborhoods with more alcohol outlets have higher rates of alcohol consumption and alcohol-related health problems and violence.[44]

As alcohol consumption fell in the 1970s and 1980s, alcohol companies looked to increase profitability by reaching new consumers and using less expensive advertising channels. Young people, especially young blacks and Latinos, were an especially attractive target, as they represented a new base of lifetime customers and their lower rates of drinking presented growth opportunities.[45]

In black and Latino neighborhoods, new forms of alcohol advertising pro-
liferated. Billboards with images of young people enjoying alcohol sprouted
throughout these communities, with several studies showing twice as many alcohol billboards in black as in white communities.[46] Magazines and radio advertisements also increased, and studies showed that black youth were more likely
to be exposed to such ads than white youth. In one study, ads for one brand, Colt
45 Malt Liquor, accounted for 32 percent of all radio alcohol advertising heard
by black youth.[47]

Blacks have long noted the role that alcohol has played in their oppression. In
1845, Frederick Douglass wrote:

> Slaveholders like to…disgust their slaves with freedom, by plunging
> them into the lowest depths of dissipation.…One plan is to make bets
> on their slaves, as to who can drink the most whiskey without getting
> drunk; and in this way they succeed in getting whole multitudes to
> drink to excess. Thus, when the slave asks for virtuous freedom, the
> cunning slaveholder, knowing his ignorance, cheats him with a dose
> of vicious dissipation, artfully labeled with the name of liberty.…So,
> when the holidays ended, we staggered up from the filth of our wallow-
> ing, took a long breath, and marched to the field—feeling, upon the
> whole, rather glad to go, from what our master had deceived us into a
> belief was freedom, back to the arms of slavery.[48]

Douglass's concerns have been echoed by black leaders over the years, all motivated by a belief that alcohol contributes to addiction, chronic disease, family conflict, community fragmentation, crime, violence, and limited economic growth.[49]

The alcohol activists that emerged to combat increased advertising to youth
in black communities squarely blamed the alcohol industry.[50] This distin-
guished them from groups like Mothers Against Drunk Driving (MADD)—a
mostly white and middle-class movement that emerged in the 1980s to reduce
drunk driving and targeted drunk drivers. Several industry practices attracted
the attention of the black activists: the marketing of malt liquor, a high-alco-
hol-content, high-sugar alcoholic beverage, to young black men; use of sexist
and violent images in alcohol advertisements and of black artists to promote
alcohol use; and a high density of retail outlets in black communities. While
no single community or organization took on all these practices, the collective
response of black communities and institutions to the targeted marketing of
alcohol demonstrates the potential for a population to act to protect itself from
corporate harm.

Malt liquors like St Ides, Colt 45, Ole English 800, Hurricane, and King
Cobra contain 6 to 8 percent alcohol, compared to less than 5 percent in other

beers. Malt liquors are sold in 40-ounce containers, often at less than $2 a bottle, a lower price than other types of alcohol. One 40-ounce container has more alcohol than four shots of whiskey. Malt liquors also contain more calories and more carbohydrates than standard beers, contributing to diet-related diseases like diabetes, already prevalent in many black communities. Almost a third of the sales of malt liquors are in black communities.[51]

In many communities, alcohol billboards became a target for activists. Beginning in the 1980s, the Chicago Citywide Coalition against Tobacco and Alcohol Billboards mobilized to urge removal of such billboards from Chicago's poor neighborhoods. The Coalition also protested at Black Expo, a business show designed to promote economic development in black Chicago that was sponsored by tobacco and alcohol companies. The Coalition demanded that local elected officials and the media stand up to companies that promoted the community's "biggest addictive killers."[52] By asking influential community leaders to choose between their community and the alcohol and tobacco industries, the coalition drew a provocative line in the sand.

In the early 1990s, after billboard owners refused to remove the large advertisements, the activists, including Michael Pfleger, a white Roman Catholic priest in an African-American parish, climbed ladders to deface the signs. Pfleger and others were charged with destruction of private property but were later acquitted by a jury.[53] In 1997, the Chicago City Council voted 46–1 to eliminate tobacco and alcohol billboards from selected areas in Chicago. Pfleger described the decision as "a tremendous victory for the children of Chicago, for our neighborhoods, especially black and Hispanic neighborhoods."[54] A few years later, when billboards advertising alcohol began to appear again, Pfleger threatened to revive the practice of painting over such billboards, if that was what it took "to get companies to respect the community."[55] Although a Supreme Court decision in another case ultimately overruled Chicago's ban, the long battle educated community members about industry influences on youth drinking.

Several years earlier, Chicago activists also played a leading role in removing from stores PowerMaster, a new malt liquor produced by the G. Heileman Brewery for marketing in Chicago's African-American neighborhoods. Father Pfleger, this time joined by another Chicago minister and activist, the Reverend George Clements, went to the brewery's corporate office in La Crosse, Wisconsin, to meet with company president Thomas Rattigan. When the clergymen were told that Rattigan was out of town and no one else would meet with them, they refused to leave and were arrested for trespassing.[56]

These activists launched a national campaign of black leaders, including Surgeon General Antonia Novella and representatives of anti-drinking groups, to protest PowerMaster. In 1991, the Bureau of Alcohol, Tobacco and Firearms informed Heileman Brewery that they were withdrawing approval of the

PowerMaster label.[57] They cited a passage in the law established by the Federal Alcohol Administration Act of 1935 that forbade the labeling or advertising of beer as being "strong, full strength, extra strength, or high test," all words that could be construed as indicators of a product's alcoholic strength.[58] After the BATF ruling, Father Pfleger observed, "When we are spiritually strong, there's no problem we cannot overcome. We have a serious alcohol problem in the African American community, and this means something worse won't be added to it. Big business better watch out if it's doing wrong."[59]

Similar campaigns took place in African-American communities in Oakland, Milwaukee, Philadelphia, Raleigh, Detroit, and Baltimore—and in some Hispanic, white, and Native American communities as well.[60] After the riots in Los Angeles in 1992, the Campaign to Rebuild South Central LA Without Liquor Stores was credited with preventing the rebuilding of 150 alcohol outlets and helping spur the conversion of 44 liquor outlets to community-friendly businesses such as laundromats.[61]

In the early 1990s, activists from several of these groups created the National Association of African Americans for Positive Imagery (NAAAPI), which aimed to help "end the excessive marketing of alcohol, tobacco, and other harmful products to communities of color." Its goals were to "mobilize the African American communities around the nation to support positive and healthy media and advertising images." NAAAPI was active for about twelve years, helping to support local and national campaigns against tobacco and alcohol marketing, train local leaders, and create a forum in which activists could share experiences.[62] After the organization dissolved, its members continued to play leadership roles in campaigns against tobacco and alcohol in African-American communities.

Today, few organizations are still actively organizing against the alcohol industry in black communities, although its alumni continue to be leaders in health and civil rights struggles. But an analysis of the rise and decline of this activism provides useful lessons. By linking resistance to alcohol marketing in black communities to the many other struggles to protect their communities against external threats, black activists were able to tap into the deep roots that have sustained the civil rights movement over the last century. By tackling marketing of both tobacco and alcohol—and more recently, unhealthy food as well, community activists raised the larger question of who benefited from promoting consumption of these products.

In doing so, they shifted the frame from giving individuals the right to choose whatever product they wanted, the corporate message, to communities having the right to protect their children and families from sickening marketing. And they showed that ordinary citizens could mobilize their communities to challenge the practices of the world's largest corporations.

The limitations also teach lessons. The lack of a national movement to challenge unhealthy alcohol industry practices forced local activists to fight defensive battles against the most offensive specific advertising campaigns or egregiously risky products. Given the industry's greater resources, activists were forced to serve as the Dutch boy with his finger in the dike, running from one industry onslaught to another. The groups also lacked the power to defend their victories in court, making it possible for the alcohol industry to overturn local successes. As the other stories in this section show, finding ways to link the energy and commitment of local activism, the capacity of national groups to exert power in Washington, and the vision of a movement that cuts across issues and sectors is an essential task for those who seek to challenge the corporate consumption complex.

CALIFORNIA AIR RESOURCES BOARD AND THE AUTO INDUSTRY: GOVERNMENT AS A FORCE FOR CORPORATE CHANGE

In the last decade, California has been regarded as the poster child of government dysfunction—huge budget deficits, irreconcilable partisan conflicts, and endless ballot initiatives on every issue imaginable. But hidden within the state bureaucracy, one small agency, the California Air Resources Board (CARB), shows another story: the ability of a government agency to use scientific evidence and a mobilized public to defend its mission against one of the world's most powerful industries. Although CARB has not won every battle with the auto industry, and critics point out serious limitations, it has been able to win concessions that set new standards for environmental and public health protection. An examination of the history and achievements of CARB shows it has contributed to safer, less polluting cars in California, the United States, and other parts of the world, illustrating the potential for government itself to be a force for corporate change.

CARB was created by the state's legislature in 1967 to limit motor vehicle pollution and promote clean air. Its creation marked an effort to reconcile Californians' long love affair with the car with the less romantic realities of smog, gridlock, and rising rates of respiratory problems. CARB's mission was, and remains, "to promote and protect public health, welfare and ecological resources through the effective and efficient reduction of air pollutants, while recognizing and considering the effects on the state's economy."[63] CARB's board, appointed by the governor, comprises experts in medicine, chemistry, engineering, business, and law, as well as representatives of California's regional air pollution control agencies.

In 1970, as Congress considered the Clean Air Act, California waged a long and successful battle to ensure that the new law left CARB with the authority to establish automobile emission standards stricter than the federal levels. The auto industry vigorously opposed this measure, but the newly emerging national environmental movement and some powerful California legislators helped over-come this opposition. In 1977, Congress extended the option of lowering stan-dard emission levels to other states.[64] In 1991, CARB was moved into the newly created California Environmental Protection Agency.

Throughout its history, CARB has joined with environmental groups, public health researchers, and health advocates to emphasize the health and economic costs of air pollution. A 2010 study by the RAND Corporation found that air pol-lution generated $200 million a year in hospital expenses in California. CARB chairwoman Mary Nichols told a *San Francisco Chronicle* reporter that people who argue that fuel regulation costs money "should think about the cost of not doing anything.... The fact that we're paying for all these hospitals and emer-gency room visits is sobering."[65] Another study estimated that CARB regulations on black carbon emissions, a short-lived but highly toxic pollutant, would lead to an 80 percent decline in California's air levels by 2020, demonstrating that its regulations protected health.[66]

One of California's biggest battles with the auto industry was over the state's right to take action to reduce global warming, seen by many public health experts as a serious threat to health as well as the environment.[67] In 2006, the state passed AB32, Global Warming Solutions Act of 2006, which set the goal of reducing 2020 greenhouse gas emissions to their 1990 levels, a 25 percent reduction. AB32 directed CARB to develop an action plan to achieve those goals by 2011 (later delayed to 2013 because of the 2008 economic crisis).[68] The plan included a cap-and-trade program in which companies buy a diminishing pool of "carbon allowances," then trade these allowances with other companies, leading to steady declines in emissions; new standards for the carbon content in fuels; requirements for increased fuel efficiency in vehicles; and mandates for communities to become more energy efficient, including by developing mass transit, walking, and biking plans.[69]

CARB's regulation attracted strong national opposition from both the automobile and energy industries. In 2004, the auto industry filed lawsuits in California and three other states to derail California's 2002 Clean Car Law, the predecessor to AB32, charging that it gave states rights reserved to the federal government. In 2007, the U.S. Supreme Court ruled against the auto-maker's main arguments, holding that greenhouse gases are a pollutant, that the EPA has the power to regulate them under existing law, and that green-house gas emission standards under the Clean Air Act are not preempted by the federal fuel economy law.[70] Advocacy groups like the Environmental Defense Fund played a role in developing the legal arguments that persuaded the Court and in public education campaigns to encourage auto companies to "innovate rather than litigate . . . in light of the serious financial challenges facing the industry."[71]

Over time, however, the automobile industry became more cooperative, perhaps in part because they recognized the inevitability of new standards. In 2011, the Obama Administration, the State of California, and major global auto companies including Ford, Chrysler, General Motors, Toyota, Nissan, and Volkswagen, agreed to a single set of greenhouse gas standards to go into effect between 2017 and 2025.[72] The Obama Administration's auto bailout was believed to have contributed to the industry's willingness to shake, rather than bite, the hand that had rescued it.

After the agreement was reached, a CARB spokesman told the *Washington Post* that "the agreement will provide strong standards that benefit the nation and recognize and build on California's leadership role in air quality and climate protection."[73] CARB's determination to move forward, its long-term perspective, and its ability to join with the federal government promised auto makers a higher degree of the regulatory certainty that enables long-term planning.

Early in 2012, CARB mandated that 15 percent of all cars sold in California should run with zero or near-zero emissions. It also mandated a 50 percent reduction from current levels of auto-generated greenhouses gases. Remarkably, U.S. car makers have been largely supportive. "It's a pretty amazing story to see how far the auto companies have come in doing their part," said Simon Mui of the Natural Resources Defense Council.[74] Using another AB32 mandate, some cities and towns have begun designing transportation systems less dependent on automobiles. Santa Rosa, for example, a town north of San Francisco, is redesigning its downtown around rail.[75]

The public debate about the costs and benefits of AB32 illustrates a common tendency of business to exaggerate the costs and minimize the benefits of public health and environmental regulation. Two business school professors from Cal State Sacramento were hired by the California Small Business Roundtable to analyze AB32. They concluded that the new law would cost small businesses $50,000 a year, and each household $3,857 a year. But an independent review of their study by a Stanford University engineering professor and a UCLA economist concluded that the study was "deeply flawed" because it excluded consideration of the economic benefits of energy savings, made unreasonable assumptions about the costs of home modification, and inexplicably counted the fuel savings new car owners would realize as a cost for older-car owners. In an editorial in the *Los Angeles Times*, the independent researchers wrote that the Cal State study overestimated costs by a factor of 10 and ignored many benefits.[76] These public debates about the evidence of the CARB's impact on air quality, health, and costs helped create the public opinion that persuaded politicians and courts to side with the state and against industry.

CARB has also been criticized by environmental justice activists. In a lawsuit against CARB, Associated Irritated Residents, a coalition of environmental justice groups, claimed that the cap-and-trade scheme will allow the state's largest emitters of greenhouse gases—mainly utilities and refineries—to purchase their way to compliance rather than reducing their own emissions.[77] Other environmental groups argued that CARB was too friendly to industry concerns and inadequately protected public health.

Despite these legitimate criticisms, it is clear that CARB's actions have protected public health and the environment. As a result of CARB's and local air district's work to limit air pollution, Californians today breathe the cleanest air since measurements have been recorded. The number of first-stage alerts in the Los Angeles area has been cut from over 200 per year in the 1970s to fewer than ten per year today. Other regions of the state also have improved air quality despite massive increases in population, the number of motor vehicles and the distances they are driven.[78]

California has also set national and international standards for regulation of auto pollution. In the last decade, thirteen states have followed California's lead and adopted the Clean Cars standards: Arizona, Connecticut, Maine, Maryland, Massachusetts, New Jersey, New Mexico, New York, Oregon, Pennsylvania, Rhode Island, Vermont, and Washington. The "California Car" has driven innovation in Detroit and helped U.S. automakers recover in part from their unsustainable addiction to the high profits that SUVs generated. Mary Nichols, the CARB chairwoman, suggested that by gearing up for California's zero-emission standards, U.S. car makers will get ready for new and profitable markets in India, China, and elsewhere.[79] Vickie Patton, the general counsel of the Environmental Defense Fund called the new 2012 zero-emission rules "a very powerful and history-making movement in which California is pushing the U.S. and the world towards pollution-free cars."[80] More broadly, another observer noted that CARBs cap-and-trade policies and emission standards serve to internalize back to the auto industry the cost of externalities such as air pollution and global warming.[81]

In a panel discussion on climate change in San Francisco's tony Commonwealth Club, Mary Nichols summarized the breadth of CARB's goals:

> We're talking about really transforming the entire transportation system. California, and actually the country as a whole, are in the business of moving things around.... But we have to figure out how to get a balance going here where we get these ultra-clean and ultra-efficient vehicles and transform the whole market for these vehicles, and, at the same time, also recognize that there were limits on them because we need to put more things and more people into mass transit.... So we're

talking about a gigantic economic transformation.... It's all connected it's just starting with the passenger cars.[82]

From the 1970s on, through campaign contributions, lobbying, the revolving door. and litigation, big corporations have repeatedly captured regulatory agencies and converted them into units that spent more effort protecting profits than the public.[83] CARB, even with its wrinkles, shows another path is possible: public health and environmental interests can claim and protect a regulatory agency, encouraging it to fulfill its public mandate. CARB also shows the potential of integrating thinking and acting at the local, national, and global levels. Its governing processes provide a forum for local officials and environmentalists, and its staff, as a result of their experience and technical expertise, have a voice in national and global deliberations on the regulation of the auto industry. As a state agency, CARB also shows the opportunities of working at that level to influence local, national, and global decisions. Given the powerful influence of corporations in Washington and the crazy-quilt pattern of United States federalism, the CARB story shows that state governments provide advocates for alternatives to corporate consumption fifty venues for action.

Of course, CARB is not immune from auto industry influence, and as a government agency it is forced to compromise with powerful stakeholders. By itself, it can never match the resources and reach of the global auto industry. But if health and environmental groups could transform more state agencies and perhaps even some federal ones into forceful proponents for public health protection, a movement for healthy and sustainable consumption would have some powerful new allies.

THE MILLION MOM MARCH AND THE GUN INDUSTRY: FROM GUN CONTROL TO PROTECTING CHILDREN

On Mother's Day in 2000, several hundred thousand people gathered at the National Mall in Washington, D.C., for the Million Mom March (MMM) for sensible gun control, the largest public gun-control event in U.S. history (see Figure 7.2). Newspaper reports estimated the crowd at between 200,000 and 750,000, and simultaneous marches in seventy other cities attracted tens of thousands of additional participants.[84] While the MMM did not achieve its legislative goals, its success at reframing America's long debate on guns and its ability to mobilize women and communities around the country to convert their anguish and anger about gun violence into political action provide important lessons for those seeking to change corporate practices that harm health. Its limitations illustrate the challenge of sustaining activism in a hostile political environment and perhaps suggest directions for a more successful gun-control movement.

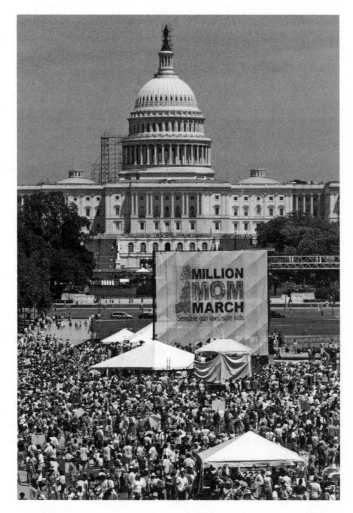

Figure 7.2 The Million Mom March in Washington, D.C., May 2000. Corbis Images.

Several events triggered the actions that led to the MMM. In the two years before planning for the march began, several high-profile shootings took place in schools in Pearl, Mississippi; West Paducah, Kentucky; Jonesboro, Arkansas; Edinboro, Pennsylvania; Springfield, Oregon; Littleton, Colorado; and Granada Hills, California. These events made it clear that gun violence was not just an urban problem; it afflicted suburban communities around the country. The shooting death of a kindergartener by a classmate in Detroit and two high school students at a zoo in Washington showed that children in cities also continued to be at risk.[85]

In explaining why the event happened when it did, one MMM participant told Lawrence Wallack and his colleagues, who studied the impact of the march,

"The time was right.... We are seeing enough people begin to understand that the gun lobby is a little bit more like the tobacco lobby.... People are getting a little bit fed up with the fact that, as parents, we feel hopeless.... Many people are beginning to rethink the ways I can [make] a difference."[86] Susan Dees-Thomases, a founder of the MMM, said her initial goal was not to change the world, but to let everyone else know what she had just learned: that handguns kill twelve children every day in America and nobody was doing anything about it.[87]

At the same time, political debates on guns in Washington and state capitals continued to be dominated by the National Shooting Sports Foundation, the gun industry trade group, and the more publicly known National Rifle Association, which was voted in a 1999 *Fortune* poll of lawmakers as the most influential lobbying group in the country.[88] The NRA's stock responses to shootings were that criminals, not guns, killed people; that child locks were an unnecessary feature on handguns; and that the Second Amendment fully protected the rights of gun owners. A few weeks before the march, a top official of the NRA boasted that if George W. Bush won the presidency in 2000, the organization would enjoy the spoils of an administration "where we work out of their office."[89] Around that time, gun manufacturers Glock and Smith & Wesson ended their negotiations with state and local officials for a code of conduct and new safeguards, expecting (correctly, as it turned out) that if Bush were elected, they would be protected from lawsuits.[90]

As communities lost lives to gun violence and the media blared these stories into living rooms everywhere, the NRA's politics-as-usual were less than convincing. Polls in 2000 showed that 72 percent of women (and 22 percent of men) favored more regulation of guns, an important finding since some politicians feared losing the votes of one gender at the expense of the other.[91]

MMM organizers crafted counter-messages designed to take advantage of this opening. One California MMM organizer, whose son has been shot and killed as a bystander during a robbery, told participants in the march, "We love our children more than the NRA loves their damn guns!"[92] Others asked, "Why should we license drivers and register cars but not handguns?" Kristen Rand, the director of federal policy for the Violence Policy Center and an adviser to MMM explained, "The gun industry is unregulated. Every other product in America, from automobiles to household items and food, is regulated by some governmental agency. The gun industry is exempt from basic health and safety regulations."[93]

Gun control is not a political issue, MMM participants insisted. Nancy Inhofe, an emergency room pediatrician, mother of two, daughter-in-law of Oklahoma's pro-gun Republican senator James Inhofe, and local coordinator for the MMM, explained, "It doesn't matter what side you're on politically. Personal experience has prompted me and people like me to want to make sure guns are safe. I've seen enough."[94] These messages, Wallack and colleagues observed, made the MMM "intellectually accessible." Their simple yet compelling themes spoke to many people in a way that earlier gun-control campaigns had not.[95] By creating messages that appealed to participants' minds and emotions, MMM offered a more satisfying experience than groups that offered only one or the other.

At the march, women who had experienced loss explained their hopes. Madelia Marsh-Williams, whose daughter Natasha had been murdered in Washington, D.C. said, "I think about Natasha all day every day....It's too late for Natasha now. But it's not too late for other kids. I have a 7-year old son, and we need to have these guns registered and we need licensing."[96] Another speaker, Dr. Michele Irwin, told the crowd:

> I come to you today wearing three hats. One as director of our nation's capital's level-one trauma center; two as a practicing emergency medicine physician; and three as the mother of a 3-year old that I send out every day and pray that she returns safely. For the 60 children that will be shot today, they will be taken, for the most part, to an emergency department. The physician working in that department is going to have to deliver bad news to that child's survivors. For eleven of those children, it will be the worst possible news that a parent could receive, the fact that their child is dead. Having worked in emergency departments, first in Chicago and now in our nation's capital, I have seen the havoc that gun violence causes in teen-on-teen violence, in domestic violence, and in adult violence as a result of easy access to guns and lack of accountability....I would welcome the decrease in business that child safety locks on guns would provide me. I would welcome knowing that I would not have to deliver that kind of bad news as frequently as I have in my career as an emergency room physician.[97]

Although the MMM reinforced traditional gender roles—women were described as "moms," "caring for children," and "apolitical"—it also challenged women's roles and elevated them above the stereotypical domestic setting. The march was in Washington, D.C., not the local playground. Organizers debated NRA spokesmen on television, lobbied Congress, and went to the White House to meet with President Clinton. This duality enabled MMM to attract women with both traditional and feminist values.

MMM was also groundbreaking in its organizational structure and methods. It was both a Washington-based interest group and a social-movement organization, a hybrid that could play hardball with legislators and take to the streets to bring new messages into the media.[98] MMM was also one of the first campaigns to use the Internet for community activism, organizing events, sharing information, and reaching women who could not make it to meetings. This emphasis on making the organization accessible to mothers and working women increased opportunities for participation.

The MMM also succeeded in creating a safe space for people who wanted to end gun violence but had varying viewpoints on guns. One participant observed that the march was:

> most remarkable... for its success at bringing together people who have many different ideas about what it means to own a gun. Certainly many attendees, such as myself, do not own a gun and have no desire to ever do so. Many others think that gun ownership itself is not a problem and just want that ownership, and the guns themselves, to be more strictly regulated. As parents with a common goal—keeping our children safe—we have to contend with these differences in beliefs about guns and the very confusing variations in gun laws from state to state, or even, in some places, from town to town. Our biggest roadblock, however, is our own ignorance about what is regulated in the first place. Most of us do not know just how much freedom the gun industry and potential gun owners really have.[99]

MMM also attracted significant media attention. In the nine months leading up to the march, 458 news stories on MMM appeared in the country's leading fourteen newspapers. In the three weeks before and after the event, 883 stories were broadcast on television. In Washington, 1,370 national and international reporters received credentials to cover the march.[100] In the thirty months after the march, the nation's newspapers carried at least 2,300 stories describing local MMM activities or members.[101] This extensive coverage provided MMM with the opportunity to educate tens of millions of people about gun violence and the gun industry.

Finally, MMM created a new generation of experienced and passionate anti-gun violence activists. One participant explained they "were women who never had anything to do with any sort of activism. We could do anything because we had no idea we couldn't do it. You know, it's like flying, because no one ever told you about gravity."[102] These women are now leaders of local groups throughout the country.

The MMM also had significant weaknesses. Despite efforts to expand their outreach into black and Latino communities and to enlist churches, MMM was a mostly white event. Unlike the previously described organizing against the alcohol industry in black communities, MMM was not able to connect to black churches or neighborhood organizations. Nor did it succeed in connecting with the growing number of gun victims groups in low-income neighborhoods, a potentially powerful ally that could have helped to make MMM more accessible to blacks.[103]

Perhaps most tellingly, MMM made little progress in achieving its legislative goals. More than a decade later, handguns still require no registration and most handgun owners do not need a license. In fact, Congress, the Supreme Court, and state legislators have offered additional protections to the gun industry and gun owners.[104] The MMM could not sustain its success in mobilizing people to maintain pressure on elected officials, nor could it overcome the powerful and relentless opposition of the NRA and the gun industry. Soon after the march, MMM merged with the Bell Campaign, another gun-control advocacy organization, a relationship that did not work out.[105] This led MMM to join the Brady Campaign to Prevent Gun Violence, a large, national, Washington-based organization. The Million Mom Chapters is now a local arm of the Brady Campaign, describing itself as a "nationwide network of grassroots volunteers who work for sensible guns laws to protect you, your family, and your community."[106] More than 100 chapters give the Brady Campaign a grassroots base that has the potential for creating more sustainable activism.[107]

Perhaps the greatest challenge facing gun-control advocates—and other corporate reform groups—as Wallack and his colleagues observe, is how to "capture the importance and excitement of the policy 'marathon' in a society that is dominated by a 'sprint' mentality."[108] To pose a more serious threat to the marketing, product design, and political practices of the gun industry, gun-control activists will need to be able to blend the mobilizing power of the MMM with the insider political savvy and clout that the NRA has been able to muster in Washington.

Twelve years after the Million Mom March, on December 14, 2012, Adam Lanza shot and killed twenty-seven people, including twenty first grade students attending the Sandy Hook Elementary School, his mother, and six others. The massacre in Newtown, Connecticut, opened yet another chapter in the sorry history of gun violence in America. Once again a mothers' organization was created, this time called Moms Demand Action; once again a March on Washington was organized; and once again a wide range of public officials from President Obama to governors and mayors across the country vowed to take action to implement policies that better protected people from gun violence.

It will take a few years to see if this new wave of activism will lead to more meaningful changes in gun policy than previous ones. While the MMM unquestionably offered those seeking to reduce gun violence new strategies, tactics, and frames, the success of future campaigns will require taking on some new challenges. First, to pass laws that actually lower gun deaths and injuries, advocates will need to contest the power of the NRA to influence Congress. As Shannon Watts, a founder of the Moms Demand Action, observed hopefully that while Congress has long been running scared of the NRA, that organization "only has

4 million members. Ask them in four weeks who they're more scared of, the NRA or a mom? It's going to be the mom."[109]

Watts may have been thinking sprint instead of marathon in her four weeks' estimate, but in the days and weeks after the Senate voted against background checks for gun buyers, Moms Demand Action saw a 30 percent increase in membership. A gun control group founded by Gabrielle Giffords, the Congresswoman shot in Arizona, raised an astonishing $11 million from 53,500 donors. Moms Demand Action has continued to hold "stroller jams" at the offices of Congressmen they hope to influence, where moms with strollers and small kids cluster in a corridor or office to make their presence felt. And Michael Bloomberg has vowed to play hardball against the NRA, promising to contribute heavily to the 2014 congressional races, supporting gun control advocates and opposing its opponents.[110]Stripping the NRA of its invincible image may help level the political playing field. In six of seven 2012 Senate races where the NRA spent more than $100,000 on the general election, the candidate supported by the NRA lost. Of twenty-six House incumbents who lost their seats in 2012, eighteen were endorsed by the NRA.[111] As one political analyst observed, "the reason for the gap between perception and reality is that, for many years, the NRA has had no real opposition. This has given the debate a strange quality: For gun-control advocates, the recent challenge has been less about persuading politicians on policy grounds and more about trying to convince them that the conventional wisdom about gun politics is wrong."[112]

Another NRA vulnerability is its sleazy financial relationship with the gun industry, a relationship in which the gun industry contributes dollars to the NRA with the understanding that it will lobby for gunmakers in settings where gun manufacturers may be less welcome or credible.[113] For example, Beretta donated $1 million to the NRA to work to overturn gun-control laws in the wake of the 2008 U.S. Supreme Court decision that found Washington D.C.'s ban on handguns unconstitutional. Many NRA members simply want to hunt or shoot targets but are also willing to restrict unlimited access to guns. Public campaigns urging these members to reject the NRA's leaders who are allied with rightwing political groups and gun makers may further diminish the gun lobby's power to veto legislation supported by a majority of Americans. More broadly, weakening the influence of the gun lobby, a task that will take years, and other similar toxic forces in Washington can open doors for other meaningful improvements in health policy and democracy.

Second, to meet the challenge of creating a marathon rather than a sprint mentality, gun violence prevention advocates will need to expand their focus from the horrific mass shootings that capture media attention to include the daily gun carnage, especially in black and Latino communities. Because sadly these events happen every day, they provide opportunities for mobilization, organizing, and education that can continue before and after the massacres. They may thus be able to provide a more stable foundation for the ongoing advocacy that will be needed to change laws.

Finally, a successful movement needs to focus more on the gun industry and its practices and products and perhaps less on the important but secondary (from the perspective of public health prevention) issues of mental health services, and violent movies and video games. Improving mental health services and reducing exposure to violent movies and games are of course worthy objectives in their own right. But the most meaningful way to reduce gun injuries and deaths is to have fewer and safer guns available to fewer people. Achieving this goal will require changing how the gun industry does business, so that should become the goal of advocacy.

HEALTH PROFESSIONALS RESIST CAPTURE BY THE PHARMACEUTICAL INDUSTRY

The pharmaceutical industry has a problem. A 2005 national public opinion poll found that 50 percent of respondents had an unfavorable view of the industry.[114] Another poll that year showed that fewer than 13 percent of American consumers believed that information provided by pharmaceutical companies is more trustworthy than similar information from other organizations. Polls also suggest that other consumers are viewed as reliable sources of information, and their influence is growing as trust in the industry falls.[115] Press coverage is also negative: in 2007, newspaper headlines on articles about the industry were almost four times more likely to be negative than positive, and articles were twice as likely to be negative.[116]

Media coverage and public debates about windfall pharmaceutical profits, inadequately tested prescription drugs, "disease mongering," aggressive advertising, pay for delay, and harmful side effects of common medications present the industry with a credibility problem that jeopardizes profits and threatens to increase regulation. To counter these threats, the pharmaceutical industry has intensified their efforts to find more credible representatives to the public. Based on their prior history and their understanding of public perceptions, their top choices for this role have been physicians and other health professionals.

To enlist providers to become proxy sales representatives, the industry carries out a variety of activities, including spending by one estimate more than $39 billion in 2004 to market to physicians and other health providers.[117] It increased spending on advertising to doctors and hired more sales representatives ("detailers") to visit and bring gifts to doctors in hopes of persuading them to prescribe their products. It sponsored "medical education" conferences, often at fancy resorts, and paid for doctors to attend. It hired prominent doctors to tout its products at professional meetings and paid others to put their names on articles ghostwritten by industry representatives for publication in medical journals. It also advertised directly to patients, encouraging them to "ask their doctor" about the advertised product—a strategy reminiscent of McDonald's ads urging children to nag their parents to buy them a Happy Meal. The industry also established databases on doctors' prescribing behavior so they could target individual physicians for additional advertising.[118] A growing research literature documented that these practices increased prescribing—and thus company profits.[119,120]

In response to these efforts to hijack the reputations and integrity of health professionals, a growing number of physician, medical student, and provider organizations began to organize to end these practices and disassociate themselves from what they regard as unethical business practices that jeopardize patient trust. No Free Lunch is one such group. It describes itself as an organization of:

> health care providers who believe that pharmaceutical promotion should not guide clinical practice. Our mission is to encourage health care providers to practice medicine on the basis of scientific evidence rather than on the basis of pharmaceutical promotion. We discourage the acceptance of *all* gifts from industry by health care providers, trainees, and students. Our goal is improved patient care.[121]

The group helped medical students organize No Free Lunch activities on their campuses and advocated institutional policies that restricted sales activities. They also encouraged doctors not to accept or dispense free drug samples (on which drug companies spent more than $10 billion in 2002), arguing their main purpose was to encourage brand loyalty, that these samples fell outside the drug safety follow-up system, and that generics and state-run prescription assistance programs provided a more sustainable way of helping low-income patients.[122]

While No Free Lunch worked primarily to educate individual physicians, other groups worked at the institutional level, seeking to persuade academic medical centers to establish guidelines that limited the influence of pharmaceutical companies on providers. Table 7.2, based on a 2004 national survey of 3,100 physicians in six specialties, shows that almost all physicians reported some potential conflicts of interest based on gifts or payments from the pharmaceutical industry.[123]

Both small and large institutions came up with strategies to reduce these types of pharmaceutical industry influence. At a small family practice in rural Oregon, the providers decided to ban all visits by drug sales representatives.[124] Their reasons were both practical—the regular visits interrupted patient

Table 7.2 **Prevalence of Various Physician and Drug Industry Relationships**

Industry Provides:	Estimated Prevalence (percent)
Meals	83
Pharmaceutical samples	78
Reimbursement for continuing medical education	26
Payment for consulting	18
Payment for serving as speaker or on a speakers' bureau	16
Reimbursement for travel, food, or lodging at professional meetings	15
Payment for serving on an advisory board	9
Free tickets to cultural or sporting events	7
Any gift or money relationship	94

Source: Campbell EG, Gruen RL, Mountford J, Miller LG, Cleary PD, Blumenthal D. A national survey of physician–industry relationships. *N Engl J Med.* 2007;356(17):1742–1750.

care—and ethical. A physician explained, "We'd all like to think that the presence of drug reps doesn't affect the way we prescribe, but they wouldn't be here if it didn't." Drug company failures to disclose side effects that they had known about added to the discomfort with detailing visits. Another doctor said, "The straw that broke the camel's back around here was Vioxx. We were heavily detailed on Vioxx…and you know the study that was designed to look at GI side effects, and found instead that it increased the risk for heart attacks." In general, patient response to the new policy was positive. One doctor recounted, "I got a handwritten thank you note [*from a patient*] that said, 'Way to take a stand.'" To make up for the perks that the pharmaceutical reps offered, the practice established monthly provider-education sessions on drugs and hosted a free meal for providers every month. After the new policy went into effect, providers believed that they had successfully disentangled themselves from a relationship they believed adversely affected patient care.[125]

The American Medical Student Association, the National Physicians Alliance, and the Prescription Project are among the national organizations that have worked to persuade academic medical centers to adopt mandatory standards for preventing conflicts of interest with pharmaceutical or medical device companies. A 2006 national survey of 125 academic medical centers' conflict of interest policies found that only 38 percent of responding institutions had developed institutional policies.[126] One reason such policies are important is that studies show that industry-sponsored research is much more likely to deem drugs effective than independently funded studies. One meta-analysis of 1,140 research studies found that industry-sponsored trials had 3.5 times greater odds of reporting pro-industry conclusions.[127] Since such sponsorship is not always disclosed, physicians may be unaware of possible biases in research studies they use to guide their practice. Requiring companies and researchers to disclose the source of funding may help providers make more informed judgements.

A 2012 survey by a medical students association scored the nation's medical schools on their conflict of interest policies. The survey found that 149 of 152 medical institutions surveyed participated in the Scorecard, a 98 percent participation rate. Of these, 18 percent received A's, 49 percent B's, 10 percent C's, 9 per cent D's and 6 percent F's, suggesting that professional and media advocacy had forced many of the country's medical schools to adopt and enforce conflict-of-interest policies.[128]

In some institutions, opponents argued that such guidelines were unnecessary because physicians do not make decisions based on "pizza and pens," as Harvard Medical School hematologist Thomas Stossel told *Lancet*. He feared that restrictions on interactions between the drug industry and physicians could obstruct biomedical advances.[129] The drug industry also thought the guidelines proposed by the Prescription Project were unnecessary. Ken Johnson, senior vice-president at the Pharmaceutical Research and Manufacturers of America, said, "A new law is not necessary when pharmaceutical marketing is already heavily regulated by the Food and Drug Administration."[130]

To challenge these ideas, the National Physicians Alliance organized a cadre called "Unbranded Doctor." Dr. Jerome Kassirer, former editor-in-chief of the *New England Journal of Medicine*, explained that, "Unbranded Doctor is unmasking the pharmaceutical industry's bogus claim that its marketing efforts are just educational ventures for physicians. By signing up physicians to renounce gifts, lecture fees, and 'education' from companies, the Alliance is championing objectivity, integrity, and professionalism."[131] The Alliance is also a member of Rx Democracy, a coalition of health organizations that seek to register voters and encourage political participation. The organization notes that "more than 2 million Americans did not vote in 2008 due to illness or disability and millions more suffer health disparities due, in part, to a lack of voice in the democratic process."[132] These activities illustrate how activists can link efforts to modify corporate practices that harm health with those that expand democracy.

Another industry practice that concerned physicians was the mining of prescription drug databases that are compiled by for-profit companies who then sell the information to drugmakers. By finding out which doctors were prescribing their drugs, companies could target doctors for advertising or offer to make payments to them to persuade others to prescribe the products. In 2010, the investigative journalism outlet *Pro Publica* began an investigation of such pharmaceutical industry payments to doctors.[133] They created a national database that showed payments totaling at least $258 million. To illustrate the abuses,

Pro Publica told the story of Pennsylvania rheumatologist Dr. James I. McMillen, whom the U.S. Food and Drug Administration ordered in 2001 to stop "false or misleading" promotions of the painkiller Celebrex, saying he minimized risks and touted it for unapproved uses. Over the next eighteen months, three other drug companies paid Dr. McMillen $224,163 to deliver talks to other physicians about their drugs. *Pro Publica* found that 250 of the doctors for whom the investigators had found records of payments from drug companies had state medical board sanctions against them, for issues ranging from inappropriately prescribing drugs, to providing poor care, to having sex with patients. Some of the doctors had even lost their licenses. One drug company, Lilly, had eighty-eight speakers who had been sanctioned, and four more who had received FDA warnings.[134]

To halt such abuses, physician groups have advocated for state laws to prevent pharmaceutical companies from mining prescription databases to identify providers for targeted advertising of their products. In 2006, for example, the Vermont Medical Society unanimously approved a resolution calling the sale and marketing use of doctors' prescribing practices without consent "an intrusion into the way physicians practice medicine."[135] By 2011, three states (Vermont, New Hampshire, and Maine) had passed laws banning the release of individual provider names in such databases, claiming that such disclosures violated patient and provider confidentiality. The pharmaceutical industry promptly sued, and in 2011, the U.S. Supreme Court declared that Vermont's law unconstitutionally restricted the free speech rights of pharmaceutical and data-mining companies.[136] The decision provides one more example of how the combination of an industry's willingness to use its deep pockets to sue public interest groups and public officials and the Supreme Court's pro-corporate bias have made it harder to use the law to protect public health.

To avoid this legal obstacle, some physician groups have supported new federal laws to protect unwarranted industry intrusion into research and practice. To promote greater transparency, the Physician Payments Sunshine Act, included as part of the 2010 Affordable Care Act, requires pharmaceutical companies to report all gifts and funds given to physicians, professional groups and teaching hospitals.[137] In an interview with *Internal Medicine News*, Allan Coukell, director of medical programs at the Pew Charitable Trust in Washington, which sponsors the Pew Prescription Project, explained that the new law is "part of the larger context of a reevaluation by the medical profession of what constitutes an appropriate relationship between prescribers and the industry that markets products."[138] He noted that the Association of American Medical Colleges, along with leaders of medical journals, high-profile academics, and professional societies, all acknowledge the need to evaluate the extent of these relationships and their potential impact on care. "I think the Sunshine Act brings some transparency to those relationships," he said, "but what will happen next is part of a larger overall shift. I do think there is something of a movement within the profession to have a little bit more of an arm's length relationship with the marketing department." The Sunshine Act went into effect in August 2013; thereafter the Department of Health and Human Services will annually post this information on a searchable online database.

These successful efforts by health care providers to reduce their ties with the pharmaceutical industry demonstrate several lessons of wider applicability. First, many professionals resent being manipulated by the industry and are willing to reject even lucrative offers to make them into sales representatives rather than independent professionals. If doctors, nurses, teachers, social workers, nutritionists, journal editors, and their professional organizations could take similar steps to avoid being used to promote any commercial product, they would both deprive the corporate consumption complex of a favored class of proxies and enhance their own credibility.

Second, successful organizing can take place at the individual, institutional, professional organization, and political levels, with action at each level reinforcing each other level. Defining these multiple levels of opportunity for education and organizing can expand the reach and intensity of campaigns to modify harmful corporate practices. It also offers more people the chance to participate.

Third, establishing clear and mandatory institutional and professional guidelines on acceptable corporate behaviors offers all parties a clear roadmap. Corporations welcome strategic ambiguity, a deliberate vagueness about the rules, because it gives them greater opportunities to recruit professionals to advance their business goals. Institutional or professional standards also give health providers who are uncomfortable with questionable industry practices in their setting a formal mechanism for complaint and reform.

Finally, professionals who organize to assert their independence from industry can become powerful spokespeople to the public, the media, and policymakers, helping to advance an agenda to reduce harmful corporate practices. Wresting such assets away from the corporate consumption complex can provide a movement for healthier alternatives with an important ally for education and communications.

GLOBALIZATION FROM THE BOTTOM UP: COMPELLING TRANSNATIONAL TOBACCO COMPANIES TO ABIDE BY THE FRAMEWORK CONVENTION

Many organizations around the world have contributed to successes in reducing the tobacco industry's global power to market premature death and preventable illness. But one, Corporate Accountability International (CAI), illustrates how a global David can take on a global Goliath—and sometimes win. CAI was created in 1977 with the name "Infant Formula Action Coalition." Its first target was the multinational food company Nestlé, then the world's largest producer and advertiser of infant formula. The coalition's activism helped persuade the World Health Organization to pass the International Code of Marketing of Breast-milk Substitutes, described briefly in Chapter 6. CAI then expanded to take on other corporate products and practices. In 1993, the organization launched their *Challenge Big Tobacco* campaign and contributed to the enactment of the Framework Convention for Tobacco Control, the world's first public health and corporate accountability treaty.

CAI also takes on tobacco companies within the United States. In the early 1990s, the organization began campaigns against Philip Morris (now Altria) and RJR Nabisco (now Reynolds American Tobacco), calling for a boycott of the food products made by Kraft, then owned by Philip Morris/Altria. The campaign exposed Big Tobacco's attempts to hide behind Kraft's family-friendly image and to disguise its political influence. The adverse publicity from the tobacco-control movement campaigns may have contributed to Altria's decisions to spin off Kraft.[139] For the past several years, Corporate Accountability International members have attended Philip Morris's annual shareholders meetings to raise health, human rights, and other issues.

The Challenge Big Tobacco campaign began with a simple goal: saving 200 million lives by 2050. Since the World Health Organization passed the Framework Convention on Tobacco Control (FCTC) in 2003, CAI has worked extensively to persuade WHO, national governments, and NGOs to compel the tobacco industry to live up to the treaty requirements, a measure that experts estimate would help CAI to meet its goals in saving lives.

On May 31, 2012, "World No Tobacco Day," Gigi Kellet, director of the CAI campaign, explained why her organization had made this campaign a priority:

> The global community is standing with...NGOs...with more resolve than ever to stand up to Big Tobacco's bullying. Civil society and governments are teaming up to launch a coordinated global campaign to challenge tobacco industry interference in order to counter Big Tobacco's billions of dollars. So on this year's World No Tobacco Day we are sending a different message than in years past. We're calling attention not only to tobacco's highly addictive and deadly effects, but also to the fact that the only thing standing in the way from tackling the greatest preventable cause of death on the planet is Big Tobacco's interference. Today's actions, focused on challenging Big Tobacco, could do

more to save lives than any other part of the treaty. We urge all countries to stand firm together.[140]

The campaign Challenge Big Tobacco offers some important lessons for those seeking to modify harmful corporate practices. It shows how CAI, a relatively small NGO and only one small player in the global anti-tobacco movement, can amplify the voices of activists around the world by creating bottom-up global networks, using international meetings and organizations to mobilize local and national action in several countries, and assisting individuals and organizations to take leadership in fights against the tobacco industry in their own countries.

At the 2011 Philip Morris annual meeting in New York City, CAI released its *Alternative Annual Report: Philip Morris International Exposed*. The report noted that each year PMI "provides its shareholders a glowing image of a company that is handsomely rewarding its shareholders by expanding into new markets, developing new products, and overcoming market and regulatory challenges." The alternative report described instead the "financial lowlights: the price paid for profits." It claimed that PMI's 2010 reported growth of 11.6 percent in profits and 4.1 percent in its cigarette shipment volume contributed to:

• One tobacco-related death every six seconds worldwide, 5.4 million people every year;
• An average loss of fifteen years of life for each smoker;
• Healthcare costs that averaged $74 for each person in the world;
• Healthcare expenses and productivity losses that cost the world economy $7.39 for every dollar of PMI revenue.[141]

To achieve these profits, CAI asserted, PMI spends nearly $5 on its so-called corporate social responsibility initiatives for every tobacco-related death—a means of distracting attention from its core business of selling a harmful and deadly product. PMI implements a range of tactics to undermine the success of public health policies that protect people from the harms of tobacco, including: litigating, particularly by leveraging international trade agreements; targeting women and children with deceptive advertising, promotion, and sponsorships; entering into strategic partnerships with governments; establishing front groups; and engaging in so-called corporate social responsibility initiatives.

At the PMI meeting, advocates from around the country, including several nurses, challenged CEO Louis Camilleri and PMI for its global abuses, and urged PMI to "Butt Out of Public Health." They later held a two-minute silent vigil in the meeting to honor those who had died from tobacco use. Later, CEO

Camilleri told a nurse who asked a question, "It's not that hard to quit" smoking, a statement for which he later apologized.[142]

CAI also seeks to apply lessons it has learned from infant formula and tobacco to other industries. At the 2011 UN High Level meeting on NCDs, CAI's Gigi Kellett noted,

> If we are to reverse the staggering rates of preventable illness and death, the WHO and UN must safeguard public health policy from conflicts of interest. A fox guarding a hen house is a fox guarding a hen house. The global community has removed the tobacco industry's seat from the tobacco control table due to its history of interference in policy. It's time we hold other industries contributing to or profiting from today's public health epidemics similarly accountable.[143]

Have the actions of CAI made a difference? Can an organization with an annual budget of about $5.5 million, sustained by contributions from individuals and foundations, compete with a corporation like PMI, with annual 2011 revenues of more than $31 billion? Some of its actions, like those at shareholder meetings, seem more symbolic than substantive. But in the opinion of global and national public health leaders, the organization has been an indispensable ally. Said Dr. Haik Nikogosian, head of WHO's Secretariat on the FCTC, "Corporate Accountability International has been an active partner not only by providing expert guidance, but also by challenging the tobacco industry directly and making sure that the Article 5.3 guidelines addressed the concerns of people around the world. I look forward to continuing our cooperation." Alexander A. Padilla, Filipino Undersecretary of Health, wrote to CAI that, "None of these changes would have been possible were it not for your grim determination to make amendments to the original [FCTC] text. You and all those responsible deserve the thanks and appreciation of future generations in ridding us of the tobacco scourge."[144] And Doras Kiptui, from the Kenyan Ministry of Health, observed, "Corporate Accountability International plays a key role in inspiring allies around the world to stand firm against the tobacco industry. With the strength of the global tobacco treaty and our allies behind us, we will ensure that public health is safeguarded from the influence of these life robbing, profit-driven corporations."[145]

Today, as we have seen, the food, alcohol, automobile, pharmaceutical, and firearms industries are following tobacco's road of assuring future profits by expanding their efforts to capture new markets in Brazil, India, Russia, China, South Africa, and other emerging nations. CAI shows that it is possible for health activists in developed nations to offer another view of globalization: one in which activism, not lethal products, is our export, and respect and mutual assistance rather than domination and manipulation is the relationship with organizations based in the Global South.

Optimism Future: The Building Blocks for Success

For organizers for a movement for a healthier more sustainable balance between public health and private profit, past and present campaigns to change risky corporate practices are like a toy chest overflowing with building blocks: strategies, tactics, successes, and failures. In the next chapter, I will consider how these blocks can provide a foundation for a movement that can stand up to the huffing and puffing of the corporate consumption complex and offer an alternative to a future of premature death and preventable illness, a deteriorating environment, and corrupted democracy.

8

Wanted

A Movement for a Healthier, More Sustainable Future

Biology, history, and the changing environment confront every stage of society with its own public health challenges. In medieval times, it was the plagues that swept through poorly nourished populations living in filthy conditions. In industrializing Europe and the United States, it was poor sanitation, inadequate water systems, and poor nutrition that caused premature death among people living in rapidly growing cities. Today the public health challenge is the domination of a system of production and consumption that has come to value profit over human well-being.

Every society is judged by its success in overcoming its unique challenges. Societies that get it right extend life, prevent premature death, and reap the benefits of improved quality of life and additional productivity. Societies that are guided by ideology rather than evidence fail to make progress and their population suffers the health consequences.

In this century, the United States faces the starkest yet most promising questions. Can what is still the wealthiest nation in the world chart a new path in which our system of production and consumption is redirected to make health, sustainability, and democracy the priorities? Can we partner with other people and nations around the world to make our enviable scientific and technical knowledge and wealth available for human improvement? Or will a few hundred global corporations continue to have first call on these assets to advance their own profits at the expense of human well-being?

These are momentous questions that a movement for healthier, more sustainable consumption must answer. Changing the business and political practices of multinational corporations—the single most correctable contributors to global premature death and preventable illnesses and injuries—will improve the lives of billions of people. Failure will mean growing epidemics of chronic disease and injuries, widening health inequalities, further deterioration in our natural environment, and continued corruption of democracy. Where is the movement that can take on this challenge? What does it need to do to be successful?

In Lewis Carroll's *Through the Looking-Glass*, the White Queen urges Alice to "imagine six impossible things before breakfast." Alice responds that "there's no use trying. One *can't* believe impossible things." "I daresay you haven't had much practice," replies the Queen. "When I was your age, I always did it for half-an-hour a day."

Building a movement that can successfully challenge the corporate consumption complex and its practice of hyperconsumption will require imagining—and then carrying out—four tasks that many would consider impossible. First, we need to evaluate past successes in changing corporate practices and extract the practical lessons that can guide the creation of a more powerful, cohesive, and successful movement. Second, we must construct and popularize an ideology of health and democracy that can successfully compete with the corporate consumption ideology and its prescription of hyperconsumption. Third, we must weaken, then dismantle, the corporate consumption complex, the powerful alliance of corporations and their supporters that dominate politics, the economy, and society to promote hyperconsumption and block efforts to institute healthier alternatives. Finally, we need to forge in practice a policy agenda that offers a vision of a healthier, more democratic future and unites the diverse strands of individuals and organizations working to change the role of corporations in our society. Following the White Queen's advice to Alice, let's practice our imagination by examining how to accomplish these four tasks that from a distance may seem impossible.

Lessons for a Movement

Creating an inclusive and effective movement that successfully reduces the harm to health that corporations impose is like cooking a meal; it requires a variety of ingredients, blended properly to create the intended effects. From the previous descriptions of past and present efforts to change corporate practices, I will extract some of the lessons for cooking up a successful movement. These lessons can guide practice for an emerging movement at three key levels: engaging people's minds and emotions, inviting new partners, and preparing leaders.

ENGAGE PEOPLE'S MINDS AND EMOTIONS

The first group of lessons offers strategies for engaging individuals via the multiple routes that move people into action: ideas, emotions, and a sense of belonging.

Make the personal political. A maxim that emerged from the Women's Movement of the 1960s and 1970s suggested that in order to fully engage participants, movements needed to make the personal political, and the political personal. Women were moved to demand changes in employment, health care, family benefits, and domestic violence policies because they understood that their daily lives and emotions were shaped by such policies. Similarly, families of dying smokers, people with diabetes, or mothers who have lost children to gun violence understand profoundly how corporate practices affect their lives. Their fights to protect the health of their families and communities are personal, emotional, and passionate, all ingredients that help to grow and sustain movements. This contrasts sharply with more traditional health education campaigns that encourage behaviors like smoking cessation, healthier eating, safe sex, and wearing seatbelts—all worthwhile activities, but not the messages that will sustain activism or by themselves significantly improve public health.

Engaging people's emotions serves another purpose: it offers an alternative to the emotional appeal of the corporate consumption complex. The realm of consumption, as Juliet Schor has noted, has "long been a 'dream world' where fantasy, play, inner desire, escape and emotion loom large. This is a significant part of what draws us to it."[1] Collective action that appeals to similar desires and emotions can fulfill deeper needs and compete more effectively with corporate marketers than those that appeal only to reason.

Suggest alternatives. It is not enough to point out the problems corporations cause. Effective campaigns for change highlight the problem and also propose alternative arrangements. Making these alternatives visible and accessible offers individuals another path into activism.

A few examples:

- The Brooklyn Food Coalition, while resisting corporate domination of the food environment, also works to create a local food economy that links regional farmers directly with consumers, schools, and communities.
- CARB requires car makers to produce vehicles that pollute less, while also assisting cities and counties to develop more robust mass transit systems.
- Beyond advocating laws and institutional policies that limit marketing and gifts to doctors, the campaigns to reduce the pharmaceutical industry's influence on medical practice also seek to expand state-supported drug assistance programs.

By proposing alternatives to hyperconsumption and disease promotion that are feasible within the current economic and political climate, these campaigns suggest a specific path to a desired outcome. They also serve as an impetus for more robust public-sector alternatives to the corporate-dominated economy. At best, the alternatives—a school/farm program, a public bicycle program, or an alcohol-free youth program—also provide new opportunities for individuals, families, and communities to participate and become more involved in activism.

Proposing alternatives to corporate-driven consumption has the additional advantage of emphasizing the links between corporate production and consumer consumption. Without major changes in our food production system, it is hard to imagine a meaningful increase in healthy food consumption as long as an industrial system for processing food for national and global markets remains the default option. By implementing even modest alternative patterns of producing food, transportation, and pharmaceuticals, a movement can gain traction that can later be built upon, picked up by other jurisdictions, and serve as a feasible example for public education.

The point is not to build boutique alternatives for a handful of individuals—an attractive but doomed effort to escape the tentacles of the corporate consumption complex. Nor can any alternative ultimately succeed absent a movement that is building the power to achieve transformative changes. Rather, the food coops, community-supported agriculture, community development corporations, and worker-owned cooperatives become models for economic and political activity not dominated by big corporations, and staging grounds for broader efforts to reclaim the common goods that have become increasingly privatized. In the coming decades, the creation of robust, democratic public-sector production of food, mass transportation, and medicines can provide a beachhead for alternatives to a corporate-dominated economy.

Target Specific Companies. First, successful movements to modify harmful corporate behavior target specific corporations and their practices. The tobacco-control movement accelerated its successes when it switched from targeting smokers to shining a spotlight on the tobacco industry itself. Corporate Accountability International focused on one company, Philip Morris International, not only because it is one of the largest global tobacco corporations, but also in order to put names and faces on those who make decisions about marketing, production, and lobbying. When tobacco executives publicly and repeatedly put profits ahead of their role in causing millions of deaths, this generates the outrage that fuels governments, citizens, and advocacy organizations to mobilize and demand reforms.

Using specific names, products, and logos to identify harmful practices also exploits one of the greatest vulnerabilities of multinational corporations: their brands. Coca-Cola, McDonald's, Marlboro, and similar brands are valuable assets that companies use as the foundation for global marketing. By changing customers' associations with these brands—from happiness, comfort, and manliness to premature death and preventable illness—health activists can threaten a company's bottom line and create an opening for change.

In 2003, an activist lawyer in California sued Kraft for marketing Oreo cookies to children under ten without disclosing what was known about the harmful effects of trans fat. In light of the media attention that the lawsuit attracted, a market research firm found that the total volume of online discussions on trans fat increased more than eightfold in the weeks that followed. Fearing this concern would jeopardize a valuable brand, Kraft announced that it would reduce or eliminate the trans fat in Oreos just one day after the media coverage about the lawsuit began. Jonathan Carson, President and CEO of BuzzMetrics, an online research firm, commented, "On-line word-of-mouth enabled a lawsuit against one company to shift into a major food-industry policy and public relations crisis."[2]

Conversely, movements that target unhealthy policies rather than specific companies or their practices see diminished results. The effort of gun-control organizations like the Million Mom March to make lax regulation the problem has made it more difficult to persuade the public that gun makers' irresponsible marketing and production practices play a major role in gun violence and deaths. The National Rifle Association's mastery of media advocacy, lobbying, and campaign contributions has made the fight seem as if it is one between groups with opposing interpretations of the Constitution's Second Amendment, rather than one between the public and gun profiteers. It is a tribute to the NRA's power that they succeeded in making the debate about varying constitutional interpretations rather than the irresponsible production and marketing practices of the gun industry.

By including the names of specific companies, executives, and products in their campaigns, organizers can frame their efforts in clear moral terms: private gains should not cause public harms. This message is easier to communicate than more generic ones about the deficiencies of the free-market system. Some argue that blaming individual companies or executives over-simplifies or unfairly vilifies these actors. In my view, however, if the causal evidence on the role of the product or practice on health is clear, naming names illuminates the actions needed for change: it focuses public attention on individual and corporate behavior, not ideology about the free market or consumer choice. Finally, holding individual companies and their managers accountable resonates with the American discourse on responsibility, which should apply to all sectors of society, not just consumers.

INVITE PARTNERS INTO THE MOVEMENT

A second set of lessons can guide efforts to broaden the movement by enlisting new organizations and individuals into campaigns to change corporate practices.

Frame Conflict to Invite Broader Participation. Successful movements frame their messages to broaden participation and connect their cause to other causes. In the 1970s and 1980s, the tobacco-control movement learned that "the right to breathe clean air" mobilized people more effectively than the tobacco industry's advocacy for individuals' "right to smoke." The campaigns against pharmaceutical companies' influence on medical practice emphasized doctors' obligation to practice medicine based on evidence, not pharmaceutical industry profit, to solicit support from medical institutions and professional organizations.

Chapter 5 outlined some of the frames that the corporate consumption complex uses to mobilize supporters and isolate opponents. Box 8.1 suggests some counter-frames that have emerged from the movements to change corporate practices. By looking for ways to link their narrower campaigns to more general messages, organizers can create a stronger alternative to corporate ideology. By connecting the specific demands of a particular campaign (e.g., "stop selling this brand of malt liquor") to the larger theme of protecting children from marketing that promotes unhealthy products, campaigns can lay the foundation for connecting their activities with similar ones elsewhere, thus magnifying the pressure for change.

Box 8.1 **Engaging Frames from the Movements to Change Health Damaging Corporate Practices**

1. In a modern, democratic society, the prerequisites for health—clean air, healthy food, safe consumer products—should be rights, not privileges.
2. Public policy should make healthy choices easy choices, not promote private gain at the expense of health.
3. A decent society protects children and other vulnerable populations from special interests that seek to profit by encouraging unhealthy behavior or lifestyles.
4. A primary goal of governments is to protect public health. Only government has the resources and mandate to fulfill this function effectively.
5. Diminishing the power of governments does not always increase individual freedom, it may simply grant more power to corporations and other special interests.
6. Protecting and expanding our democratic rights gives people more opportunities to shape the decisions that affect their lives; diminishing these rights transfers these opportunities to others, especially corporations.

Operate at Multiple Levels. Successful movements develop the capacity to operate on multiple levels, from the local to the global. The Treatment Action Campaign, described in Chapter 6, simultaneously organized free clinics for people with AIDS in South African townships, pressured their own government and multinational drug companies doing business in South Africa to change policies, and developed alliances with global NGOs. Meanwhile, with the help of U.S. activists, TAC organized demonstrations that persuaded U.S. politicians to end their support for patent rights that benefited drug company profits at the expense of drug access for people with HIV in South Africa. Similarly, the Brooklyn Food Coalition, the Million Mom March, and Corporate Accountability International's campaign "Challenge Big Tobacco" operated between local and global levels as the issues demanded and opportunities arose. The campaigns to reduce the inappropriate influence of pharmaceutical companies on doctors' medical practice also operated at multiple governmental levels, with victories at each level reinforcing and opening the doors for success at other levels. Of significance, when movements operate globally, it is more difficult for corporations to shift marketing of unhealthy products to developing and emerging nations without public reaction.

The power of corporations depends in part on their ability to operate forcefully at multiple levels, from inside the consumer's head to within global trade forums. By matching corporations' ability to operate on small and large scales, a movement can create multiple pathways into activism and challenge corporations in a variety of settings. The California Air Resources Board's dexterity in this regard allowed it to confront the auto industry in multiple settings, keeping the pressure up even when, for example, a more auto industry-friendly Congress and White House looked to delay stricter regulations of auto emissions. While corporations will use their lobbying and legal resources to attempt to preempt state or local action to strengthen public health protection against risky practices, adept public health advocates can sometimes find opportunities to take the fight to another level or branch of government.

Engage Government. In the stories in Chapter 7, governments played different roles: opponent, ally, or instigator of change. In each case, government was a critical player by virtue of mere involvement; the stature and reach of government served to influence the outcome of changing corporate practices. CARB, for example, a government agency, has been able to continue to set new standards for the auto industry in that state for several decades because it has the active support of elected officials, other state agencies, an energized environmental movement, and the residents of California. The Brooklyn Food Coalition articulated a vision of a healthier food system, then reviewed the New York City mayor's food policy proposals, deciding whether to propose revisions or support them as written.

Learning how to analyze the positions and interests of the heterogeneous individuals and agencies that populate government in the United States and in other countries is a critical skill for movement organizers. Viewing government as a monolithic entity that either promotes or opposes corporate interests is a simplistic perspective that can misdirect strategy. Rather, the goal should be to identify and nurture those sectors of government that will act to protect public health. At the same time, government officials or agencies that have been captured by corporate interests or see their role as a mediator between the 99 percent and the 1 percent, rather than a protector of the public interest and democracy, should be isolated and discredited.

But campaigns to change corporate practices also give and receive resources, information, and political support from government allies. The exchanges go beyond money—they include research that provides scientific evidence to justify policy change, public demonstrations that support or protest new policies, threats of disruption or civil disobedience, and earned media coverage of the issues. Contributions from government to campaigns include public hearings that educate policymakers and the public, research reports that document the prevalence of the problem, and enforcement actions that demonstrate the problem. By finding ways to strengthen these reciprocal relationships, those seeking to modify corporate practices can build more powerful and sustainable partnerships.

Promote Democracy. A movement for a healthier world is a movement for more democracy. As Amartya Sen argues, having personal and collective agency gives people the power to seek well-being.[3] Democratic processes also invite participation. For many people, the opportunity to participate in movements to rectify injustices serves as an antidote to the isolation and alienation modern life often imposes. A leader of the Brooklyn Food Coalition explained, "Many of our members first join to find the sense of community they long for."[4] Similarly, the Million Mom March and Moms Demand Action offered its participants an opportunity to feel like they were making a difference.

Promoting democracy can also counter corporate efforts to undermine democratic participation. In the tobacco and pharmaceutical industries, advocates have used litigation to force companies to reveal what they know about the health effects of their products. Media coverage of such revelations can help to generate outrage and demands for more effective public oversight.

According to one academic analyst, the *Citizens United* Supreme Court decision that expanded corporations' rights to contribute to electoral campaigns without limits has "galvanized citizens groups and some members of Congress to try to ameliorate the ruling's expansion of corporate financial influence on election campaigns."[5] These voices of dissent, through their legal, legislative, and media actions, have helped educate people about the ruling's consequences and brought activists from many sectors together to propose ways to counteract the corrosive influence of *Citizens United* on electoral politics.

Unquestionably, the campaigns to modify corporate behavior have changed policies, attitudes, and company practices. But even while they have saved hundreds of thousands of lives, it will always be difficult to attribute outcomes such as longer life to any specific campaign or series of campaigns. The fact that we lack the scientific ability to prove that advocacy or policy changes had a measurable impact on health should not obscure their contributions.

In addition to mobilizing masses of people to take action against dangerous corporate practices, these public health campaigns have established ongoing monitoring of the health practices of specific companies or entire corporate sectors over extended periods of time. A few of the many groups that conduct such monitoring are listed in Box 8.2. These and similar organizations provide the public and social movements with the ongoing information needed to guide advocacy and target policy change. These campaigns have likewise inspired more researchers to study health-related corporate practices and to make their findings known to the public and policymakers. Some organizations that produce and distribute the evidence that advocates can bring to the policy arena are listed in Box 8.2. Finally, the campaigns have supported and been supported by a number of national organizations that have the potential to create and sustain a more cohesive national movement. One valuable resource is the growing number of investigative journalism organizations whose independence from corporate sponsors allows them to pursue leads that mainstream media often ignore. The International Consortium of Investigative Journalists and the Center for Public Integrity's investigation of the global tobacco industry, described in Chapter 1, and the Pro Publica's exposé of pharmaceutical industry payments to doctors to prescribe their medicines, described in Chapter 2, illustrate these contributions.

In these and other ways, the campaigns to change harmful corporate practices have created some of the important building blocks that social movement scholars identify as crucial: a repertoire of tested tactics and strategies, a cadre of experienced activists, and defined grievances and carefully crafted messages to communicate those perceived injustices to the public.[6] Together, the resources shown in Box 8.2 offer the emerging movement for healthier corporate practices the expertise and organizational support needed to become a more powerful force for change.

At the same time, the campaigns have exhibited weaknesses that can limit their future growth and effectiveness. To date, no cohesive national agenda has linked the activities of activists working in different industries (e.g., pharmaceutical, food, and tobacco) or different geographic regions. No clearly defined ideology serves to counter the powerful ideas promoted by the corporate consumption complex, and too often, even people who want to reject hyperconsumption are

Box 8.2 **Selected Resources for a Movement**

Organizations That Monitor Industry Practices	Alcohol industry—Alcohol Justice, Center on Alcohol Marketing and Youth at Johns Hopkins University Automobile industry—Center for Auto Safety Firearms Industry—Brady Campaign to Prevent Gun Violence, Harvard Injury Control Research Center, Violence Policy Center Food Industry—Center for Science in the Public Interest, Rudd Center at Yale University, Food and Water Watch Infant formula industry—International Baby Food Action Network Pharmaceutical Industry—Public Citizen Health and Safety Tobacco Industry—Center for Tobacco Control Research and Education at University of California-San Francisco Marketing to Children—Campaign for a Commercial-Free Childhood Trade—Center for Policy Analysis on Trade and Health
National Organizations That Consider Several Industries	Corporate Accountability International—food, tobacco, water CorpWatch—corporate malfeasance and multinational corporate accountability Environmental Working Group—toxic contaminants in food, water and other media Public Citizen Health Research Group—automobiles, infant formula, pharmaceuticals, and others Union of Concerned Scientists—automobile, climate change, energy, food, transportation
Global Resource Organizations	Alcohol—Global Alcohol Policy Alliance, World NGO Network on Alcohol and Health Firearms—Control Arms, International Action Network on Small Arms Food—International Association of Consumer Food Organizations Tobacco—Framework Convention Alliance General—People's Health Movement, Social Forum, Third World Network

unable to find attractive and accessible alternatives. Few national leaders are visible and attractive across the diverse populations that are the constituencies for a movement to change corporate practices. Other harmful consequences of corporations on our society—such as income inequality, subverted democracy, and environmental degradation, have been underemphasized by those working on health, limiting the potential for broader alliances. These limitations constitute the to-do list for an emerging movement.

BUILD LEADERS

A final and vital lesson from past campaigns is the importance of creating leaders who have the vision, skills, and political savvy to build a long-term movement. Successful movements need strong local, national, and global leaders—individuals who can strategize, build, inspire, and fund-raise. Successful organizations develop ways to cultivate such individuals. Leadership development can occur at all levels of organizations, from the local church to the global NGO. In the United States, organizations such as Highlander Center, the Midwest Academy, and the Center for Third World Organizing have long offered training for community organizers. Some schools of public health are beginning to offer courses on investigating the health consequences of industry practices, but none yet offer organized programs to train public health leaders to take on this task. Few national organizations have specifically prepared leaders for campaigns against corporations, a gap that needs filling.

Many movements have found that victims of injustice or personal loss make the most effective (and affecting) leaders. Mothers who lost children to gun violence, individuals whose family members died of tobacco or alcohol-related causes, or people whose diabetes was exacerbated by unhealthy foods make compelling leaders for grassroots campaigns against harmful corporate practices. More broadly, including individuals who have been most harmed by such practices ensures that their voices will be heard and lends the movement a motivated foundation. As one activist in the New York City food justice movement explained, "If people of color and poor people are not leading the food movement, then once again our needs will be overlooked."[7]

Create a New Ideology for Health and Democracy

For many people around the world, hyperconsumption is the norm, the very definition of modern society. Alternatives are seen as primitive, abstemious, undesirable, or at best utopian and unattainable. In this view, since few would choose to give up this lifestyle voluntarily, the only possible route to a different future is the dreaded "Nanny State," in which government hectors its citizens and deprives them of life's pleasures. It is a tribute to the corporate consumption complex that these beliefs are so common. To persuade people that a lifestyle that brings many of its adherents premature death, painful illness, and preventable injuries is highly desirable is a remarkable achievement. Any movement that wants to mount a successful challenge to hyperconsumption must offer attractive alternative patterns of consumption.

Creating alternatives to hyperconsumption requires two simultaneous processes: reducing the demand for unhealthy products, the ideological task discussed here, and dismantling the corporate consumption complex, the strategy to reduce the supply of unhealthy products discussed in the next section. Movement organizers often debate which should be primary, but in my view, the most effective approach is to pursue reducing both the demand for and supply of unhealthy products and practices concurrently, with successes on one front reinforcing advances in the other.

From a health perspective, alternatives to hyperconsumption need to meet two criteria. First, they should promote population and individual health. Second, they should be sustainable—practically, environmentally, and economically. Followers need to be able to stick with a lifestyle, not try it out, then abandon it like a fad diet. This requires thinking about how the proposed changes will fit within the lives of real people in different parts of the world.

Environmental sustainability is often defined as the use of resources that allows future generations to enjoy the same benefits as the previous generations. Patterns of consumption that deplete natural resources, damage the environment, or create health burdens for future generations are not sustainable. For this discussion, I define healthy and sustainable consumption as patterns of living in which people produce and consume in ways that sustain health, protect the well-being of future generations, and maintain the Earth's capacity to support life.

What would healthy, sustainable consumption look like, and how would it differ from hyperconsumption? A few statistics help show the way:

- An Australian researcher estimated that if present trends on smoking in Australia continue, all female smoking will end by 2029, and male smoking will be virtually eliminated the next year. Australia has the world's strongest tobacco-control policies and the lowest rates of smoking.[8] By restricting the places where people can smoke and ending the tobacco industry's right to market tobacco (but *not* prohibiting its use), other cities, states and nations may be able to bring adult smoking rates down to negligible levels, usually defined as less than 5 percent of the adult population.[9]

- The New Mexico county with the highest alcohol-related chronic disease death rate has a rate almost 40 times higher than the county with the lowest level. Four counties in New Mexico have death rates lower than the U.S. average, but twelve have rates more than twice the US average.[10] These data show wide variations in alcohol-consumption-related death rates in a single state, suggesting that modifying policies, enforcement and other environmental factors could help states and counties with higher rates reduce deaths. Bringing New Mexico's alcohol-related chronic diseases death rate down to the U.S. rate could prevent 2,500 premature deaths in a decade.
- In Sweden, improved design of cars and highways has dramatically reduced motor vehicle accidents. In 2004, 50 Swedes per 1 million died in motor vehicle accidents, compared to about 240 per 1 million in the Russian Federation.[11] Sweden's success in regulating car safety, designing safer roadways, and changing driver behavior show that other nations could take similar actions that would prevent millions of deaths and injuries.
- The average American's daily consumption of added sugars increased by 149 percent between 1977 and 2006,[12] a result of changes in the products manufactured and marketed by the food industry. Higher consumption of added sugars is associated with several important risk factors for cardiovascular and metabolic diseases. Returning to the 1977 level—hardly a time of sugar deprivation—could help millions of people from becoming overweight and prevent tens of thousands from developing diet-related diseases.

For markers of hyperconsumption such as excess consumption of sugar, fats, salt, tobacco (in the developing world) or alcohol (among women), a return to the societal levels of just a few decades ago would bring substantial health benefits. This fact contradicts the belief that healthy consumption requires prohibiting unhealthy products or a return to a Stone Age hunting and gathering lifestyle.

Sustainable consumption also entails reducing our demand for natural resources, particularly non-renewable resources. According to one research group, if all 7 billion people on Earth lived like the average American, we would require five planets to support human life.[13] Many strategies exist to reduce the demand for resources: limiting the increasing consumption of meat; developing more sustainable, local and less resource-intensive agricultural practices; encouraging energy conservation; and promoting mass transit, walking, and bicycling rather than individual car transport. Each would significantly reduce resource depletion, and shrink humanity's carbon footprint. And each is already in practice somewhere, providing testing grounds for what works and evidence on how to scale up successful models.

Each of these changes would also contribute to reducing chronic disease and injury. Eating less meat and less processed food (each generators of many food miles, the distance food travels between farm and mouth) while increasing intake of fruits and vegetables reduces obesity, heart disease, cancer, and diabetes. While passive transportation burns non-renewable energy and fuels obesity, mass transit has been shown to contribute to improved health. A study in North Carolina found that, after two years, riders on a new commuter light-rail transit system had an 18 percent reduction in body mass index compared to those who kept driving to work.[14] Showing how changes in consumption can improve health and protect the environment can win support for healthier policies. As one international research team observed, "climate preservation and the improvement of health for people everywhere are inextricably linked. Coherent and sensitively designed cross-sectoral policies and programs in agriculture, energy use, and urban planning may produce major potential co-benefits for people and planet."[15]

Who can lead the world to the values and lifestyle that support healthy sustainable consumption? Many constituencies have the qualifications to serve as guides. In the United States and other Western nations, candidates for its promotion include ethical consumers, alternative lifestyle sub-populations, corporate social responsibility groups, and perhaps a few responsible corporations. Finally, in the large, emerging nations of Africa, Asia, and Latin America, governments and non-governmental organization are exploring new ways to think about consumption and sustainable development.

ETHICAL CONSUMERS

"Ethical consumers," a term coined in the United Kingdom in the late 1980s, are people who make purchasing decisions based on their assessment of the values and practices of producers, not simply the prices or qualities of the products. In 2005, Datamonitor, a market research firm, found that "67 percent of consumers in the US and Europe claim to have boycotted a food, drinks, or personal care company's goods on ethical grounds."[16] In the United States, making decisions about what to buy or boycott is as old as the first Boston Tea Party, in which patriotic consumers organized and participated in boycotts of British goods and encouraged coordinated consumer action. While many more people tell pollsters that they make ethical purchasing decisions than sales data suggest, with almost 70 percent of GDP driven by what the U.S. government calls "personal consumption expenditures," even modest changes in purchasing could influence corporate decisions—and health.[17]

The Council on Economic Priorities, an ethical consumption advocacy group, explains the rationale:

> Your choice of what car, washing machine, computer, or even breakfast cereal to buy may make more difference than you think, especially if

you let companies know that social and environmental records affect your choices. Companies wield tremendous power, but individuals can influence corporate practices and can actually help change the world. It's the simple, positive activism of casting your economic vote conscientiously.[18]

Critics of ethical consumption claim it is a "panacea for middle-class guilt ... an individualistic form of politics, a means through which neoliberal governments encourage consumers to become 'responsibilised' amidst the atrophying of wider social safety nets."[19] Its value, perhaps, is not as a stand-alone individual strategy but as one component of a panoply of responses to hyperconsumption. In addition, conscious consumption can serve as an antidote to "upscaling"—the notion that to stay in place consumers constantly need to buy more and bigger.[20] Contesting the psychology of upscaling can help undermine hyperconsumption.

A recent U.S. variant of ethical consumption is "conscious consuming," also known as "downshifting" or "voluntary simplicity." "Simplifiers" look to spend less time working and buying and more with friends and family. They seek more authentic connections to people and possessions and to contrast their lifestyle from the mainstream. At the farther end of the simplifying continuum, some choose to live off the power grid, seeking to demonstrate their independence from the corporate economy. Few have an explicitly political agenda.[21] Simplifiers and other sub-populations experimenting with alternative consumption practices usually constitute only a fraction of the population. But their experiences can serve as a laboratory for testing new ideas, a springboard for more generalizable efforts, and a demonstration that even in corporate-dominated economies, alternatives are available.

Can individual efforts to adopt healthier patterns of consumption be linked to larger political efforts? The GROW campaign of Oxfam, a British charity, illustrates one approach. GROW seeks to change the food buying and preparation habits of women in developed nations to drive changes in the global food system. By strengthening the emotional connection women feel to the producers of their food, they hope to recruit support for policy change. "Corporations and governments are not the only power in the system," Oxfam argues. "Those of us that buy, cook and eat the food are more powerful than we might think. If together we can say we want this rather than that, we become a force that affects the system.... They can either adapt to meet our demands, or someone else will fill their place."[22] The creation of "transitional towns" in Europe and North America is another example. In this campaign, grassroots citizens groups pressure local governments to take action to slow climate change and enable patterns of consumption that reduce reliance on the corporate economy.[23]

CORPORATE SOCIAL RESPONSIBILITY

Corporate social responsibility (CSR) groups believe that corporations can be persuaded to adopt more responsible practices through a combination of market, political, and moral pressure. They argue that all corporations should pay attention to the "triple bottom line"—their economic, social, and environmental impact. CSR strategies include ethical investing, shareholder activism, boycotts, and multifaceted corporate campaigns. The concept of CSR has been used widely to reform corporate labor and environmental practices and to remedy human rights violations; it has been used less often to modify practices that harm the health of consumers.

Between 1995 and 2010, professionally managed assets that were invested by organizations such as Calvert Investments, Trillium Asset Management, and others that followed socially responsible guidelines increased by 380 percent to $3.07 trillion—a bigger increase than the overall 260 percent increase in all professionally managed assets.[24] Social responsibility funds have helped investors avoid tobacco and alcohol stocks and supported environmentally responsible energy and automobile companies, but have been less active in distinguishing between healthy and less healthy food companies.

A more recent CSR variant is impact investing, in which investors seek both financial and social returns. Whereas earlier CSR efforts focused on withdrawing investor dollars from socially destructive investments, impact investing seeks to redirect these dollars to more constructive uses. *New York Times* business writer Paul Sullivan describes impact investing as "a private equity fund for social change."[25] A J.P. Morgan analyst predicts that by 2020, there could be between $400 billion and $1 trillion invested this way, generating cumulative profits over ten years of between $183 billion and $667 billion.[26] The Spring Creek Foundation, an Ohio-based philanthropy group, has proposed a model for using impact investing to create healthier, more sustainable food systems, offering small growers and retailers an alternative to reliance on agribusiness and mainstream financial institutions and investors an opportunity to make money while doing good.[27] Similarly, a group of public health researchers at University of California-Berkeley have suggested the creation of Health Impact Bonds, through which government and entrepreneurs can partner to invest in creating healthier environments, with part of the savings in health care costs returned to investors.[28]

For both traditional CSR funds and impact investing, institutional asset owners (pension funds, endowments, insurers) are potential partners for increasing the volume and impact of responsible investment. A 2012 report concluded that, with total assets of more than $20 trillion, these anchor investors "play a fundamental role in the domestic U.S. and world capital markets.

For advocates of impact investing, engagement of institutional asset owners is one key to growing markets that create measurable social and environmental benefits."[29]

One such arrangement is the Carbon Disclosure Project (CDP), a consortium of more than 300 institutional investors with more than $57 trillion in assets in 2008. Participants include Barclays Group, California Public Employees' Retirement System, Goldman Sachs, Merrill Lynch, Morgan Stanley, and UBS, among others. Since 2002, the CDP has asked the world's 500 largest companies every year to disclose their greenhouse gas (GHG) emissions, risks, opportunities, and management strategies, illustrating the potential for institutional investors to influence disclosure and environmental practices of major companies.[30]

At the policy level, tax and regulatory policies can encourage institutions to invest in measures such as healthier food production or transportation alternatives. At the institutional level, workers and unions can demand that their pension, endowment, or insurance funds invest in companies that encourage healthier and sustainable consumption and disinvest from those that fail to do so. In 2000, the board of the California Public Employees' Retirement System ordered the fund to divest from all tobacco companies, overriding the recommendation of staff who warned that getting rid of tobacco stocks would lower the return on investment. In 2008, some members concerned about the value of their pensions tried but failed to reverse this decision.[31] In 2013, a few weeks after the Connecticut school shootings, the California State Teachers Retirement System voted to withdraw its $500 million investment in Cerberus Capital Management, the owner of Freedom Group, the maker of the Bushmaster assault rifle used to kill twenty-seven people in Newtown.[32] In the future, debates about institutional investment decisions can provide health advocates in universities and hospitals with a platform to discuss healthier, more sustainable patterns of consumption.

Corporate campaigns were first developed by unions as a supplement to traditional worker organizing. Using organizing techniques developed by Saul Alinsky, corporate campaigns mobilized people to pressure companies into changing practices, including labor or environmental practices.[33] Their tactics seek to make it more difficult for corporate managers to resist change than to make concessions. Corporate Accountability International's campaigns— against Nestlé for marketing infant formula, against Philip Morris for undermining national tobacco-control programs and policies, and against McDonald's for marketing unhealthy fast food to children—are examples of corporate campaigns with a health focus. Their role is to educate the public about the adverse health consequences of risky products and to shame companies into reducing their promotion of unhealthy consumption. One listing of 173 corporate campaigns that were carried out between 1960 and 2012 identified only eight that had consumer health as a primary focus.[34] Expanding such efforts may help "de-market" unhealthy consumption and create space for healthier alternatives.

Despite their potential to influence the investment of trillions of dollars, several factors limit the potential of these various streams of CSR to contribute to alternative patterns of consumption. First, many companies continue to use CSR more as a public relations tool than as a serious effort to change the social impact of their operations. PepsiCo and Coca-Cola, for example, cite their philanthropic contributions to physical activity programs as an example of their responsibility for reducing obesity. Independent observers regard these donations as an effort to distract media attention from the role their products play in super-sizing the world's children.[35] Second, many of the industries and companies that contribute to chronic diseases and injuries have irresponsible practices at the core of their business model—marketing tobacco to young adults, for example, or making cheap, poorly made handguns widely available. CSR is unlikely to convert tigers into giraffes.

Finally, companies that make social responsibility commitments often abandon them when economic conditions change. In 2007, market changes led Ford to drop the partnership it had with the Sierra Club to promote the Mercury Mariner Hybrid, a more eco-friendly SUV, and to revert to heavy promotion of its more profitable (but polluting) Explorer.[36] As I described previously, when PepsiCo shareholders complained that its increased marketing of "good-for-you" snacks was resulting in lost market share for sugary beverages, Pepsi promptly upped its advertising budget for soda, and other fun-for-you (but-make-you-sicker-quicker) products.

With these limitations, is there a place for CSR as a vehicle for changing consumer minds and corporate practices related to hyperconsumption? I am skeptical that by itself CSR can have much influence on business practices, absent deeper transformations of government–market relationships. But as a platform for public education, CSR challenges the cornerstone belief of free-market fundamentalism that profit always comes first. If more people and policymakers accept the notion that corporations have *any* social responsibility beyond maximizing return for investors, then the debate becomes not if but how: Who draws the line between private gain and public benefit, and where? As investors, institutional pension funds and CSR advocacy groups struggle to make corporations more accountable, the public health consequences of corporate practices bring an added outcome that can widen public discussion on the appropriate role for corporations in our society. In this view, CSR can become a vehicle to recruit the tens of thousands of people who want to make more ethical decisions on their investments into a movement for healthier, more sustainable consumption.

SUSTAINABLE CORPORATIONS?

Can corporations themselves, even without the external pressure of CSR activists, play a role in creating healthier, more sustainable patterns of consumption? The simple answer is "Yes, but." The yes acknowledges that many companies have found ways to make money by selling healthier, "greener" products. Companies like Organic Valley, a farmer-owned cooperative of 1,687 family farms, or Electric Vehicles International, a manufacturer of electric trucks and cars for government and businesses, can make it easier for consumers to find and afford the products or transportation that protect health and the planet. Public policies and consumer purchases that support these types of businesses can strengthen alternatives to hyperconsumption.

The reservations about a corporate role in sustainable consumption spring from some fundamental rules of capitalism. Making a profit usually depends on selling more, whereas protecting health and the environment generally requires consuming less. Additionally, successful small companies are often bought up by bigger companies, ones whose commitment to health or environmental values may be more limited. A *New York Times* investigation found that as the market for organic food multiplied over the last decade, giant agri-food corporations such as Coca-Cola, Cargill, ConAgra, General Mills, Kraft, and M&M Mars have "gobbled up" most of the nation's organic food industry.[37] These big companies now play a major role in setting standards for organic food and, as the *Times* reported, routinely make decisions that favor their interests over those of small producers and the health of eaters.

In summary, if corporations are to play a significantly expanded role in producing healthier products, the rules of the game will need to change. As long as maximizing profits is the bottom line, opportunities for promoting health will be limited. Changing the incentives to reward producing health and the penalties to deter harming well-being requires political decisions, not business ones.

BRICS FOR SUSTAINABLE CONSUMPTION

Emerging nations like Brazil, Russia, India, China, and South Africa (known as BRICS) can also make contributions to offering alternatives to hyperconsumption. In China, Peggy Liu, the leader of the Joint U.S.-China Collaboration on Clean Energy (JUCCE), an NGO that seeks to accelerate the greening of China, told delegates at the 2012 Rio+20 United Nations Conference on Sustainable Development about her organization's vision of the "China Dream"—an alternative to the high-consumption American Dream of the later twentieth century. Noting that China's population will add the equivalent of another one-and-a-half U.S. populations in the next 13 years, Liu argues that now is the time for China to forge a new sustainable consumerism that offers both a path to prosperity and an end to global resource devastation.[38] She urges the creation of a sustainable lifestyle that "excites people" and taps into consumers' desires and aspirations.

Clearly, China recognizes the importance of domestic consumption—now the main driver of economic growth, having surpassed government investment in 2012.[39] The economic slowdown in China makes the nature of its domestic consumption even more important. And the Chinese government understands the choices it faces: Xie Zhenha, the Minister for Climate Policy, has observed that "if we allow China's per capita carbon emissions to rise to U.S. levels, it will be a disaster for the world."[40] Preventing such a disaster in a nation that is now the largest automobile market in the world, and in which automobiles symbolize success, presents the government with some tough decisions. JUCCCE's China Dream, which includes a variety of corporate and NGO partners, seeks to use government policy, Chinese cultural values, social media, and corporate initiatives to create a widespread desire for a sustainable life.

Whether the China Dream campaign can overcome inevitable corporate and government opposition remains to be seen. As Liu notes, "The window of opportunity for a new lifestyles to take hold won't last forever. If we wait too long, the emerging middle class will have already developed their tastes and habits. It will be too late to steer the masses to greener pastures."[41] She concedes that "few sustainable consumerism campaigns have succeeded to date," but notes that "the elements that can enable societal change are now aligning.... People are more open than ever to lifestyle change. The current economic squeeze leaves consumers eager for alternatives to conspicuous consumption." How China resolves competing demands for cleaner air, healthier lives and more democracy with those for more Western-style consumption, more opportunities for investment, and more government control will have a critical influence on the future of global hyperconsumption.

Brazil can also play a role in changing global patterns of consumption. Brazilian public health researchers Carlos Montiero and Geoffrey Cannon have observed that country has substantial remaining natural resources; capable governments at the federal, state, and national levels; a commitment to a strong public sector; and extensive experience using public policy to ensure that its food and pharmaceutical sectors serve the public interest and promote health. "In Brazil," Montiero and Cannon note, "protection of public health still remains a prime duty of government that has not eroded as it has in other countries."[42] Moreover, Brazilian social and labor movements have continued to push their government to resist corporate-managed globalization. As an illustration, Brazilian law entitles all schoolchildren to one daily meal at school. At least 70 percent of the food supplied to schools must be fresh or minimally processed, and a minimum of 30 percent must be sourced from local family farmers. These policies serve both to promote child health and to restrict the role multinational food companies and the highly processed foods they manufacture can play in an important sector of the food economy.

India, another emerging nation, is debating whether to make free medicine available to its citizens in all public hospitals. The plan would provide hundreds of essential drugs free to patients in government-run hospitals and clinics at a cost of nearly $5 billion over five years.[43] Since the government would buy only inexpensive generic versions of drugs, the plan would jeopardize the profits Western drug makers hope to realize from brand-name drugs in emerging markets like India. By putting massive purchasing power in the hands of government, the plan would diminish the power of drug multinationals to set the rules for the market while also reducing marketing and use of inappropriate, dangerous, or ineffective drugs.

BRICS nations will face huge resistance to sustainable consumption policies from the corporate consumption complex—and their own wealthy élites. Since most of the world's largest corporations depend on these nations for twenty-first-century profitability, reduced demand threatens their future. But since at least some leaders and some citizens groups in each of these countries understand the dire national consequences of hyperconsumption, their collective power is one of the most promising resources for a healthier approach to economic development and consumption.

This review of potential players in promoting healthy sustainable consumption suggests that no lone constituency, organization, or nation can create viable alternatives to hyperconsumption at a scale that would make a health difference. The various strands I have described here operate independently, sometimes in conflict, and lack an infrastructure of power that can match the corporate consumption complex. Today, consumption takes place in many settings and forms—home, school, community, shopping mall, Internet. So far, no scholar or movement has developed an integrated theory of consumption across settings that can unite the efforts to create a coherent alternative. In the long run, however, many more of the world's people and nations will benefit from healthier more sustainable patterns of consumption than those who profit from the current consumption regime.

A comprehensive political and economic agenda to advance healthy, sustainable consumption forces us to address other fundamental problems facing the United States and other wealthy nations. Most significantly, to create the millions of new jobs that are the foundation for real economic growth requires rethinking where these jobs will come from.

Here, a vision of an economy based on healthy sustainable consumption can suggest new directions. A food economy more rooted in local production, processing, and distribution of food has the potential to create new jobs that produce healthier food, impose less of a burden on the environment, and support bottom-up economic development. A transportation system that encourages mass transit and active transportation has the potential to produce new manufacturing, construction, and service jobs. A healthcare system that uses drugs judiciously and helps those at risk of chronic illnesses to better prevent or manage the disease can create new entry-level jobs while reducing the cost of healthcare and pharmaceuticals. Already the environmental movement has stimulated the creation of "green jobs" that promote growth and environmental protection by retrofitting old buildings to become more energy-efficient, building new, more environment-friendly housing, and cleaning up brownfields, polluted industrial sites that if properly decontaminated can be reclaimed for commerce, housing, or recreation.[44]

In the nineteenth and early twentieth centuries, social movements created a politics of production that informed worker activism and led to new protections against corporate abuse. Today, as Juliet Schor has observed, a new critical politics of consumption is urgently needed to address the "profound failures of the current consumption regime."[45] Weaving the alternative strands of the critiques of hyperconsumption into a cohesive fabric that can support a new activism of consumption will require imagining two more of the White Queen's impossible tasks.

Dismantle the Corporate Consumption Complex

As long as corporations occupy our minds, our media, our shopping malls, and our political processes, they will have an advantage in shaping patterns of consumption and discouraging healthier, more sustainable alternatives. Thus, evicting corporations from their privileged positions is an essential task.

Let's consider strategies for serving "eviction notices" in three separate arenas where the corporate consumption complex now exercises its power: Our consciousness, our communities and our political processes. The goal of these strategies is to reduce the power of corporations to shape the environments, behaviors, and lifestyles that influence health.

EVICTING CORPORATIONS FROM OUR MINDS

In the last three decades, the number of advertisements the average American city dweller is exposed to daily has increased from 2,000 to 5,000. "We never know where the consumer is going to be at any point in time," Linda Kaplan Thaler, chief executive at the Kaplan Thaler Group, a New York ad agency, told the *New York Times*, "so we have to find a way to be everywhere. Ubiquity is the new exclusivity."[46] From infancy through death, corporations bombard us with messages via television, radio, billboard, print, Internet, and texting. Is it surprising that the jingles, logos, products, values, and lifestyles that corporations promote have become embedded in our consciousness?

Deprogramming our minds is both an individual and a collective task. At the individual and family levels, protecting children from corporate penetration can bring current and future payoffs. Most child development experts agree that children are not equipped to make informed decisions about what to buy and consume. Based on a review of the relevant literature, Jennifer Pomeranz at Yale's Rudd Center for Food Policy and Obesity summarizes the emerging consensus that "the accumulation of evidence reveals a true deficit in young children's ability to comprehend the intent of marketing techniques, which makes them vulnerable to both unintentional deception and deliberate overreaching by advertisers."[47] Older children may have the cognitive capacity to judge messages but lack the experience or knowledge to evaluate the plausibility of advertisers' claims. According to some public health lawyers, advertising to customers unequipped to judge its veracity is "inherently misleading," making such messages ineligible for First Amendment protection.[48]

Another reason to protect children is that they have become, as Juliet Schor observes in *Born to Buy*, "conduits from the consumer marketplace into the household, the link between advertisers and the family purse."[49] Schor notes that "young people are repositories of consumer knowledge and awareness. They are the first adaptors and avid users of many of the new technologies. They are the household members with the most passionate consumer desires, and are most closely tethered to products, brands and the latest trends."[50] Severing these links removes the marketer–in-chief from inside the household and delays identification with corporate values until young people are better equipped to evaluate commercial message both cognitively and emotionally.

By protecting children from advertising as much and for as long as possible, removing commercial influences from schools, and minimizing the time their children spend in high-intensity marketing zones, (e.g., shopping malls, fast food outlets, children's television programs, and corporate-sponsored Internet sites), parents can delay the corporate intrusion into their children's minds. These delays can postpone initiation into the lifetime unhealthy consumption habits for which corporate marketers recruit.

But in the long run, parents need community and government support to protect their children and adolescents against the nannies who truly threaten our children: corporations like McDonald's, Pepsi, Coke, Budweiser, and Philip Morris that expose children to messages that encourage life-shortening habits.[51,52] One such protection is publicly supported counter-advertising campaigns. Counter-advertising offers viewers images and messages that contradict or undermine corporate ads. One study found that viewing an anti-smoking ad before seeing movie characters smoke "temporarily tainted the image of smoking" among fourteen to fifteen year old teenagers. "Subjects who saw the anti-smoking advertisement spontaneously generated negative thoughts about the movie characters."[53] In 1967, under the Fairness Doctrine, the Federal Communication Commission ruled that television stations had to air anti-smoking advertisements at no cost to the organizations providing such messages. The new mandate led to widespread exposure to anti-smoking education and sharp declines in smoking rates.[54] Part of the reason the tobacco industry accepted the 1971 ban on television advertising of cigarettes is they feared continued exposure to anti-tobacco ads would reduce their business and profits. In 1987, the Fairness Doctrine, which required holders of television and radio broadcast licenses to present controversial issues of public importance, honestly and equitably was formally rescinded, another victim of Reagan era deregulation.

The Truth Campaign, a health education initiative launched by the Legacy Foundation, the nonprofit creation of the tobacco Master Settlement Agreement, brought young people the message that the tobacco industry sought to profit by addicting them to a deadly substance. Rather than preaching to teens to follow their parents' guidance on tobacco, the truth message, directed especially at the rebellious teens most likely to smoke, was, "Don't let tobacco executives fool you so they can get rich off you." Evaluations studies showed that the Truth Campaign's anti-corporate message was more successful than traditional anti-smoking programs in preventing young people from taking up smoking and getting them to quit. One systematic evaluation study found that by 2004, the truth campaign had prevented about 450,000 U.S. adolescents from trying smoking.[55] The tobacco industry sued to get the messages off the air but failed in court. Similar campaigns led by health departments or voluntary health organizations could help to counteract promotion of unhealthy food, problem alcohol use, ineffective or risky medications, and polluting cars, immunizing people against advertisers' inducements. With the advent of lower-cost social media campaigns, the high cost of Legacy's mainstream media Truth Campaign, the main deterrent to replication, has been significantly reduced.

Counter-advertising that supports healthier, more sustainable consumption will never be able to reach as many viewers, listeners, or clicks per impression as do corporate advertisers. More subversively, however, these campaigns can help audiences critically analyze advertising messages and substitute images that challenge hyperconsumption rather than glorify it. Their most valuable role may be in triggering face-to-face and online discussions that over time diminish the corporate consumption complex's control over our minds.

EVICTING CORPORATIONS FROM OUR INSTITUTIONS AND COMMUNITIES

At the community level, the corporate consumption complex dominates retail space, the digital environment, and increasingly, public spaces such as schools and hospitals, thus converting more public space into selling space. To counter this corporate intrusion into public space, jurisdictions have taken action. In 2008, Los Angeles approved a one-year moratorium on new fast food outlets in the city's poorest neighborhoods, a limit later extended indefinitely. Observers believe that the moratorium encouraged the development of food co-ops, community gardens, and healthier, non-chain food outlets. "I don't think those ideas and initiatives would have taken hold if we were continuing to allow of the development and establishment of fast food outlets," said one organizer.[56] In Philadelphia, the city banned alcohol advertisements on city-owned or controlled property.[57] In Boston, the state transit agency ended alcohol advertising on the city's mass transit system.[58] Many hospitals have decided to remove McDonald's outlets from their facilities, worrying that their presence sent a bad message to parents and the many patients with diet-related diseases.[59] By campaigning to create more commercial-free zones in our communities, schools, and hospitals, health advocates can both protect people from health-damaging influences and stimulate public discussion of appropriate restrictions on using public space to promote private gain.

Today, corporations and their marketing allies are also the main source of health education for most Americans. Through their social media sites; their advertisements on television and Channel One, the school-based television network; their support for professional organizations like the Academy of Nutrition and Dietetics, the professional association of nutritionists and dietitians; and their sponsorship of sporting events and entertainment, corporations like Pepsi, McDonald's, Altria, and Anheuser-Busch InBev spend more time influencing our children and young adults than any health teacher or counselor. By restoring this task to the parents, teachers, doctors and others whose mandate is to protect the well-being of our youth and removing it from corporations whose main goal is to extract cash from their customers' pockets, our society can provide young people with the knowledge and skills they need to make more informed decisions about health.

EVICTING CORPORATIONS FROM OUR POLITICAL SYSTEM

The most important and difficult step in dismantling the corporate consumption complex is reining in its power to shape our politics. As long as tens of thousands of corporate lobbyists and billions of dollars in corporate campaign contributions distort our democracy, it will not be possible to advance an alternative to hyperconsumption and the health burdens it imposes. There is no dearth of good ideas by which to restore more democratic processes to our political system. In recent years, democracy activists have organized to:

- Reverse the *Citizens United* Supreme Court decision by legislation or constitutional amendment in order to limit special interest contributions to legislative or electoral campaigns;[60]
- Strengthen or create new public campaign financing as exists in some states and cities (e.g., Arizona, Maine, Connecticut, and New York City). In some places this is achieved by mandating or subsidizing media outlets to provide equal-time access to major political candidates. Joanna Diamond of the American Civil Liberties Union explained that "Public financing would make public officials more accountable to voters in general and less beholden to the often-narrow economic interests of a few big contributors. It would also allow public officials to do their jobs instead of raising money."[61]
- Put wedges in the revolving doors between industry and government to reduce conflicts of interest and the exchange of inside information between government and industry officials. Between 1998 and 2006, 43 percent of members who retired from Congress later took jobs as federal lobbyists. According to Public Citizen, a watchdog organization, those individuals made an average annual salary of around $2 million. The Center for Responsive Politics issued its own report that found a total of 370 former members now work in some capacity of the "influence-peddling" business.[62] In 2011, Republican congressman Bill Posey introduced legislation to extend the post-employment restrictions on lobbying by members of Congress and officers and employees of the legislative branch.[63] A website that accepts bets on the likelihood of proposed legislation succeeding gave the bill a 3 percent chance of passing.
- Create new vehicles for democratic participation such as participatory budgeting, in which ordinary people decide how to allocate part of public budgets and town meetings, at which citizens discuss and vote on local and national policy ideas (e.g., whether or not to pass a constitutional amendment to reverse the *Citizens United* decision). These and other democratic processes create opportunities for citizens to gather and discuss in public what they want from government and markets.

The problem is not imagining alternatives, but putting them into practice at a scale that can make a difference.

A few examples of communities and jurisdictions claiming new rights to say no to the corporate consumption complex illustrate how the power of the complex can be curtailed. The federal Emergency Planning and Community Right-to-Know Act of 1986 encouraged and supported emergency planning efforts at the state and local levels and provided the public and local governments with information concerning potential chemical hazards in their communities.[64] Communities could use this knowledge to identify hazardous exposures from local chemical plants and force environmental agencies to better regulate. While never fully implemented, the principle that citizens have a right to know—and the parallel duty of corporations to disclose what they know about the health effects of their products and practices—could become powerful tools for promoting democracy and health.

Recent battles to require food companies to disclose whether or not their products included genetically modified organisms (GMOs) show the potential of mobilizing people to demand to know more about what they buy. Monsanto's vociferous opposition to GMO labeling further shows how much corporations do not want be forced to disclose facts that might reduce sales.[65]

Even more forceful is the right to act and to refuse. In Philadelphia, a coalition of community groups demanded in the early 1990s that Reynolds Tobacco Company abandon its plans to test-market Uptown Cigarettes, a brand created to appeal to black consumers in their community. As Charyn Sutton, a spokesperson for the campaign, explained,

> The Uptown struggle was one of "taking back" the issue of choice and redefining it in a larger community context, rather than an individual context. Excessive tobacco advertising in African American communities push[es] tobacco products in a way that takes away choice.... The Coalition believed that African Americans were exercising their right of free choice—by rejecting Uptown.[66]

In this case, Reynolds decided to abandon this product rather than risk national protests to withdraw the new brand and the loss of its valuable African American market.

Restoring the democratic rights that corporations have usurped is a long-term project that will require participation from many sectors of society, motivated by differing concerns. By understanding its centrality to changing the corporate practices that now damage health and by adding their voices and issues to the battle, health professionals and activists can accelerate progress.

Another important reason for the continued dominance of the corporate consumption complex is the parallel weakening of government and the public sector. Effective challenges to corporate power require restoring a better balance between government and markets. Several broad policy initiatives that are playing out across the world can help to achieve this goal.

Rewriting Corporate Charters. Corporate charters, issued by state governments, specify the rights and responsibilities of corporations. In the past, states granted charters for a limited time and could revoke them if corporations violated laws; every state except Alaska has the statutory authority for such revocations. Over time, however, business-friendly courts and legislatures narrowed the scope of charters and weakened public oversight. Now some reformers seek to reinvigorate the charter to better protect the public from corporate excesses.[67]

One approach has been to propose a "Three strikes and you're out" rule. In 1998, a coalition of thirty citizens' groups in September petitioned the attorney general of California to begin charter revocation proceedings against Union Oil Company of California (Unocal), charging the company with numerous legal violations, including environmental pollution, unfair and dangerous labor practices in the United States and its foreign operations, and collaboration in military actions with the dictatorship in Burma. The California attorney general dismissed the petition within a week. In 2003, California state senator Gloria Romero introduced a corporate three-strikes bill that would punish corporate repeat offenders. The bill would have declared a corporation that commits three or more major violations of law within a ten-year period a "corporate repeat offender." Such offenders would not be permitted to be incorporated or to transact intrastate business in California.[68] The bill did not pass.

In 2009, Ralph Nader and other consumer activists asked U.S. Attorney General Eric Holder to beef up the Justice Department's pursuit of corporate criminals, broaden citizens' rights to bring legal actions against corporations, and proposed legislation that would strengthen consumer protection by creating a criminal sanction for corporations that knowingly distribute life-threatening products.[69] Attorney General Holder did not respond.

The failure of these actions suggests that, to date, the approach to use the law to revoke the charters of irresponsible corporations has been mostly symbolic. But how law is used changes slowly. It took more than three decades for litigation against the tobacco industry to succeed, with changes in judges' decisions following rather than leading public opinion. Revoking the charters of corporations that routinely violate the law seems to appeal to American ideals of fairness and responsibility. It deserves further consideration.

Taking Corporations to Court. Other legal approaches have been used to challenge risky corporate practices.[70] Fears of legal liability can motivate corporations to change practices, and the determined efforts of the fast food, gun, and pharmaceutical industries to pass state and federal legislation that protects them from legal liability shows their understanding of its potential. Forcing companies to assume responsibility for the costs their health-damaging practices externalize onto the public can serve as a trigger to change. Litigation has been used both by government and private parties. State attorneys-general have been active in taking alcohol, firearms, food, and pharmaceutical companies to court.[71] Private groups, both non-governmental organizations and classes of consumer brought together for civil action against companies, have also used the courts to claim that corporations violated their rights or owe them damages.

Like any strategy, using the law to change corporate practices faces big obstacles—industry opponents will always have more resources, federal courts increasingly favor business over public interests, and the rules for the law are set by defenders of the status quo. But as two experienced public health lawyers concluded, public health litigation "can deter dangerous activities and play an important role in advancing the political and social struggle for public health."[72] More broadly, it can create still more opportunities for public discussion on what rules should govern the appropriate balance between private profit-seeking and protecting public health.

Reinvigorating Regulation and Corporate Crime Law Enforcement. Smart regulations save lives, and the business effort to weaken regulations since the 1970s is a powerful contributor to the growth in corporate practices that harm health. As I have shown, the public generally supports regulations that protect health and the environment, which on the whole provides a political opportunity to challenge corporate deregulatory pressure. What is needed to restore a more robust regulatory stance?

First, public health researchers need to conduct the studies that document the health and economic benefits of regulation and communicate these findings to the public and policymakers. Businesses routinely exaggerate the costs of regulation and minimize its health and environmental benefits. For example, when the EPA conducted economic impact analyses of the Toxic Substances Control Act, its estimates of the cost of compliance were 25 times lower than the estimate of the private corporation Dow Chemical. An independent review by the Government Accountability Office found the Dow numbers to be unreliable, yet because they existed and had been submitted into the rule-making record, they had to be part of EPA consideration.[73] More evidence on the public health benefits of regulation could arm advocates for the political battles that strengthening regulations require. Closer scrutiny of the dubious claims that corporations make about the costs of regulation could counter misleading allegations.

Second, regulatory agencies need to be provided with the staff and resources needed to do their job right. As Phillip Cooper explains in his book *The War Against Regulation*, a favorite tactic of corporations and their political supporters is to slash the budgets of regulatory agencies, then accuse them of being ineffective.[74] In 2011, a coalition of health and consumer groups protested an

11 percent cut in the budget of the U.S. Food and Drug Administration proposed by the House Republicans. They noted that

> cutting the FDA budget is like robbing Peter to pay Paul—the result will cost the federal government much more than it saves, because of increased costs of Medicare, VA medical care, medical care for our armed services, Medicaid, and other federally-supported health care programs. In addition, the delays in getting FDA approval and the recalls that will become necessary because of unsafe food and medicine will cost companies in every state in our nation billions of extra dollars each year.[75]

In the current budget battles in Washington, advocates can make the case that cutting spending on public health regulations now imposes health burdens and costs on our children and grandchildren, a consequence deficit hawks claim to want to avoid.

Third, legislative bodies—and public advocates—need to provide not only the resources, but also the mandates for oversight that will ensure that regulatory agencies are acting effectively. The failures of the financial regulatory agencies contributed to several dimensions of the 2008 economic crisis, including lack of oversight of predatory mortgage lending, risky bank investments, and commodities speculation. In 2011, the bipartisan Financial Crisis Inquiry Commission concluded that regulators "lacked the political will" to scrutinize and hold accountable the institutions they were supposed to oversee, and failed to require big banks to hold more capital to cushion potential losses and halt risky practices. The commission found that regulatory agencies were "caught up in turf wars" that led them to ignore their missions.[76] As damaging as these financial regulatory failures were, inadequate or ineffective regulation of industries such as food, tobacco, alcohol, and automobiles leads to premature death and preventable illnesses for current and future generations. If elected officials were to hold regulatory officials and corporate leaders accountable for their records, they could provide new incentives for truthfulness and due diligence.

As well as the specific need to strengthen the regulation of each of the consumer industries that contributes to chronic diseases and injuries, advocates need to consider new ways to regulate corporate decision-making more broadly. The 2008 economic crisis highlighted the adverse consequences of deregulating financial institutions and failing to enforce the anti-trust laws that might have prevented the rise of "too-big-to-fail" banks. These same risks result from non-enforcement of antitrust rules in industries that produce consumer goods.

Mark Cooper, director of research for the Consumer Federation of America, told a congressional committee in 2009, "Capitalism without bankruptcy is like

Catholicism without hell. It lacks a sufficiently strong motivational mechanism to ensure good behavior."[77] By giving the message that big corporations will not be allowed to fail, government gives them license to take risks that society, not their investors or managers, will pay for. Weak antitrust enforcement also enables economic concentration, a trend that reduces citizens' and consumers' power to act on their interest. As I described in previous chapters, economic concentration in the food, alcohol, tobacco, and pharmaceutical industries reduces competition and its price-lowering impact and allows companies to invest more in marketing and research and development of more profitable, often unhealthier products.

Another approach is to strengthen enforcement and penalties for corporate crime. As long as corporate executives can count on simply being fined rather than jailed for violating regulations, they can pass the costs of law-breaking onto their consumers. But Lanny Breuer, chief of the Justice Department Criminal Division, has observed that "the strongest deterrent against corporate wrongdoing is the prospect of prison time."[78] If corporate managers understood that making decisions that they knew would lead to premature death or preventable illnesses or injury could put them behind bars, they might be deterred from such behavior.

In recent years federal prosecutors have offered many corporate law breakers deferred prosecution agreements in which, in exchange for a fine and promise of good behavior, charges are dropped. In criticism of this practice, David Uhlmann, a professor at the University of Michigan Law School and former head of the Environmental Crimes Section at the Justice Department, observed,

> It is one thing when a first-time offender commits a minor drug offense and is told by prosecutors that she will not face criminal charges if she performs community service and does not commit any future violations. It is an entirely different matter when a large corporation is allowed to avoid criminal prosecution, by agreeing to pay millions—or billions—in civil penalties. Apart from the ethical questions deferred prosecutions raise, they send a terrible message—if corporations agree to pay the government enough money, they can avoid criminal charges.[79]

Reducing the use of deferred-prosecution agreements for corporate crime is another step that could strengthen compliance. A significant legal barrier to reclaiming public space is the increasing protection that corporate commercial and political speech has won from business-friendly courts. Challenging this relatively recent reinterpretation of the First Amendment both legally and politically can become another battleground for reducing corporate influences.

For the foreseeable future, defining appropriate roles for government and the corporations that act as executive agents for our market system is likely to be one of the central political questions dividing the nation. Progress in strengthening public oversight will undoubtedly be slow, and activists will need patience and a willingness to learn by trial and error.

Another, perhaps more idealistic, approach is suggested by sociologist Fred Block. He suggests that instead of debating whether more market or more state is better, we should instead ask how government and markets can together create a moral economy, one that operates to improve the well-being of people.[80] In a moral economy, writes Block, "the continuous exercise of democratic self-governance...reforms our institutions to make both the economy and the government work better to achieve our shared objectives."

By insisting that the appropriate balance depends on the outcome of government and market interactions, not ideological beliefs about which is better, those who believe a better world is possible can change the terms of the debate. Referring to Franklin D. Roosevelt, the New Deal, and the civil rights, student, and environmental movements, Block also argues for the power of a moral language to mobilize people to take action "to align our economic and political institutions with our deepest moral commitments." Here, too, health can provide a powerful frame for rethinking how governments and markets ought to interact. By persuading the American people that any relationship that leads to premature death and avoidable illnesses and injury cannot be moral, advocates for healthier more sustainable society can win over new supporters.

Create a Unifying Policy Agenda

The final "impossible" task for a movement that can succeed in reducing harmful corporate practices is to forge a policy agenda that unifies the many strands of activism now in motion. Such an agenda needs to be broad enough to attract and engage the many social forces concerned about the impact of corporations on society: Those seeking to restore democracy, shrink inequality, and develop fairer trade and other types of relations among rich, poor, and emerging nations. The agenda also should be specific enough that the thousands of organizations working on health and justice at local, regional, national, and global levels can find something to link their struggles with those of others. The agenda should be a tool that these organizations can use to better enable them to educate and engage their members, find new allies, and win victories.

This agenda can only emerge from practice, from repeated interactions among the general public, activists, movement leaders, policymakers and scholars. The overall agenda will inevitably change over time as it is field-tested in actual campaigns, with successful strands expanding and less successful ones being dropped. What I propose here (summarized in Box 8.3) is an effort to

---

Box 8.3 **A Policy Agenda for a Movement for a Healthier Future**

The movement for a healthier, more sustainable future supports policies that will:

1. Expand consumers' right to know and corporations' duty to disclose the health consequences of corporate practices and products.
2. Require corporations to pay for the health and environmental consequences of their products and practices.
3. Establish global health standards for product design and marketing.
4. Restore public ownership of science and technology.
5. Restore the visible hand of government in public health protection.
6. Prevent corporations from using their money and power to manipulate democratic processes.

---

create such an agenda, meant to serve as a spark for discussion and to illustrate possible content.

Let's examine each of these in more detail and explore which constituencies might take the lead in advancing each goal.

EXPAND CONSUMERS' RIGHT TO KNOW AND CORPORATIONS' DUTY TO DISCLOSE THE HEALTH CONSEQUENCES OF CORPORATE PRACTICES AND PRODUCTS

Right to know and duty to disclose policies appeal to a sense of fairness and basic market principles. Free market ideology assumes that all parties to commercial transactions have equal information. In practice, however, "Buyer beware" is too often the norm. Strengthening the weak right-to-know and duty-to-disclose rules for consumer products could provide a legal framework for redefining consumer rights and better balancing the obligations of government and markets.

In the case of the tobacco industry, the legal cases forced the tobacco industry to make public the thousands of documents that showed what (and when) big tobacco companies knew of the harmfulness of their products. This information played a critical role in changing public attitudes towards the corporate executives and companies that prospered from selling products they deliberately made increasingly lethal. The documents helped to persuade a federal judge that, by suppressing research, destroying documents, manipulating the use of nicotine so as to increase and perpetuate addiction, and distorting the truth about low-tar and light cigarettes to discourage smokers from quitting, the tobacco industry had "abused the legal system in order to achieve their goal—to make money with little, if any, regard for individual suffering, soaring health costs, or the integrity of the legal system."[81]

Providing consumers with the rights to demand similar investigations from other industries can help to provoke the public debates that will be needed to redefine the rights and responsibilities of corporations and consumers. Should advocates seeking to bring about changes in the food, firearms, pharmaceutical, and alcohol industries get access to similarly detailed documents in the coming decade; their power to create new sanctions for industries that knowingly act to harm public health grow.

France has come up with a modest starting point for the right to know, known as the *Loi Evin*. This 1990 law requires alcohol companies to restrict their marketing to verifiable factual statements about their products.[82] If the United States is not yet ready for right to know, perhaps starting with the right not to be lied to or misled could move us in the right direction.

REQUIRE CORPORATIONS TO PAY FOR THE HEALTH AND ENVIRONMENTAL CONSEQUENCES OF THEIR PRODUCTS AND PRACTICES

The ability of corporations to shift health and environmental costs to consumers or taxpayers has long been a major obstacle to reducing corporate harms. Policies that remove the right to externalize these costs can change the calculus of corporate decision-making.

Strategies for reducing negative externalities include litigation by governments or health care institutions to recover the costs of corporate-induced harm;[83] "performance-based regulation," in which companies are required to reduce adverse health consequences of their products but can do so in any way they devise;[84] taxes on unhealthy products, sometimes used to subsidize healthier ones;[85,86] and eliminating subsidies for unhealthy products such as high-fructose corn syrup or corporate tax breaks for practices such as advertising fast food and soda to children. An important priority for policymakers and health researchers is to generate evidence on the efficacy and political feasibility of these various approaches.

ESTABLISH GLOBAL HEALTH STANDARDS FOR PRODUCT DESIGN AND MARKETING

As long as multinational corporations can evade regulations in one country by marketing unhealthy products in another, public health advocates will end up shifting health problems from wealthier, more developed nations to less developed ones. The Universal Declaration of Human Rights (approved in 1948), the International Covenant on Civil and Political Rights (1966), the Convention on the Elimination of All Forms of Discrimination against Women (1979), the Convention on the Rights of the Child (1989), and several other UN treaties have firmly established universal rights in many dimensions. In this century, new universal rights are needed to protect individuals against the most powerful force of this era, multinational corporations.

The Framework Convention on Tobacco Control, the proposed Sydney Principles on food marketing to children, and the Arms Trade Treaty that emerged from the UN in 2013 are examples of international standards that can serve as models for global health standards. The FCTC, the first and oldest global health treaty, provides a more level playing field for challenging the tobacco industry, even though it has not yet ended tobacco industry efforts to exploit the vulnerabilities of markets in poor and emerging nations.

What does seem clear from an accumulating body of evidence is that industry-generated standards are not adequate to protect public health.[87,88,89,90] Rather, effective global standards require governments and international bodies to have enforcement powers sufficient to ensure compliance.

Another arena for global standards is truth-in-advertising and product labeling. New evidence shows that consumers' ability to understand such information varies widely, depending in part on their health literacy.[91,92] Advertisers manipulate such vulnerabilities by, for example, making misleading health claims.[93] Making such practices unacceptable not only in developed nations but in the emerging nations now targeted by multinational corporations could protect billions of people from harmful exposures to risky products.

RESTORE PUBLIC OWNERSHIP OF SCIENCE AND TECHNOLOGY

The public health advances of the past 150 years resulted from researchers, social movements and governments in developed nations working together to apply new insights from science and technology to provide clean water, sanitation, safer food, and immunizations to the masses. In this era, corporations have appropriated science and technology to their quest for higher profits. In so doing, they have amplified rather than helped to control today's epidemics of chronic diseases and injuries. Restoring public ownership of science and technology so that their fruits can benefit rather than damage public health is an essential task.

Industry campaigns to withhold damaging scientific data and to create scientific uncertainty have undermined efforts to protect public health. When the gun industry and the National Rifle Association joined forces to persuade Congress to end federal funding for research on gun violence,[94] or when the pharmaceutical industry pays researchers to conduct studies designed to show the benefits but not the harms of its products, both science and public health suffer.

Our society and our elected officials depend on objective evidence to make decisions about public health and environmental policy and regulations. Universities that establish partnerships with corporations that allow profit rather than truth or social need to dictate research deprive the public of such evidence.[95] Corporate-sponsored research that includes secrecy or non-disclosure clauses allows corporations to review or censor findings before publication. The practice of paying scientists for profitable discoveries forces scientists to violate basic concepts of scientific integrity and face unacceptable conflicts of interest. From a policy perspective, it reduces the credibility of the scientific enterprise and the trust the public places in science and scientists. Professional organizations that want to maintain their integrity need to oppose this corporate takeover of science.

Policy remedies that can return science to the people and reduce corporate intrusion include clear institutional and professional conflict-of-interest-policies; restrictions on giving for university research that limit the strings corporations can attach to their gifts; and increased academic and legal sanctions for companies, universities, and researchers that violate these standards.[96] By changing institutional norms and cultures, it may be possible to make it easier for scientists to resist such pressures and to educate the public about the pernicious role of corrupt science. By seizing such opportunities to restore public ownership of science, researchers and universities can contribute new resources to the effort to improve global health.

RESTORE THE VISIBLE HAND OF GOVERNMENT IN PUBLIC HEALTH PROTECTION

Protecting the health of the public is one of the most basic functions of government. Its erosion by the neoliberal idea that markets can solve all social problems is a clear and present danger to global health. At every level of government, health authorities can take action to protect health by reducing risky corporate practices. The corporate campaign to undermine these government functions by claiming that voluntary standards are sufficient is not based on credible scientific evidence. By linking the disparate advocacy campaigns to protect government's public health function into a coherent alternative vision of the proper balance between government and markets, a movement can offer a concrete alternative to the "market knows best" philosophy.

Strengthening government's ability to protect health has to occur at the global and national levels. A study by researchers at the University of California-Berkeley found that the global production and consumption patterns that multinational corporations have created have a disproportionately adverse health and environmental impact on poor and middle-income nations.[97] Wealthy nations have a moral responsibility, if not yet a legal one, to ensure that companies headquartered in their nation are not contributing to global health inequalities.

PREVENT CORPORATIONS FROM USING THEIR MONEY AND POWER TO MANIPULATE DEMOCRATIC PROCESSES

The greatest obstacle that social movements face is the current ability of corporations to dominate our political processes. As long as movements are forced to fight on a playing field so tilted they roll to the bottom, only limited victories are possible. The American people have a long history of mobilizing to fight unfair corporate power; current movements will need to mine that history to find the right paths for today. Health movements can contribute a powerful voice to the fights to restore democracy by creating fairer rules on lobbying, campaign finance, the revolving door between government and corporate employment, and voter registration.

Other avenues to restoring democracy and justice include more vigorous prosecution of corporate crimes, especially those that result in illness and death, and a reconsideration of the political rights of corporations. On one hand, corporate America and its representatives on the Supreme Court argue that corporations are people, with the same rights to speak and influence politics as flesh and blood people. On the other hand, they still insist that corporations have limited liability for their crimes and no moral obligations except to their shareholders. This self-serving contradiction seems ripe for challenge and a vehicle for bringing together the many campaigns against corporate privileges.

This agenda is a starting point for building a more unified and coherent movement to reduce the threats that corporations pose to our future, but it makes sense to also acknowledge its limitations. Neither this agenda nor any other can serve as a roadmap for a movement. Roadmaps emerge from practice, not the minds of researchers. The agenda is not a substitute for the detailed policy analyses that are needed to translate its broad policy goals into concrete proposals that specific campaigns advocate. To assist readers to make these translations, Box 8.4 lists some of the specific demands that groups described in this book have made in each of the six policy goals. These illustrate the breadth of issues that a broad agenda can bring together.

Finally, the agenda focuses on policy goals. It does not speak to how to achieve these goals nor does it address other vital movement imperatives I have described previously: the need to engage people's emotions, to offer a sense of community, or to sustain involvement over time.

Box 8.4 **Selected Campaigns That Illustrate Policy Agenda Goals**

1. Expand consumers' right to know and corporations' duty to disclose the health consequences of corporate practices and products.
   • Mandatory package warning on tobacco products
   • Calorie labeling and useable nutrition labels
   • Mandatory GMO (genetically modified organisms) labeling
2. Require corporations to pay for the health and environmental consequences of their products and practices.
   • Master Tobacco Settlement Agreement
   • Lawsuits (unsuccessful to date) against gun manufacturers and fast food outlets
   • Increased excise taxes on alcohol
   • Financial penalties against drug companies for illegal off-label promotion of their products
   • Guidelines that prevent pension funds and other institutional investors from investing in corporations that persistently damage health
3. Establish global health standards for product design and marketing.
   • Framework Convention for Tobacco Control
   • International Code of Marketing of Breast-milk Substitutes
   • Proposed Sydney Principles on Food Marketing to Children
   • Arms Trade Treaty
4. Protect science and universities from corporate intrusion.
   • No Free Lunch, Unbranded Doctors, and other campaigns to limit pharmaceutical marketing to healthcare providers
   • University and healthcare institutional conflict of interest policies
   • University decisions not to accept any contributions from tobacco industry
   • Increase public funding for scientific research
5. Restore the visible hand of government in public health protection.
   • New rules requiring fast food outlets to post calorie information
   • Added FDA role in regulation of tobacco products
   • Los Angeles moratorium on new fast food outlets in high-obesity neighborhoods
   • Bans on trans fatty acids
   • Require alcohol companies to withdraw dangerous products from market
   • Set strong standards for auto fuel efficiency, safety, and emission control

(continued)

Box 8.4 **(Continued)**

- Support and provide infrastructure to creating public-sector alternatives to private food, transportation, and pharmaceutical markets
- Regulate gun product safety
6. Prevent corporations from using their money and power to manipulate democratic processes.
    - Health professional organizations support for constitutional amendment to overturn *Citizens United*
    - Strengthen limits on revolving door between industry and government
    - Require legislative approval and public health participation in setting health and environmental standards in trade treaties
    - Tax speculative financial transactions to create fund for public heath innovation

---

From Impossible Tasks to Tipping Points

One reason the four tasks facing the emerging movement seem so difficult is that the corporate consumption complex has succeeded in making so many believe that there is no alternative. As the movement begins to succeed in these tasks, however, this lack of imagination may dissipate. As organizers learn how to broaden and deepen their appeals, the movement will reach tipping points that create new opportunities for success. Movements never grow in linear, predictable fashions.

In his novel *The Magician's Nephew*, C. S. Lewis wrote: "One moment there had been nothing but darkness; next moment a thousand, thousand points of light leaped out." Today thousands of organizations around the world are lighting up the many paths that can lead to an end to the corporate practices that promote hyperconsumption, premature death, and preventable illnesses and injuries. We don't yet know which paths are dead ends and which will lead to the transformative tipping points that will show another world is possible.

What we do know is that business as usual will ensure growing health burdens, increasing inequality, rising environmental damage, and deteriorating democracy. Will our society grasp its opportunity to chart a different future? The choice is ours.

Afterword

The World That Is Possible
New York City, October 2034

I wrote *Lethal but Legal* more than 20 years ago because I was worried about humanity's survival. Growing epidemics of chronic diseases and injuries, escalating environmental damage, increasing concentration of corporate power and wealth, and declining democracy and government protection of health were converging towards a dangerous tipping point. After the book's release, I had many conversations about these fears with readers, researchers, activists, health professionals, and students. What struck me most was that although most agreed that the rise of the corporate consumption complex and its relentless marketing of hyperconsumption threatened public health and democracy, even those persuaded by the book's arguments were pessimistic that another future was possible. Corporations were too powerful, they said, and opposition too weak. Acquiescence was more popular than resistance, and any possibility of a real alternative seemed hopelessly naïve.

Two decades later hindsight provides new insights. Today, a global movement for a healthier and more sustainable world thrives, expanding its influence and impact, winning many small and medium-sized victories that hold the promise for a transformed world in which human well-being, rather than profit alone, is an acknowledged goal. Of course threats remain. Perhaps a closer look at some of the changes in the specific industries I described in the book will help us to understand the ingredients that led to successes and the obstacles we can expect to face in coming years.

Automobiles

After the 2022 recession, the federal government again took over General Motors (by then General Motors Chrysler) when bankruptcy once more threatened. This second failure had been precipitated by new limits on sales of private automobiles in China and India, where lung disease from auto pollution was bankrupting health care systems; huge damage settlements in the recurring multiple lawsuits on the safety problems that GM had covered up for three decades; and the market failure of GMC's new super-sized SUV, the Rhinoceros XL, the polluting, accident-prone but lucrative product that GMC had hoped would restore profitability.

After the bailout this time, however, instead of handing the company keys back to management, the federal government retained a 40 percent stake in GM and insisted on more changes. Half the companies' new products and profits were to come from mass transit vehicles, CEO salaries were capped at 30 times the wage of production workers (in 2013, GM CEO Mary Barra had made 329 times the pay of the average auto line worker),[1] and the company invested in new auto-sharing franchises that were estimated to cut the demand for new cars by another 20 percent in the 2040s. Within five years of the bailout, GMC was again turning a profit, and the profits on the federal share had been invested in a research fund to find further ways to cut air pollution and improve mass transit systems around the world.

What led to the different outcome than the one after the 2009 bailout? A powerful alliance of labor unions, environmentalists, and health advocates led a national campaign to persuade elected officials and voters that GM did not deserve another financial rescue without making substantial concessions on health, safety, and the environment. The growing global climate-change movement made some elected officials more willing to say No to auto and energy company lobbyists. GM's willingness to pay a fine of more than $900 million to settle its role in a cover-up of ignition switch problems that had caused at least 124 deaths further damaged the company's credibility.[2] Voters were more skeptical of the auto industry's threat that any concessions would lead to job loss and economic disaster—in part persuaded by the evidence showing that in many markets producing new mass transit vehicles created more jobs and better promoted sustainable development. Several national governments in Asia, Africa, and Latin America promised to buy these new trains and buses, which were safer, less polluting, and cheaper than the available alternatives, thanks to technologies developed in the previous decade.

A successful lawsuit against the National Highway Transport and Safety Administration by several state attorneys-general found that for decades an understaffed NHTSA had failed to adequately monitor auto safety, which had resulted in thousands of preventable deaths.[3] A better-staffed NHSTA found more problems and forced more recalls. Similarly, the U.S. Environmental Protection Agency's revelation in 2015 that Volkswagen had deliberately installed software that falsified emission results reported to regulators led to the forced resignation of its CEO and more stringent enforcement of emissions controls in the United States and Europe.[4] Media coverage of these scandals contributed to a change in public opinion that supported more federal oversight of an auto industry perceived to insufficiently value the lives and safety of its customers.

Tobacco

Twenty years ago, the tobacco industry hoped that e-cigarettes—electronic nicotine delivery devices—would be its savior, providing an opportunity to hook another generation to nicotine and more time to find new ways to market addicting products and thwart public health regulation. Unfortunately, in the United States, this strategy has proved at least partially successful. The FDA was reluctant to regulate e-cigarettes forcefully and tobacco industry opposition, reinforced by anti-regulatory business and political allies, made it difficult to develop strong state and local regulations. Today, the U.S. regulatory response to e-cigarettes and tobacco products is a patchwork quilt, with some state and cities acting successfully to reduce tobacco and nicotine use and others struggling to keep up with new digital and viral marketing strategies.

Globally, however, many countries, including Australia, Brazil, South Africa, and Uruguay, have led vigorous national campaigns that have virtually eliminated tobacco use and nicotine addiction. In those nations, less than 5 percent of the population now uses tobacco and the burden of future premature deaths and preventable illnesses from tobacco diseases is considerably lighter than two decades ago. Even China and India are showing steady drops in smoking rates. The Framework Convention on Tobacco Control, for many years a somewhat fragile counterweight to the tobacco industry, is now the platform for a robust global organization that includes governments and civil society groups. When the United States finally ratified the FTCT on its twentieth anniversary in 2023, it contributed $5 billion over the next 10 years to strengthen the capacity of participating nations and groups to enforce its provisions. The U.S. government also signed on to a World Health Organization resolution to urge ministries of health in all member nations to avoid any interactions with the United States Chamber of Commerce and its more than 100 international affiliates until that group ended its lobbying to thwart public health regulation of tobacco.[5]

Food

A turning point in the battle to control marketing of unhealthy food was the Million Families March for Healthy Food and Healthy Kids on Washington. Led by the mothers and fathers of children with diabetes, the 2020 march had three "simple" demands: stop advertising unhealthy food to children, require food companies to contribute to paying for care for the diseases their products and marketing promote, and end corporate activities to undermine public health measures to encourage healthier eating. Two keynote speakers at the March were a teenager with fatty liver disease, a condition that had grown exponentially in the first two decades of this century,[6] attributed largely to diets of highly processed foods and soda, and a mother who led the Retire Ronald Coalition that forced McDonald's to abandon its marketing scheme designed to persuade kids to pester their parents to take them to McDonald's. Another speaker, a former marketing director for Coca-Cola, apologized to the millions of people with fatty liver disease and diabetes and their families for his role in contributing to these global epidemics. "Coca-Cola urged you to open happiness in order to increase its profit," he said, "but instead so many of you opened a floodgate of pain and suffering. It's time to end the marketing of sickening products."

It took another 10 years to force Congress to pass and the president to sign the Stop Marketing Sickening Foods to Kids Act, and the Sunshine on Corporate Campaign Contributions and Lobbying Expenses Act. In the interval, the Million Families March sparked a flurry of grass-roots organizing in both the black and Latino communities hardest hit by diet-related diseases and the suburban neighborhoods where parents had more resources to protect their children's health.

The March also birthed a new national organization, Communities & Families for Healthy Food. Communities & Families for Healthy Food brought together national organizations like Corporate Accountability International, Center for Science in the Public Interest and the Union of Concerned Scientists; food justice coalitions from New York, Los Angeles, Chicago, and Detroit; and health professional and teachers' organizations. Another founding member, Black Lives Matter, recognized that reducing the inequitable racialized burden of diet-related deaths required taking action to change the quality, healthfulness and prices of food available in Black communities. Despite their ideological and organizational differences, members of Communities & Families for Healthy Food agreed to make implementation of the three demands a priority. They also played an active role in the 2024 national elections, helping to elect candidates who said improving children's health would be their priority.

To achieve the March's third goal of stopping industry activities that harm health, a cadre of public health lawyers borrowed from the successes of the tobacco industry to file dozens of class action lawsuits against McDonald's, Coke, Pepsi, Kellogg's, Mars, and other big food companies. In the first decades of this century, these cases consistently lost. By the third decade, however, the rising cost of care for diabetes and other chronic diseases and the growing public distaste for global food companies that profited by exacerbating epidemics persuaded judges and juries to act differently.

In one court case in Texas, plaintiffs forced the disclosure of documents that showed that for decades soda companies had knowingly designed and marketed their products to hook children on sugary beverages known to cause health problems. Extensive media coverage of these cases led some hedge funds and institutional investors to move their capital to safer companies, thus increasing the pressure on big food to settle cases that threatened to become even bigger liabilities. By 2028, the 10 biggest food companies were willing to accept an offer from the Justice Department to establish a Healthy Food Fund of $1 trillion, to be paid out over 30 years, to reimburse Medicaid and Medicare for the some of the costs of caring for people with diabetes and other diet-related diseases. The fund now subsidizes fruit and vegetable production and supports a national cooperative of farmer-owned markets and public food markets in low-income communities across America. With this level of support, some urban neighborhoods have converted their food deserts and swamps into food oases, where for the first time in decades it is easier to find affordable healthy food outlets than fast-food chains and convenience stores.

Pharmaceuticals

Two seemingly unrelated events triggered the changes in the global pharmaceutical industry now under way. The first was a global pandemic of extensively drug-resistant tuberculosis (XDR TB) that began in Lithuania, Kazakhstan, and Latvia but soon spread to other former Soviet republics, then to India, China, South Africa, and ultimately even to the poor in high-income nations like the United States and the United Kingdom. The second was the failure of the World Health Organization to achieve its goal of 25 by 25—a 25 percent reduction in premature mortality from noncommunicable diseases by 2025, 15 years after the UN High Level Meeting on NCDs.

XDR-TB describes strains of TB that are resistant to first and second line treatment drugs. By 2013, XDR TB had been identified in 100 countries.[7] Between 2009 and 2013, the number of people diagnosed with multi-drug resistance (MDR) TB, defined as resistance to at least two common TB drugs, and XDR-TB, tripled, reaching 136,000 worldwide. In 2015, a spokeswoman for Médecins Sans Frontières told *The Guardian* that "the alarming spread of drug resistant TB in the former Soviet Union is of critical concern.... This dismal news must serve as a wake-up call for governments, donors and drug companies to step up and improve the drug-resistant TB response today.... We have to be aware that a TB problem anywhere is a TB problem everywhere because it is air-borne and we live in a world where people move much more freely now."[8]

Unfortunately, many, including the pharmaceutical industry, slept through that wake-up call. In 2012 Pfizer, in 2013 AstraZeneca, and in 2014 Novartis, three of the world's largest pharmaceutical companies, had announced that they were closing their TB drug discovery programs.[9] For drug companies, develop-ing new TB drugs was less profitable than developing drugs for diseases that affected wealthier populations. Several other industry practices had contributed to the spread of XDR TB and other drug-resistant disease strains: promoting antibiotics aggressively for humans and animals, leading to overuse, environ-mental contamination and resistance; producing insufficient supplies of drugs used to treat MDR and XDR TB, resulting in incomplete treatment and further spread of these strains; and charging prices for these drugs that put them out of reach of many governments and patients fighting resistant strains of TB.[10]

The recession of the early 2020s, like its 2007 predecessor, had led many countries to impose austerity measures in efforts to revive their economies. Several former Soviet republics cut public health spending by more than 40 percent, leading to a rapid rise of the already prevalent XDR TB. As the people of these struggling nations left home to look for better opportunities in Western Europe, North America, and Australia, they brought their XDR TB with them, challenging these countries' public health systems that had also fallen vic-tim to austerity budgets. By 2025, the economist Jim O'Neill's 2015 predic-tion that antimicrobial resistance would kill 300 million people and reduce economic output by as much as $100 trillion by 2050 already proved a gross underestimate.[11]

In 2025, the World Health Organization acknowledged that it had failed to cut premature mortality from NCDs by 25 percent, the goal it had set in in 2012.[12] The plan had identified nine targets to accomplish this reduction, two of which required action by drug companies. The first stated that at least 50 percent of eli-gible people should receive drug therapy and counseling to prevent heart attacks and strokes and the second that 80 percent of the world's population should have available the affordable basic technologies and essential medicines, includ-ing generics, required to treat major NCDs in both public and private facilities.

But until recently, the proportion of the world's population with access to essential medicines for NCDs and other conditions has shrunk, not grown.

Added protection for drug companies' intellectual property rights provided by the Trans-Pacific Partnership and the Transatlantic Trade and Investment Partnership had allowed global transnational drugmakers to extend the time they could keep lower-price generics off the market and to charge even higher prices, putting the products out of reach of many in low- and middle-income nations as well as the poor in high-income countries. The merger of Pfizer, AstraZeneca, and Novartis into PANHealth gave that and other consolidated drug companies even more power in negotiating with national governments and global organizations, a power they used to keep prices high and alternatives off the market. As the industry became ever more consolidated, even the pooled procurement approaches that Global Fund to Fight AIDS, TB, and Malaria, the Clinton Foundation HIV/AIDS Initiative, and the WHO had used to negotiate prices and quality with suppliers of drugs for those conditions had only a limited effect on price, quality, and safety for NCD drugs.

Five years ago, an unusual cast of characters gathered in Oslo, Norway, to find new ways to expand access to essential medicines for MDR TB, chronic diseases, and other conditions. The meeting was called by Médecins Sans Frontières and the Treatment Action Group, two global non-governmental organizations, and included senior health officials from India, South Africa, China, and Brazil, nations that by 2020 were home to more than 3 billion people, as well as representatives of Norway's Government Pension Fund Global, the Abu Dhabi Investment Authority, and the China Investment Corporation, three of the world's largest sovereign wealth funds. Advising the group were three former executives of PANHealth, who had left the company after their proposal to lower prices and invest more in research on essential medicines had been rejected.

The participants at the Oslo meeting created a new company, EssentialMeds4All Inc., a hybrid company intended to lower the costs of health care in BRICS and other middle-income nations. The motivation for these nations was to reduce the burden of paying for ever more expensive drugs for ever more people with chronic diseases, costs that were bankrupting their health care systems.

The company also funds research on essential medicines, and seeks to return a profit to its institutional and individual investors. With an initial investment of $50 billion from its founders and a promise of $5 billion a year for research for the next decade, EssentialMeds4All was able to buy up several small drug companies and begin producing high quality, low cost medicines for the communicable and chronic diseases most afflicting BRICS nations. The U.S. Department of Justice kicked in another $1.5 billion a year, revenues generated from the fines that drug companies paid for off-label promotion of drugs and violations of other consumer safety laws. The company used this stream to subsidize prices of drugs purchased by Medicaid and Medicare, saving U.S. taxpayers $2 for every dollar contributed.

By 2040, pharmaceutical industry analysts estimate, the company will be among the largest pharma companies in the world and will be returning an average of 10 percent a year to investors, less than Big Pharma's windfall profits of 20 percent or 30 percent of earlier decades but enough to continue to attract capital. It will also generate more than $2 billion annually for research. As its health and financial successes grow, other sovereign wealth and institutional investment funds and private investors are expected to put their money in EssentialMeds, allowing it to compete even more successfully with traditional private sector drug companies.

Alcohol

The 2026 Framework Convention for the Control of Alcohol (FCCA), now endorsed by 85 nations representing 80 percent of the world's population, marks a turning point in the campaign to reduce alcohol-related deaths, injuries, and diseases. At the end of the first decade of the twenty-first century, alcohol caused an estimated 3.8 percent of all global deaths and 4.6 percent of global disability-adjusted life-years (DALYS), a measure of impact on premature deaths, injuries, and illnesses attributable to alcohol. The costs associated with alcohol amounted to more than 1 percent of the gross national product in high-income and middle-income countries.[13] In 2030, alcohol use disorders were the fourth leading cause of DALYs in high-income nations.[14]

Faced with these high and growing costs, governments, health organizations, and citizen groups looked to the successes of the Framework Convention on Tobacco Control and the tobacco control movements for lessons. An important first step was barring alcohol industry executives from shaping global or national alcohol control policy. The revelations that the world's largest alcohol producers had hired business groups like the U.S. Chamber of Commerce and scientists who failed to disclose their industry support to lead the opposition to the FCCA made this decision easier. A WikiLeaks disclosure, apparently from an alcohol industry whistle blower, had revealed "dark money" campaign contributions and bribes to leading politicians in the United States, the United Kingdom, Germany, Australia, and China, and to charges that eventually led to prison time for several senior executives. After that, alcohol executives, like their colleagues in the tobacco industry, became pariahs at public health policy forums on alcohol. Free of their obstruction, health officials went on to pass the FCCA, a groundbreaking success in reducing the disease burden from alcohol.

In response to these disclosures, a dozen sports and entertainment celebrities who had endorsed products made by Anheuser Busch InBev, Diageo, and

SAB Miller severed their connections with these companies and donated time to make counter-ads for the Global Alcohol Policy Alliance. Founded in 2000 as a global network of advocates for healthier alcohol policy, the alliance used these stars to create an international social media campaign to challenge the alcohol industry's manipulative advertising strategies, its use of sexist, risk-enhancing messages and images, and its continued reliance on problem drinkers to make its profits. Within two years, young-adult demand for sweetened, flavored alcoholic beverages fell by 20 percent, presenting a similar threat to Big Alcohol as the one that Big Soda had faced two decades earlier.[15]

In the United States, federal legalization of marijuana in 2022 paradoxically also contributed to public support for stronger regulation of alcohol. Global tobacco and alcohol companies, looking for new profit centers, bought out the aging hippie entrepreneurs and young pothead hedge funders who first brought marijuana to legal markets. Big Alcohol and Tobacco then used their marketing savvy and their extensive distribution outlets to promote marijuana to all the populations where use was low, leading to a rapid rise in the rare but serious side effects of marijuana use: sudden-onset psychosis, addiction, and hallucinations. As the multiple health problems associated with three of America's favorite drugs—alcohol, nicotine, and marijuana—converged among the same vulnerable populations, the public and their elected officials recognized the merit of coordinated policy responses that set strict limits on the promotion and commercial distribution of these substances, a strategy that emphasized public health protection rather than criminal prosecution of users.

Firearms

In 2010, guns took the lives of 31,076 Americans in homicides, suicides, and unintentional shootings and another 73,505 Americans were treated in hospital emergency departments for non-fatal gunshot wounds. In 2030, guns killed only 20,000 people and sent fewer than 50,000 to the hospital, an especially impressive achievement given the increase in the U.S. population. What accounted for these dramatic reductions?

Was it the election in 2024 of a president who had lost a daughter to gun violence, giving the new leader both the backbone and the moral credibility to win legislation that imposed much tighter regulation on the gun industry? Since Lyndon B. Johnson had used the Kennedy brothers' assassinations to pressure Congress into standing up to the gun lobby, no President had been able to convince Congress to act so decisively.

Was it the Hundred Hunters Against Gun Violence's sit-in in Congress, in which ardent hunters' dressed in camouflage refused to leave the House chambers until Congress passed new legislation ending loopholes in gun registration? Speaking for the silent majority of gun owners who favor sensible rules to reduce gun violence, the hunters said that the best way to ensure that their children could continue hunting and sports shooting was to monitor gun sales more carefully and restrict access to weapons of war such as the automatic assault rifles often used in mass shootings.

Or was it the creation of a new national coalition, Communities, Docs and Cops Against Gun Violence? For the first time, a multi-racial coalition of families of victims of gun violence, law enforcement officials, and health professionals developed the capacity and will to match the savvy and clout of the NRA and its backers in the gun industry. Or perhaps it was a growing recognition of the economic costs of gun violence, perhaps more tangible to some than the human costs. One estimate put the 2012 annual cost of gun violence at $229 billion, about $700 for every man, woman, and child in the United States.[16]

In fact, neither the media nor researchers have been able to figure out why, quite suddenly, the United States seemed to come to its senses in taking action to reduce gun violence. What is clear is that the benefits of stronger public protections, the diminished power of the gun lobby, and the ongoing trend of fewer households owning and using guns has left all Americans safer from gun death and injuries. This year for the first time, the United States was not in the top ten nations in rates of gun deaths, and this is the first decade in which the disparity between gun death rates between blacks and whites contracted rather than expanded.

Common Causes

On the one hand, these recent changes in the practices of the industries I wrote about 20 years ago are relatively modest. Each of the six industries still exists. Profit is still their driving motive and the corporate consumption complex still has a powerful voice in our society.

On the other hand, each of these changes will in the next decade or so prevent tens of thousands of premature deaths or avoidable illnesses or injuries in the United States, and millions more around the world. Each demonstrates that new alliances and skillful framing of the issues can succeed in modifying harmful corporate practices. Each shows that in fact another world is possible. (It is also true that had these modest changes been instituted in 2000 or 2010 or 2020 many more lives would have been saved.) So what explains these changes now and what can we learn by analyzing their common causes?

CRISES TRIGGER REFORM

Epidemics and disasters have long precipitated public health reform, and that's true today too. The epidemics of XDR TB, the dramatic rise in adult onset diabetes and fatty liver disease in children and teens, and continuing injuries and deaths from defective auto parts—each contributed to changes in the pharmaceutical, food and beverage, and automobile industries.

But for crisis to lead to change, social movements and reformers have to be able to put feasible alternatives on the political agenda. Groups like Médecins Sans Frontières and the human rights advocates who demand that access to essential medicines is a right, not a privilege, and the Million Families March for Healthy Food, who told the food industry, "Don't sicken our kids for your profits," helped to transform critiques of the status quo into practical proposals for alternatives. Through campaigns that both evoked emotions and provided evidence, these movements helped to mobilize public opinion that made public officials fear that inaction was riskier than action. The results: less marketing of unhealthy food to kids, better access to affordable fruits and vegetables, lower-cost essential medicines, and more public transit options, each contributing to fewer chronic diseases and fewer hospitalizations.

In *Shock Doctrine* Naomi Klein explained how ruling elites use disasters to advance their agenda.[17] Today social movements have learned to turn that strategy on its head: using public health and environmental crises to mobilize support for improving well-being rather than to reinforce acquiescence.

TO EXTEND HEALTH CARE REFORM, PUT PREVENTION FIRST

Another impetus for change was the growing realization that the reforms brought about by the Affordable Care Act were insufficient either to achieve significant efficiencies in the health care sector or to move the United States out of the basement of international health rankings among developed nations, where it had languished since the 1970s.[18] True, the ACA had helped millions of Americans who had been uninsured to get coverage, had restricted the most flagrant abuses of the health insurance industry, and had stabilized the rising cost of health care, all important accomplishments. But what it did not and could not do was to slow the flood of sick people into doctors' offices, emergency rooms, and hospitals.

To improve the shorter, sicker lives that characterized the United States—to make prevention a priority rather than an afterthought—requires analyzing what makes people sick in the first place and interrupting that process well before they need medical care. As health care costs resumed their rise after the 2022 recession, a new alliance of labor unions, millennials concerned about their future, environmentalists, consumer rights and progressive political groups, and civil rights and immigrant organizations emerged with the demand Put Prevention First.

With the changing demographics of the American electorate, and with coordinated electoral and social movement strategies, politicians endorsed by the alliance won control of the House in 2024 and the Senate and White House in 2028. What followed was a spate of legislation as impressive as the accomplishments of the late 1960s and early 1970s.

The Hide No Harm Act, first introduced in 2015 in response to the General Motors cover-up of auto safety defects,[19] makes it a crime for corporations to conceal dangerous defects from the public, and sends corporate violators to prison. The Stop Marketing Illness and Injuries to Children Act prohibits any child-targeted advertising of products that reasonable scientific evidence demonstrates to be associated with child illness and injuries. The Public Airways for Public Health Act restores elements of the Fairness Doctrine promulgated by the Federal Communications Commission in the 1970s that required network broadcasters to offer free time to groups with contrasting views on controversial matters of public interest.[20] The new Act requires TV, radio, and Internet providers to offer free time to groups with contrasting views on message promoting products and lifestyles for which reasonable evidence shows harm. For the first time in a century, these accurate, often edgy health education messages can compete with the corporate advertising that has been the main source of information on food, drugs, alcohol, and tobacco for most Americans. The Disclose Dark Money in Elections and Lobbying Act requires corporations and individuals to report all contributions to any organization that seeks to influence legislation or elections.

Of course, each act required painful compromises in order to win passage. By themselves they do not solve the problems caused by lethal but legal corporate practices. What they have done, however, is reversed the long slide towards government abandonment of corporate oversight.

Another contributor to putting prevention first was the creation of the Prevention Fund in 2025. This national fund, fed by streams of revenue from taxes on alcohol, tobacco, sugar, and ultraprocessed food, fines collected by the Department of Justice and state attorneys general from companies convicted of violating public health regulations, and a transaction tax on financial speculation supported robust prevention activities around the nation. These included developing edgy youth-friendly counter-marketing campaigns on unhealthy food, alcohol, and tobacco that the new Federal Communications Commission ruling required TV, radio, and Internet providers to offer for free; sponsoring independent scientific groups to monitor the health impact of corporations; and beefing up enforcement of public health protections in poor communities. Next year, the European Union and several other high-income nations plan to join with the Prevention Fund to create a Global Prevention Fund, charged with supporting activities and research that will reduce the harmful impact of transnational corporations on the health of people living in low- and middle-income countries.

A LITTLE HELP FROM THE SUPREME COURT

Some major Supreme Court decisions also helped level the playing field for those who wanted to use conventional political strategies to limit corporate power. In 2014, many had believed that a corporate-friendly Supreme Court was as inevitable as the ocean's tides. But with the electoral changes of the last decade and the resignation and deaths of several Supremes, a solid court majority has started to reconsider the expansion of corporate rights that had begun in the 1970s. In her majority opinion overturning the 2010 *Citizen's United* decision, the new Chief Justice rejected its findings that money equals speech, and that corporations have the same right to free speech as individuals. Quoting Justice Stevens' dissent from the earlier case, the decision declared that "the financial resources, legal structure, and instrumental orientation of corporations raise legitimate concerns about their role in the electoral process. Our lawmakers have a compelling constitutional basis, if not also a democratic duty, to take measures designed to guard against the potentially deleterious effects of corporate spending in local and national races."[21]

The Court's upholding of The Stop Marketing Illness and Injuries to Children Act and the Hide No Harm Act further expanded consumers' rights to safe products and government's right to act to prevent deaths, rather than to simply compensate victims. These and similar decisions also remind activists that the Supreme Court can and does reverse itself (for example, in the past century on the minimum wage, free speech rights of teachers, sex between consenting adults, interracial marriage, and separate but equal schools)[22] and that Court opinions often follow rather than lead changes in public opinion, as the 2015 decision guaranteeing the right to same-sex marriage had shown.

CHANGING PUBLIC OPINION CREATES OPPORTUNITIES TO CHANGE POLICY

As public opinions on corporations, the role of government, and inequality changed, a political climate that encouraged more forceful government action emerged. In 2014, 47 percent of Americans had said that they had little or no trust in major corporations' ethical behavior.[23] By the end of 2015, a diverse crowd including Thomas Piketty, Pope Francis, Bono, Beyoncé, Barack Obama, Joseph Stiglitz, and, according to one poll, six out of ten Americans,[24] argued that the government should do more to reduce the gap between the rich and the poor.

The 2008 and 2023 recessions showed that markets alone were unable to sustain economies that benefitted most people or protected their well-being, and that government intervention could help curb the most egregious corporate practices. After the 2008 recession, business leaders had successfully resisted more forceful public sector action to solve the economy's problem. After the more recent downturn, increased numbers of people insisted "fool me twice, shame on me," an attitude that contributed to wide political support for the public stake in General Motors Chrysler and the new legislation on more active government oversight of corporations.

NEW ROLES FOR PROFESSIONAL ORGANIZATIONS AND UNIVERSITIES

Professional organizations and universities have also changed their ways. After several major professional organizations including the American Psychological Association, the Academy of Nutrition and Dietetics, and the American Academy of Family Practice were revealed to have made agreements with government agencies or corporations that put the interests and values of the outside groups ahead of those of the profession and the public, most organizations developed stricter conflict of interest and transparency rules. In some cases, where the professional organization had moved slowly, thousands of members resigned and created more activist alternatives, jeopardizing the revenue streams and clout of the mainstream group.

Today alliances like Health Professionals and Researchers for Social Responsibility monitor professional organizations, rate their conflict of interest policies, and help develop ethical standards that discourage professionals from becoming corporate marketing agents for food, pharmaceutical, or other companies. This public oversight has hampered corporations' ability to freely use researchers and health professionals for credibility engineering, long a mainstay of maintaining popular support.[25]

Universities have also changed. An embarrassing series of scandals, in which well-regarded scientists were found to have surreptitiously accepted corporate money or fabricated research results to advance business interests, led many institutions to develop and enforce stronger conflict of interest rules. In addition, as declining federal funding for research had led some American universities to turn to corporations to make up the shortfall, new controversies had erupted. Could corporations insist that researchers keep findings secret? Should universities cooperate with or accept money from businesses that used their intellectual property rights to advance profits at the expense of public health? These questions have not yet been settled but the earlier view that university corporate partnerships were the salvation for academia are no longer unchallenged, and universities have become an important forum for debating the proper role of corporations in our society.

Universities—and medical centers—have also provided a platform for another national debate on corporations. With the success of the campaign to force universities to divest from carbon-based energy industries, a larger question arose: should universities and medical centers profit from activities that harm health? Should their endowments and pension funds have higher standards—ones that incorporate the principle of "do no harm"? A few years ago Health Professionals and Researchers for Social Responsibility proposed that no university or medical center should accept contributions from or invest in companies that violated human rights, promoted products associated with premature deaths, or contributed to campaigns that undermined democracy. University presidents and fund-raisers were apoplectic, arguing they would be unable to raise money or find suitable investments to support their institutions. "Doesn't that show that universities' current business model is incompatible with a commitment to an independent academy that supports the basic values of health, democracy and human rights?" asked the activists.

Now every Ivy League campus and many other universities have a group of students, faculty, and staff that monitor investments and contributions, organize teach-ins, and attend Board of Trustee meetings. Their campaign Towards a Moral University identifies specific steps their institution can take to contribute to better health, a safer environment, and more democracy.

CHANGING PHILANTHROPY

Another change that contributed to the growth of movements for a healthy sustainable future was the new priorities of some philanthropists. The billionaire philanthropists of the late twentieth and early twenty-first centuries—Gates, Soros, Turner, Buffet, Bloomberg, and others—supported some worthy causes but for the most part did not challenge the fundamental causes of ill health and health inequities, and thus their impact was limited. Some scholars argued that "philanthrocapitalism" had become a new wedge to open markets, enhance corporate credibility, and weaken governments.[26]

The progressive grandchildren of the billionaires and a few other hedge fund babies and heirs of the one percent coming of age in the last decade have a different perspective. Learning from the successful right-wing foundations of the

1970s and 1980s, they are now providing long-term general support to the movements and their support organizations, enough time to establish a track record and begin to make a difference. Many of the previously mentioned coalitions and alliances, including Communities for Healthy Food and Healthy Children, Communities, Docs & Cops against Gun Violence, and Professionals and Researchers for Social Responsibility, are supported by these new philanthropists. Mainstream health foundations change their priorities every few years, insist on measurable changes within a few years for health conditions that took decades to develop, and often expect grantees to enter public private partnerships with the very corporations that caused the targeted health problem. The new funders understand that their most productive investments are in the robust, rooted social movements that for the last two centuries have been the most reliable instigators of change.

GLOBALIZATION FROM THE BOTTOM UP

For many years, supporters of corporate-managed globalization argued that this was the only and inevitable road to a global future. In response, critics sometimes rejected globalization altogether, claiming it inevitably hurt the poor and benefited the rich. Today, that simplistic dichotomy has been replaced by more sophisticated questions: What are the different paths to a more global world? Who benefits and who loses from each? Who decides which path to take? Essential Medicines4All, for example, is a global organization that benefits the poor and advances equity.

Another alliance, Health Before Profits, emerged after the passage of the Trans-Pacific and Atlantic Trade Agreements. Determined to reject any more trade treaties that damaged health and the environment and undermined the mandates of national governments and the World Health Organization to protect public health, it brought together civil society groups like the Social Forum, the People's Health Movement, health ministers of several low- and middle-income nations, labor unions, and environmental groups. Their defeat of the Middle East and Trans-African Trade Treaties showed global alliances can provide an alternative to corporate globalizers.

STRATEGIC, TACTICAL AND IDEOLOGICAL FLEXIBILITY CAN OPEN DOORS

As progressive forces began to win more victories against corporate power, the defensive, "my way or the highway" mentality of many reform groups began to dissipate. In the past, each faction had insisted its strategy was the right one. In the food movement, those who believed that empowering small farmers was the way to fix our broken food system argued against those who wanted to focus on child obesity who in turn castigated the anti-hunger groups for accepting corporate money. Is it surprising that big food companies often won food policy fights because they understood the power of the divide and conquer strategy?

On the tactical side, public health lawyers insisted that litigation was the most effective way to win concessions from corporations, while corporate social responsibility groups, campaign finance advocates, and community organizers each asserted their approach was the most reliable. Now, however, experience has shown the synergistic and cumulative impact of multiple initiatives. For example, two decades of media advocacy against Citizens United, multiple state legislative efforts to limits its scope, and an unsuccessful effort to amend the Constitution all led to changing public opinion, victories for congressional candidates who supported limits on corporate money in politics, new Supreme Court Justices, a reversed decision, and, ultimately, a more level playing field for supporters of a more equitable democracy. We'll never know how much of the credit for this change can be attributed to any one activity but so what?

New leaders, less constrained by ideologies and egos, have been in the forefront of this more flexible approach—and their political successes reinforce their choices, a virtuous circle of widening influence and power. The global climate movement also contributed to this change. Its embrace of new constituencies (labor unions, youth, indigenous people), diverse strategies (divestiture, electoral campaigning, demonstrating), and multiple issues (fracking, support for global treaties, farmland protection) enabled this movement to capture public and media attention and to make progress in convincing growing numbers of people that the transnational energy companies represented a clear and present danger to the survival of humanity.

MANY ECONOMIC ALTERNATIVES TO MARKET FUNDAMENTALISM

After the collapse of the Soviet Union in the 1980s, "there-is-no-alternative" had been applied not only to political systems but also to economic ones. If state socialism couldn't survive and the various Third World economic experiments seemed either floundering or ready to cuddle up with global capitalism, what were the real-world options?

Today, a dozen variants are emerging. General Motors Chrysler is a publicly traded corporation with 40 percent owned by the taxpayers and is thus compelled to contribute to the public goals of reducing air pollution and global warming and making mass transit more available and affordable. EssentialMeds4All is a hybrid corporation, owned by a global consortium of governments and financial institutions, operated in the public interest but open for public investment.

In agricultural regions around the world, cooperatives of small farmers have organized to sell their food directly to retail distributors, bypassing several links on the value chain, and thus retaining more profit on the healthier, less-processed food they produce. Worker owned cooperatives produce everything from food to health care and manufactured goods. In the United States alone, by 2014, more than a million farmers and ranchers belonged to 3,000 farmer cooperatives.[27]

In many places, a public sector has grown to challenge the dominant private sectors. Many cities and states have created public food markets where healthy affordable food is available to poor people, either through public markets or publicly supported restaurants or food trucks. In some cases the public sector provides the infrastructure, in other cases it runs these outlets itself. Public sectors have also emerged in transportation, housing, and pharmaceuticals, illustrating an alternative to the market economy and serving as competitors, forcing private companies to vie for customer allegiance, thus improving quality and lowering prices. In health care and education, the public sector has long had competitive advantages, now other sectors are learning from these experiences.

Not surprisingly, these many alternative economic models have not yet provided the evidence that can answer the age-old questions of philosophers and political activists of all stripes: "What's the best system for governing human affairs?," "How can we balance growth and fairness?," or "What are the respective responsibilities of government and markets?" What these varying models have done, however, is contradict the arrogant belief that only the political and economic system that dominated the world in the late twentieth and early twenty-first century could solve the problems of our era.

Conclusion

In 2014, many people questioned whether a world not dominated by corporations was possible. Today, many other worlds seem possible, and a new set of questions have come to the fore: Which of these alternatives do we want? How can we best choose which of the many paths to take to get to those alternative worlds? Which paths are most sustainable? What role does concern for health play in lighting up the available paths?

As long as humans survive, each generation will chart its own path to longer, better lives and healthier, more just communities. Today the bleak prospects that our health, environment, and democracy faced in 2014 seem a bit brighter; another world was in fact possible. Our children and grandchildren will decide how to use that illumination to write the next chapter of the history of public health.

Notes

Preface

1. Olshansky SJ, Passaro DJ, Hershow RC, et al. A potential decline in life expectancy in the United States in the 21st century. *N Engl J Med* 2005;352(11):1138–1145.

Chapter 1 Manufacturing Disease: Unhealthy Products Become Ubiquitous

1. World Health Organization. Global status report on noncommunicable diseases, 2010. Description of the global burden of NCDs, their risk factors and determinants. Geneva, Switzerland: WHO, 2011.
2. Beaglehole R, Bonita R, Horton R, Adams C, Alleyne G, Asaria P, et al. and Lancet NCD Action Group; NCD Alliance. Priority actions for the non-communicable disease crisis. *Lancet.* 2011;377(9775):1438–1447.
3. Stuckler D, McKee M, Ebrahim S, Basu S. Manufacturing epidemics: the role of global producers in increased consumption of unhealthy commodities including processed foods, alcohol, and tobacco. *PLoS Med.* 2012;9(6):e1001235.
4. Fuller GW. *New Food Product Development: From Concept to Marketplace.* 3rd ed. Baton Rouge, FL: CRC Press; 2011:20.
5. Supermarket Facts: Industry Overview 2010. Food Marketing Institute. Available at: http://www.fmi.org/facts_figs/?fuseaction=superfact. Accessed August 8, 2012.
6. Zimmerman FJ. Using marketing muscle to sell fat: the rise of obesity in the modern economy. *Annu Rev Public Health.* 2011;32:285–306; p. 293.
7. McDonald's Corporation. McDonald's USA ingredients listing for popular menu items. Available at: http://nutrition.mcdonalds.com/getnutrition/ingredientslist.pdf. Updated August 7, 2012. Accessed August 8, 2012.
8. Avena NM, Gold MS. Variety and hyperpalatability: are they promoting addictive overeating? *Am J Clin Nutr.* 2011;94:367–368.
9. Kessler D. *The End of Overeating. Taking Control of the Insatiable American Appetite.* New York: Rodale, 2009.
10. Kessler D. *The End of Overeating. Taking Control of the Insatiable American Appetite.* New York: Rodale, 2009, p. 18.
11. What are the ingredients of a Cinnabon cinnamon roll? Answers.com. Available at: http://wiki.answers.com/Q/What_are_the_ingredients_of_a_cinnabon_cinnamon_roll. Updated November 12, 2007. Accessed August 8, 2012.
12. Cinnabon. Cinnabon Nutritional Information. Cinnabon Website. Available at: http://cinnabon.com/media/21554/cinnabon_nutrition.pdf. Updated October 24, 2011. Accessed August 8, 2012.

13. Power ML, Schulkin J. *The Evolution of Obesity*. Baltimore, MD: Johns Hopkins University Press; 2009.

14. Lieberman DE. Evolution's sweet tooth. *New York Times*. June 6, 2012: A27.

15. Blundell JE, Finlayson G. Food addiction not helpful: the hedonic component—implicit wanting—is important. *Addiction*. 2011;106(7):1216–1218.

16. Smith TG. All foods are habit-forming—what I want to know is which will kill me! *Addiction*. 2011;106(7):1218–1219.

17. Johnson PM, Kenny PJ. Dopamine D2 receptors in addiction-like reward dysfunction and compulsive eating in obese rats. *Nat Neurosci*. 2010;13(5):635–641.

18. Volkow ND, Wang GJ, Fowler JS, Telang F. Overlapping neuronal circuits in addiction and obesity: evidence of systems pathology. *Philos Trans R Soc Lond B Biol Sci*. 2008;363(1507):3191–200.

19. Blundell JE, Finlayson G. Food addiction not helpful: the hedonic component—implicit wanting—is important. *Addiction*. 2011;106(7):1216–1218.

20. Fuller GW. *New Food Product Development: From Concept to Marketplace*. 3rd ed. Boca Raton, FL: CRC Press; 2011:23.

21. Keynes, JM. A Treatise on Money Volume 2: The Applied Theory of Money. Cambridge: MacMillan, 1971. 8th ed.:133.

22. Fuller GW. *New Food Product Development: From Concept to Marketplace*. 3rd ed. Boca Raton, FL: CRC Press; 2011:29.

23. Associated Press. Hardee's, Carl's Jr. see profit in big patties: fast-food chains focus on what people want to eat, not what is healthy. June 27, 2006. Available at: http://www.msnbc.msn.com/id/13581901/ns/business-retail/t/hardees-carls-jr-see-profit-big-patties/. Accessed August 8, 2012.

24. NBC News. Hardee's serves up 1, 420-calorie burger. November 17, 2004. Available at: http://www.msnbc.msn.com/id/6498304/ns/business-us_business/t/hardees-serves-calorie-burger/#.UBKOYKBtCSo. Accessed August 8, 2012.

25. Gibson R. McDonald's skinny burger is a hard sell. *Wall Street Journal*. April 4, 1993:1.

26. Zimmerman FJ. Using marketing muscle to sell fat: the rise of obesity in the modern economy. *Annu Rev Public Health*. 2011;32:285–306.

27. Elliott C. Assessing "fun foods": nutritional content and analysis of supermarket foods targeted at children. *Obes Rev*. 2008;9(4):368–377.

28. U.S. Federal Trade Commission. A Review of Food Marketing to Children and Adolescents, 2012 update. Washington, DC: FTC, 2012, p. 7.

29. U.S. Federal Trade Commission. A Review of Food Marketing to Children and Adolescents, 2012 update. Washington, DC: FTC, 2012:9.

30. Frazao, E. America's Eating Habits: Changes and Consequences. U.S. Department of Agriculture, Economic Research Service, Food and Rural Economics Division. Agriculture Information Bulletin No. 750. Available at: http://www.ers.usda.gov/publications/aib750/aib750.pdf, p. 222. Published May, 1999. Updated May 26, 2012. Accessed August 8, 2012.

31. Poti JM, Popkin BM. Trends in energy intake among US children by eating location and food source, 1977–2006. *J Am Diet Assoc*. 2011;111(8):1156–1164.

32. Brownell KD, Frieden TR, Ounces of prevention—the public policy case for taxes on sugared beverages. *J Med*. 2009;360:1805–1808.

33. United States Department of Agriculture. Profiling Food Consumption in America. In: Agriculture Fact Book, 2001–2002. United States Department of Agriculture, Office of Communications. Available at: http://www.usda.gov/factbook/chapter2.pdf. Published March, 2003. Accessed August 8, 2012.

34. Centers for Disease Control and Prevention. Vital signs: food categories contributing the most to sodium consumption—United States, 2007–2008. *MMWR*. 2012;61(05):92–98.

35. Strom BL, Anderson CM, Ix JH. Sodium Reduction in Populations: Insights from the Institute of Medicine Committee. *JAMA*. 2013;310(1):31–32.

36. Russo M. Apples to Twinkies: comparing federal subsidies of fresh produce and junk food. U.S. PIRG Education Fund. Available at: http://uspirg.org/sites/pirg/files/

reports/Apples-to-Twinkies-web-vUS.pdf. Published September, 2011. Accessed August 8, 2012.

37. U.S. Federal Trade Commission. A Review of Food Marketing to Children and Adolescents, 2012 update. Washington, DC: FTC, 2012:ES-15.

38. Food and Beverage Industry Global Report–2010. IMAP. Available at: http://www.imap.com/imap/media/resources/IMAP_Food__Beverage_Report_WEB_AD6498A02CAF4.pdf, p. 9. Published August 10, 2010. Accessed August 9, 2012.

39. Food and Beverage Industry Global Report–2010. IMAP. Available at: http://www.imap.com/imap/media/resources/IMAP_Food__Beverage_Report_WEB_AD6498A02CAF4.pdf, p. 9. Published August 10, 2010. Accessed August 9, 2012.

40. Nestlé subsidiary to settle FTC false advertising charges; will drop deceptive health claims for BOOST Kid Essentials [press release]. Federal Trade Commission; July 14, 2010. Available at: http://ftc.gov/opa/2010/07/Nestlé.shtm. Accessed August 9, 2012.

41. Bauerlein V. PepsiCo chief defends her strategy to promote "good for you" foods. *Wall Street Journal*. June 28, 2011. Available at: http://online.wsj.com/article/SB10001424052702303627104576412232408827462.html. Accessed August 9, 2012.

42. Esterl M, Bauerlien V. PepsiCo wakes up and smells the cola. *Wall Street Journal*. June 28, 2011:B1.

43. Esterl M, Bauerlien V. PepsiCo wakes up and smells the cola. *Wall Street Journal*. June 28, 2011:B1.

44. PepsiCo. PepsiCo welcomes our newest billion-dollar brands. Ad, *New York Times*, January 26, 2012:B5.

45. Nettleton JA, Lutsey PL, Wang Y, Lima JA, Michos ED, Jacobs DR Jr. Diet soda intake and risk of incident metabolic syndrome and type 2 diabetes in the Multi-Ethnic Study of Atherosclerosis (MESA). *Diabetes Care*. 2009;32(4):688–694.

46. Esterl M, Bauerlein V. PepsiCo wakes up and smells the cola. *Wall Street Journal*. June 28, 2011:B1.

47. Associated Press. PepsiCo, revamping in China, takes a loss. *New York Times*. July 26, 2012: B10.

48. Lupton JR. Scientific substantiation of claims in the USA: focus on functional foods. *Eur J Nutr*. 2009;48(suppl 1):S27–S31.

49. Mariotti F, Kalonji E, Huneau JF, Margaritis I. Potential pitfalls of health claims from a public health nutrition perspective. *Nutr Rev*. 2010;68(10):624–638.

50. Moore A. Indra Nooyi's Pepsi challenge: CEO puts her own brand on new products and global goals. *Marketwatch*. December 6, 2007. Available at: http://www.marketwatch.com/story/indra-nooyi-puts-her-brand-on-pepsis-pressing-global-challenges?pagenumber=1. Accessed August 9, 2012.

51. Kantar Media reports U.S. advertising expenditures increased 6.5 percent in 2010 [press release]. Kantar Media; March 17, 2011. Available at: http://kantarmediana.com/intelligence/press/us-advertising-expenditures-increased-65-percent-2010. Accessed August 9, 2012.

52. McGinnis JM, Gootman JA, Kraak VI, eds. Food Marketing to Children and Youth: Threat or Opportunity? Washington, DC: Committee on Food Marketing and the Diets of Children and Youth, Institute of Medicine, National Academies Press; 2005.

53. McKay B. Downsize this! After years of supersizing, food makers shrink portions (and fatten profit margins). *Wall Street Journal*. January 27, 2004: B1.

54. Aizenman NC. Former Coke executive slams "share of stomach" marketing campaign. *Washington Post*. June 7, 2012. Available at: http://www.washingtonpost.com/national/health-science/former-coke-executive-slams-share-of-stomach-marketing-campaign/2012/06/07/gJQAKwgKMV_story.html. Accessed August 9, 2012.

55. Zimmerman FJ. Using marketing muscle to sell fat: the rise of obesity in the modern economy. *Annu Rev Public Health*. 2011;32:285–306; 292.

56. Young LR, Nestle M. The contribution of expanding portion sizes to the US obesity epidemic. *Am J Public Health*. 2002;92(2):246–249.

57. Young LR, Nestle M. Portion sizes and obesity: responses of fast-food companies. *J Public Health Policy*. ;28(2):238–248.

58. U.S. Federal Trade Commission. A Review of Food Marketing to Children and Adolescents, 2012 update. Washington, DC: FTC, 2012:ES-3

59. Story M, French S. Food advertising and marketing directed at children and adolescents in the US. *Int J Behav Nutr Phys Act.* 2004;1:3. doi:10.1186/1479-5868-1-3.

60. Simon M. PepsiCo and public health: Is the nation's largest food company a model of corporate responsibility or a master of public relations? *CUNY Law Review.* 2011;15:101–118.

61. Weller LN. Pepsi refreshes Alton parochial school's computers. *The Telegraph* (Illinois). August 20, 2010. Available at: http://commercialfreechildhood.blogspot.com/2010/08/back-to-school-with-pepsico-stealth.html.

62. Thompson, C. There's a sucker born in every medial prefrontal cortex. *New York Times Magazine.* October 26, 2003. Available at: http://www.nytimes.com/2003/10/26/magazine/26BRAINS.html?pagewanted=all. Accessed August 9, 2012.

63. O'Guinn TC, Muniz, Jr. AM. The social brand: towards a sociological model of brands. In: Loken B, Ahluwalia R, Houston MJ, eds. *Contemporary Perspectives in Branding Research.* New York: Taylor and Francis; in press. Available at: http://research3.bus.wisc.edu/pluginfile.php/1227/mod_page/content/1/papers/towards_a_sociological_model_of_brands.pdf. Accessed August 9, 2012.

64. Pendegrast M. *For God, Country, and Coca-Cola: The Unauthorized History of the Great American Soft Drink and the Company That Makes It.* New York: Scribner; 1993:22.

65. Nielsen Acquires NeuroFocus [press release]. Nielsen; May 26, 2011. Available at: http://www.nielsen.com/us/en/insights/press-room/2011/nielsen-acquires-neurofocus.html. Accessed August 9, 2012.

66. Penenberg A. NeuroFocus uses neuromarketing to hack your brain. *Fast Company.* September 2011. Available at: http://www.fastcompany.com/magazine/158/neuromarketing-intel-paypal. Accessed August 9, 2012.

67. Penenberg A. NeuroFocus uses neuromarketing to hack your brain. *Fast Company.* September 2011. Available at: http://www.fastcompany.com/magazine/158/neuromarketing-intel-paypal. Accessed August 9, 2012.

68. Vasu E. Frito Lay (Cheetos): the orange underground. No date. Available at: http://cargocollective.com/EMILIE. Accessed August 9, 2012.

69. Harris G. Colorless food? We blanch. *New York Times.* April 3, 2011:WK3.

70. Pinochet MO. Is your advertising more than just a green slice of life? Down to Earth. Available at: http://downtoearth.sequoialab.com/2012/01/18/is-your-advertising-more-than-just-a-green-slice-of-life/. Published January 2, 2012. Accessed August 9, 2012.

71. Cheyne A, Dorfman L, Gonzalez P, Mejia P. Food and beverage marketing to children and adolescents: an environment at odds with good health. A research synthesis. Robert Wood Johnson Foundation. Available at: http://www.rwjf.org/files/research/20110411herfoodmarketing.pdf. Published April, 2011. Accessed August 9, 2012.

72. Kraak VI, Story M, Wartella EA, Ginter J. Industry progress to market a healthful diet to American children and adolescents. *Am J Prev Med.* 2011;41(3):322–333.

73. Harris JL, Schwartz MB, Brownell, KD, Sarda V, Ustjanauskas A, Javadizadeh J et al. Fast food f.a.c.t.s.: evaluating fast food nutrition and marketing to youth. Yale Rudd Center for Food Policy and Obesity. Available at: http://fastfoodmarketing.org/media/FastFoodFACTS_Report.pdf. Published November 2010. Accessed August 9, 2012.

74. Harris JL, Schwartz MB, Brownell, KD, Sarda V, Ustjanauskas A, Javadizadeh J et al. Fast food f.a.c.t.s.: evaluating fast food nutrition and marketing to youth. Yale Rudd Center for Food Policy and Obesity. Available at: http://fastfoodmarketing.org/media/FastFoodFACTS_Report.pdf. Published November 2010. Accessed August 9, 2012.

75. U.S. Federal Trade Commission. A Review of Food Marketing to Children and Adolescents, 2012 update. Washington, DC: FTC, 2012.

76. U.S. Federal Trade Commission. A Review of Food Marketing to Children and Adolescents, 2012 update. Washington, DC: FTC, 2012.

77. Interview with Stan Sthanunathan, Vice President, Marketing Strategy & Insights, The Coca-Cola Company. Presented at: The Market Research Event, Research Insighter Podcast Series; November 7–9, 2011; Orlando, FL. Available at: http://www.iirusa.com/upload/wysiwyg/2011-M-Div/M2328/Podcast/TMRE_Insider_CocaCola.pdf, pp. 2, 6. Accessed August 9, 2012.

78. Malik VS, Popkin BM, Bray GA, Després JP, Willett WC, Hu FB. Sugar-sweetened beverages and risk of metabolic syndrome and type 2 diabetes: a meta-analysis. *Diabetes Care.* 2010;33(11):2477–2483.

79. Turow J. *The Daily You: How the New Advertising Industry is Defining Your Identity and Your Worth.* New Haven, CT: Yale University Press; 2011:2.

80. Restaurant. Harris Interactive Website. Available at http://www.harrisinteractive.com/Industries/Restaurant.aspx. Accessed on December 23, 2012.

81. Products: Red Bull Energy Drink. Red Bull USA. Available at: http://www.redbullusa.com/cs/Satellite/en_US/red-bull-energy-drink/001242989766321. Accessed August 9, 2012.

82. Yaqoob M. The red bull marketing strategy. TRCB.com. March 24, 2009. Available at: http://www.trcb.com/business/marketing/redbull-marketing-strategy-7375.htm. Accessed August 9, 2012.

83. Energy drink market experiences a jolt in sales, but stalls in attracting new customers, reports Mintel. Mintel Press Release, August 11, 2010. Available at: http://www.mintel.com/press-centre/press-releases/584/energy-drink-market-experiences-a-jolt-in-sales-but-stalls-in-attracting-new-customers-reports-mintel Accessed December 23, 2012.

84. Meier B. Caffeinated drink cited in reports of 13 deaths. *New York Times*, November 24, 2012:B1.

85. Richardson J, Harris JL. Food marketing and social media: findings from fast food FACTS and sugary drink FACTS. Presented at: American University Digital Food Marketing Conference; November 5, 2011. Available at: http://www.yaleruddcenter.org/resources/upload/docs/what/reports/FoodMarketingSocialMedia_AmericanUniversity_11.11.pdf.

86. U.S. Federal Trade Commission. A Review of Food Marketing to Children and Adolescents, 2012 update. Washington, DC: FTC, 2012.

87. Messinger PR, Narasimham C. Has power shifted in the grocery channel? *Mark Sci* 1995;14(2):189–223.

88. Lichtenstein N. *The Retail Revolution: How Wal-Mart Created a Brave New World of Business.* New York: Metropolitan Books; 2009:p. 42.

89. Lichtenstein N. *The Retail Revolution: How Wal-Mart Created a Brave New World of Business.* New York: Metropolitan Books; 2009:43.

90. Lichtenstein N. *The Retail Revolution: How Wal-Mart Created a Brave New World of Business.* New York: Metropolitan Books; 2009:58.

91. Quartier K, Christiaans H, Van Cleempoel K. Retail design: lighting as an atmospheric tool, creating experiences which influence consumers' mood and behaviour in commercial spaces. Presented at: Undisciplined! Design Research Society Conference 2008; July 16–19, 2008, Sheffield, UK. Available at: http://shura.shu.ac.uk/496/1/fulltext.pdf. Accessed August 9, 2012.

92. Arndt M. McDonald's 24/7. *Bloomberg Businessweek.* February 4, 2007. Available at: http://www.businessweek.com/stories/2007-02-04/mcdonalds-24-7. Accessed August 9, 2012.

93. Copple B. Shelf-determination. Forbes.com. April 15, 2002. Available at: http://www.forbes.com/forbes/2002/0415/130_print.html. Accessed August 9, 2012.

94. Slotting fees. CBU Marketing. Available at: http://cbumarketing.wikispaces.com/Slotting+Fees. Updated March 17, 2010. Accessed August 9, 2012.

95. Nestle M. *What to Eat: An Aisle-by-Aisle Guide to Savvy Choices and Good Eating.* New York: North Point Press; 2006:349.

96. Nelson E, Ellison S. In a shift, marketers beef up ad spending inside stores. *Wall Street Journal.* September 21, 2005:A1.

97. Robinson TN, Borzekowski DL, Matheson DM, Kraemer HC. Effects of fast food branding on young children's taste preferences. *Arch Pediatr Adolesc Med.* 2007;161(8):792–797.

98. Food Markets and Prices: Retailing and Wholesaling, Retail Trends. USDA Economic Research Service. Available at: http://www.ers.usda.gov/topics/food-markets-prices/retailing-wholesaling/retail-trends.aspx. Updated May 26, 2012. Accessed August 9, 2012.

99. Lichtenstein N. *The Retail Revolution: How Wal-Mart Created a Brave New World of Business.* New York: Metropolitan Books; 2009:42.

100. Martinez S. The U.S. Food Marketing System: Recent Developments, 1997–2006. U.S. Department of Agriculture, Economic Research Service, Economic Research Report No. 42. Available at: http://www.ers.usda.gov/publications/err42/err42.pdf. Published May, 2007. Accessed August 9, 2012.

101. World Health Organization. WHO report on the global tobacco epidemic, 2008—The MPOWER package. Geneva: World Health Organization. Available at: http://www.who.int/tobacco/mpower/2008/en/index.html. Published January 18, 2008. Accessed August 9, 2012.

102. Shenon P. New limits set over marketing for cigarettes. *New York Times.* August 18, 2006. Available at: http://www.nytimes.com/2006/08/18/washington/18tobacco.html. Accessed August 9, 2012.

103. Altria Group. Source watch. http://www.sourcewatch.org/index.php?title=Altria_Group. Updated July 10, 2012. Accessed August 9, 2012.

104. Schwartz J. Phillip Morris to change name to Altria. *New York Times.* November 16, 2001:A1.

105. Smith EA, Malone RE. Thinking the "unthinkable": why Philip Morris considered quitting. *Tob Control.* 2003;12(2):208–213.

106. Murray WR. The background. September 1990. Philip Morris. Available at: http://legacy.library.ucsf.edu/tid/fno24e00. Accessed August 9, 2012.

107. Dollisson J. Public affairs campaigning or reflections on the tobacco wars. October 15, 1990. Philip Morris. Available at: http://legacy.library.ucsf.edu/tid/rth46e00. Accessed August 9, 2012:19.

108. Notebook—GLS Plan. March 1990. Philip Morris. Available at: http://legacy.library.ucsf.edu/tid/nos65e00. Accessed August 9, 2012.

109. Smith EA, Malone RE. Thinking the "unthinkable": why Philip Morris considered quitting. *Tob Control.* 2003;12(2):208–213.

110. Brandt AM. *The Cigarette Century.* New York: Perseus; 2007.

111. Brandt AM. FDA regulation of tobacco—pitfalls and possibilities. *N Engl J Med.* 2008;359:445–448.

112. CDC. Cigarette smoking among adults and trends in smoking cessation—United States, 2008. *MMWR.*2009;58(44):1227–1232.

113. Cigarette Report for 2007 and2008. US Federal Trade Commission. Available at: http://www.ftc.gov/os/2011/07/110729cigarettereport.pdf. Published August 1, 2011. Accessed August 9, 2012.

114. *U.S. v. Philip Morris USA, Inc., et al.,* No. 99-CV-02496GK (U.S. Dist. Ct., D.C.), Final Opinion, August 17, 2006, available at: http://www.tobaccofreekids.org/reports/doj/FinalOpinion.pdf. Paragraph 3296.

115. Cigarette Reports for 2004 and 2005. US Federal Trade Commission. Available at: http://www.ftc.gov/reports/tobacco/2007cigarette2004-2005.pdf. Published April 26, 2007. Accessed August 9, 2012.

116. Navellier L. Light up with Reynolds, Americans' high dividend. *Investor Place.* December 28, 2011. http://www.investorplace.com/2011/12/reynolds-american-high-dividend-payout-rai/. Accessed August 9, 2012.

117. Altria Group Inc. (MO) profitability analysis. Stock analysis on the net. http://www.stock-analysis-on.net/NYSE/Company/Altria-Group-Inc/Ratios/Profitability. Accessed August 9, 2012.

118. World Health Organization. WHO Framework Convention on Tobacco Control. Geneva: World Health Organization. Available at: http://www.who.int/fctc/signatories_parties/en/index.html. Accessed December 24, 2012.

119. Sandoval Palos R. Smoke screen: Big Tobacco's global lobbying: the tobacco lobby goes global. *International Consortium of Investigative Journalists.* November 15, 2010. Available at: http://www.icij.org/project/smoke-screen-big-tobaccos-global-lobbying/tobacco-lobby-goes-global. Accessed August 9, 2012.

120. Anin R. Part One: Moscow's open revolving door for Big Tobacco. *International Consortium of Investigative Journalists.* November 15, 2010. Available at: http://www.icij.org/project/smoke-screen-big-tobaccos-global-lobbying/moscows-open-revolving-door-big-tobacco. Updated June 9, 2011. Accessed August 9, 2012.

121. Anin R. Part One: Moscow's open revolving door for Big Tobacco. *International Consortium of Investigative Journalists.* November 15, 2010. Available at: http://www.icij.org/project/smoke-screen-big-tobaccos-global-lobbying/moscows-open-revolving-door-big-tobacco. Updated June 9, 2011. Accessed August 9, 2012.

122. Anin R. Part One: Moscow's open revolving door for Big Tobacco. *International Consortium of Investigative Journalists.* November 15, 2010. Available at: http://www.icij.org/project/smoke-screen-big-tobaccos-global-lobbying/moscows-open-revolving-door-big-tobacco. Updated June 9, 2011. Accessed August 9, 2012.

123. Meyer H. Philip Morris, BAT, Japan Tobacco battle Putin's anti-smoke plan. Bloomberg.com. Available at: http://www.bloomberg.com/news/2012-05-31/philip-morris-bat-battle-putins-russian-smoking-crackdown.html. Published May 31, 2012. Accessed August 9, 2012.

124. Alpert LI. Kremlin cracks down on Big Tobacco. *Wall Street Journal.* October 16, 2012:B1.

125. Anin R. Part One: Moscow's open revolving door for Big Tobacco. *International Consortium of Investigative Journalists.* November 15, 2010. Available at: http://www.icij.org/project/smoke-screen-big-tobaccos-global-lobbying/moscows-open-revolving-door-big-tobacco. Updated June 9, 2011. Accessed August 9, 2012.

126. Von Bertrab AX, Gutierrez J. Smoke screen: Big Tobacco's global lobbying: A troubled model for reform in Mexico. *International Consortium of Investigative Journalists.* November 15, 2010. Available at: http://www.icij.org/project/smoke-screen-big-tobaccos-global-lobbying/troubled-model-reform-mexico. Accessed August 9, 2012.

127. Von Bertrab AX, Gutierrez J. Smoke screen: Big Tobacco's global lobbying: A troubled model for reform in Mexico. *International Consortium of Investigative Journalists.* November 15, 2010. Available at: http://www.icij.org/project/smoke-screen-big-tobaccos-global-lobbying/troubled-model-reform-mexico. Accessed August 9, 2012.

128. Von Bertrab AX, Gutierrez J. Smoke screen: Big Tobacco's global lobbying: A troubled model for reform in Mexico. *International Consortium of Investigative Journalists.* November 15, 2010. Available at: http://www.icij.org/project/smoke-screen-big-tobaccos-global-lobbying/troubled-model-reform-mexico. Accessed August 9, 2012.

129. Von Bertrab AX, Gutierrez J. Smoke screen: Big Tobacco's global lobbying: A troubled model for reform in Mexico. *International Consortium of Investigative Journalists.* November 15, 2010. Available at: http://www.icij.org/project/smoke-screen-big-tobaccos-global-lobbying/troubled-model-reform-mexico. Accessed August 9, 2012.

130. Von Bertrab AX, Gutierrez J. Smoke screen: Big Tobacco's global lobbying: A troubled model for reform in Mexico. *International Consortium of Investigative Journalists.* November 15, 2010. Available at: http://www.icij.org/project/smoke-screen-big-tobaccos-global-lobbying/troubled-model-reform-mexico. Accessed August 9, 2012.

131. Von Bertrab AX, Gutierrez J. Smoke screen: Big Tobacco's global lobbying: A troubled model for reform in Mexico. *International Consortium of Investigative Journalists.* November 15, 2010. Available at: http://www.icij.org/project/smoke-screen-big-tobaccos-global-lobbying/troubled-model-reform-mexico. Accessed August 9, 2012.

132. Von Bertrab AX, Gutierrez J. Smoke screen: Big Tobacco's global lobbying: A troubled model for reform in Mexico. *International Consortium of Investigative Journalists.* November

15, 2010. Available at: http://www.icij.org/project/smoke-screen-big-tobaccos-global-lobbying/troubled-model-reform-mexico. Accessed August 9, 2012.

133. Paolillo C. Smoke screen: Big Tobacco's global lobbying: Uruguay vs. Philip Morris. *International Consortium of Investigative Journalists.* November 15, 2010. http://www.icij.org/project/smoke-screen-big-tobaccos-global-lobbying/uruguay-vs-philip-morris. Accessed August 9, 2012.

134. Paolillo C. Smoke screen: Big Tobacco's global lobbying: Uruguay vs. Philip Morris. *International Consortium of Investigative Journalists.* November 15, 2010. http://www.icij.org/project/smoke-screen-big-tobaccos-global-lobbying/uruguay-vs-philip-morris. Accessed August 9, 2012.

135. Wilson D. Cigarette giants in global fight on tighter rules. *New York Times.* November 14, 2010:A1.

136. Baier SL, Bergstrand JH, Eggers P. The new regionalism: causes and consequences. *Economie Internationale* 2007:1(109):9–29.

137. Bloomberg M. Tobacco industry targets Uruguay's gold standard anti-tobacco laws. MikeBloomberg.com. Available at: http://www.mikebloomberg.com/index.cfm?objectid=5146E113-C29C-7CA2-FE0158F94D33A02E. Published November 15, 2010. Accessed August 9, 2012.

138. Baldomir L. Philip Morris closes Uruguay plant, affecting 62 employees. Bloomberg.com. October 21, 2011. http://www.bloomberg.com/news/2011-10-21/philip-morris-closes-uruguay-plant-affecting-62-employees.html. Accessed August 9, 2012.

139. Friends of the Earth Uruguay. *It Could Have Been Avoided.* RadioMundo July 12, 2013. Available at http://radiomundoreal.fm/6906-it-could-have-been-avoided?lang=es Accessed on July 25, 2013.

140. Harsono A. Public health suffers as Indonesia ignores calls for tobacco reform. *iWatch News,* Center for Public Integrity. September 9, 2011. http://www.iwatchnews.org/2011/09/09/6062/public-health-suffers-indonesia-ignores-calls-tobacco-reform. Accessed August 9, 2012.

141. Country profile: Indonesia. Philip Morris International website. Available at: http://www.PhilipMorrisi.com/marketpages/pages/market_en_id.aspx. Accessed August 9, 2012.

142. Deutsch A. Philip Morris faces tougher rules in Indonesia. *Financial Times.* August 11, 2010. Available at: http://www.ft.com/intl/cms/s/0/ec2521fe-a498-11df-8c9f-00144feabdc0.html#axzz234y040Td. Accessed August 9, 2012.

143. Meyersohn D, Harris D. From age 2 to 7: why are children smoking in Indonesia? *20/20,* ABC News. September 9, 2011. Available at: http://abcnews.go.com/Health/age-children-smoking-indonesia/story?id=14464140#.TyQUf4Hg2do. Accessed August 9, 2012.

144. Williams CT, Grier SA, Marks AS. "Coming to town": the impact of urbanicity, cigarette advertising, and network norms on the smoking attitudes of black women in Cape Town, South Africa. *J Urban Health.* 2008;85(4):472–485.

145. Amosa A, Haglund BM. From social taboo to "torch of freedom": the marketing of cigarettes to women. *Tob Control.* 2000;9:3–8. doi:10.1136/tc.9.1.3.

146. World Health Organization. WHO Global Infobase: Tobacco Use Prevalence, South Africa. Available at https://apps.who.int/infobase/Indicators.aspx. Accessed August 9, 2012.

147. World Health Organization. Global Health Observatory: World Health Statistics 2012. Available at: http://www.who.int/gho/publications/world_health_statistics/2012/en/index.html. Accessed August 9, 2012.

148. Dawson DA, Grant BF. The "gray area" of consumption between moderate and risk drinking. *J Stud Alcohol Drugs.* 2011;72(3):453–458.

149. Mukamal KJ, Rimm EB. Alcohol consumption: risks and benefits. *Curr Atheroscler Rep.* 2008 Dec;10(6):536–43.

150. Lim SS, Vos T, Flaxman AD, Danaei G, Shibuya K, Adair-Rohani H, et al. A comparative risk assessment of burden of disease and injury attributable to 67 risk factors and risk factor clusters in 21 regions, 1990–2010: a systematic analysis for the Global Burden of Disease Study 2010. *Lancet.* 2013;380(9859):2224–2260.

151. Lim SS, Vos T, Flaxman AD, Danaei G, Shibuya K, Adair-Rohani H, et al. A comparative risk assessment of burden of disease and injury attributable to 67 risk factors and risk factor clusters in 21 regions, 1990–2010: a systematic analysis for the Global Burden of Disease Study 2010. *Lancet.* 2013;380(9859):2224–2260.

152. Rehm J, Mathers C, Popova S, Thavorncharoensap M, Teerawattananon Y, Patra J. Global burden of disease and injury and economic cost attributable to alcohol use and alcohol-use disorders. *Lancet.* 2009;373(9682):2223–2233.

153. McKee M, Shkolnikov V, Leon DA. Alcohol is implicated in the fluctuations in cardiovascular disease in Russia since the 1980s. *Ann Epidemiol.* 2001;11(1):1–6.

154. Brewer B. Public health impact of excess drinking. Centers for Disease Control and Prevention. 2012. Available at: http://www.cdc.gov/about/grand-rounds/archives/2012/pdfs/GR_Alcohol_ALL_FINAL_Mar21.pdf Accessed on December 24, 2012.

155. Bouchery EE, Harwood HJ, Sacks JJ, Simon CJ, Brewer RD. Economic costs of excessive alcohol consumption in the U.S., 2006. *Am J Prev Med.* 2011;41(5):516–524.

156. Alcohol and Public Health: Alcohol-Related Disease Impact (ARDI). Centers for Disease Control and Prevention. Available at: http://apps.nccd.cdc.gov/DACH_ARDI/Default/Default.aspx. Accessed August 10, 2012.

157. Jernigan D. Alcohol Marketing as a Risk Factor for Underage Drinking. Centers for Disease Control and Prevention. Available at: http://www.cdc.gov/about/grand-rounds/archives/2012/pdfs/GR_Alcohol_ALL_FINAL_Mar21.pdf Accessed on December 24, 2012.

158. Boffetta P, Hashibe M. Alcohol and cancer. *Lancet Oncol.* 2006;7(2):149–156.

159. Rehm J, Mathers C, Popova S, Thavorncharoensap M, Teerawattananon Y, Patra J. Global burden of disease and injury and economic cost attributable to alcohol use and alcohol-use disorders. *Lancet.* 2009;373(9682):2223–2233.

160. Rehm J, Baliunas D, Borges GL, Graham K, Irving H, Kehoe T, et al. The relation between different dimensions of alcohol consumption and burden of disease: an overview. *Addiction.* 2010;105(5):817–843.

161. Jernigan DH. The global alcohol industry: an overview. *Addiction.* 2009;104(Suppl 1):6–12.

162. Jernigan DH. The global alcohol industry: an overview. *Addiction.* 2009;104(Suppl 1):6–12.

163. De La Merced M, Scott M. Anheuser-Busch InBev Buys Rest of Grupo Modelo, Maker of Corona Beer. *Dealbook,* NYTimes.com. Available at: http://dealbook.nytimes.com/2012/06/29/the-beer-wars-heat-up-with-modelo-deal/. Published June 29, 2012. Accessed August 12, 2012.

164. Jernigan DH. The global alcohol industry: an overview. *Addiction.* 2009;104(Suppl 1):6–12.

165. Lopes TDS. The growth and survival of multinationals in the global alcoholic beverages industry. *Enterprise Society.* 2003;4:592–598.

166. Jernigan D. The extent of global alcohol marketing and its impact on youth. *Contemporary Drug Problems.* 2010;37:57–89.

167. Smith LA, Foxcroft DR. The effect of alcohol advertising, marketing and portrayal on drinking behaviour in young people: systematic review of prospective cohort studies. *BMC Public Health.* 2009;9:51.

168. Foster SE, Vaughan RD, Foster WH, Califano JA Jr. Estimate of the commercial value of underage drinking and adult abusive and dependent drinking to the alcohol industry. *Arch Pediatr Adolesc Med.* 2006;160(5):473–478.

169. Foster SE, Vaughan RD, Foster WH, Califano JA Jr. Estimate of the commercial value of underage drinking and adult abusive and dependent drinking to the alcohol industry. *Arch Pediatr Adolesc Med.* 2006;160(5):473–478.

170. Mosher JF. Joe Camel in a bottle: Diageo, the Smirnoff brand, and the transformation of the youth alcohol market. *Am J Public Health.* 2012;102(1):56–63.

171. Schettler, R. New kick on the block: will spiked lemonades pick up where wine coolers left off? *Washington Post.* September 13, 2000:F01.

172. Statement of George A. Hacker, Director, Alcohol Policies Project, CSPI. Presented at: Center for Science in the Public Interest Press Conference on the Marketing of "Alcopops"

to Teens. May 9, 2001. Available at: http://www.cspinet.org/booze/alcopops_statement. htm. Accessed August 10, 2012.

173. Mosher JF. Joe Camel in a bottle: Diageo, the Smirnoff brand, and the transformation of the youth alcohol market. *Am J Public Health.* 2012;102(1):56–63.

174. Alcopops: Summary of findings. What teens and adults are saying about alcopops. Center for Science in the Public Interest. Available at: www.cspinet.org/booze/alcopops_summary. htm. Published May 2001. Accessed August 10, 2012.

175. Jernigan DH, Ostroff J, Ross C, O'Hara JA 3rd. Sex differences in adolescent exposure to alcohol advertising in magazines. *Arch Pediatr Adolesc Med.* 2004;158(7):629–634.

176. McClure AC, Stoolmiller M, Tanski SE, Engels RC, Sargent JD. Alcohol marketing receptivity, marketing-specific cognitions, and underage binge drinking. *Alcohol Clin Exp Res.* 2012 Dec 19. doi: 10.1111/j.1530-0277.

177. National Institute on Alcohol Abuse and Alcoholism (NIAAA), National Institutes of Health. Alcohol—An Important Women's Health Issue, NIH Publication No. 03–4956. Washington, D.C: US Dept. of Health and Human Services; July 2004, revised 2008. Available at: http://pubs.niaaa.nih.gov/publications/brochurewomen/women.htm. Accessed August 10, 2012.

178. Johnston AD. "Pinking" the wine and spirits market: When did the alcohol market become so sweet and squishy? *Toronto Star.* November 21, 2011:A1.

179. Johnston AD. "Pinking" the wine and spirits market: When did the alcohol market become so sweet and squishy? *Toronto Star.* November 21, 2011:A1.

180. Popova S, Giesbrecht N, Bekmuradov D, Patra J. Hours and days of sale and density of alcohol outlets: impacts on alcohol consumption and damage: a systematic review. *Alcohol.* 2009;44(5):500–516.

181. Erickson P. The high cost of cheap alcohol. Campaign for a Healthy Alcohol Marketplace. Available at: http://www.healthyalcoholmarket.com/pdf/HighCostFinalP.pdf. Published April 17, 2011. Accessed August 10, 2012.

182. Elder RW, Lawrence B, Ferguson A, Naimi TS, Brewer RD, Chattopadhyay SK, et al. The effectiveness of tax policy interventions for reducing excessive alcohol consumption and related harms. *Am J Prev Med.* 2010;38(2):217–229.

183. SAB Miller. Tackle tax havens, Tax Justice Programme. Available at: http://www.tackletax-havens.com/the-problems/sabmiller/. Accessed August 14, 2012.

184. Health Promotion Agency Establishment Board announced [press release]. New Zealand Governmental website: November 17, 2011. Available at: http://www.beehive.govt.nz/release/health-promotion-agency-establishment-board-announced. Accessed August 14, 2012.

185. UK Government proposes deal with drinks industry to tackle alcohol harm. *Globe* (London); 2011;1:5. Available at: http://www.eurocare.org/library/eurocare_updates/uk_government_proposes_deal_with_drinks_industry_to_tackle_alcohol_harm. Accessed August 14, 2012.

186. Jernigan DH. The global alcohol industry: an overview. *Addiction.* 2009;104 (Suppl 1):6–12.

187. Smith SW, Atkin CK, Roznowski J. Are "Drink responsibly" alcohol campaigns strategically ambiguous? *Health Commun.* 2006;20(1):1–11.

188. World Health Organization. Global status report on alcohol and health. Geneva: World Health Organization. Available at: http://www.who.int/substance_abuse/publications/global_alcohol_report/msbgsruprofiles.pdf, p. 8. Published 2011. Accessed August 14, 2012.

189. LaVallee R, Yi HY. Apparent Per Capita Alcohol Consumption: National, State and Regional Trends, 1977–2009, Surveillance Report no. 92. U.S. Department of Health and Human Services, National Institute on Alcohol Abuse and Alcoholism. Available at: http://pubs. niaaa.nih.gov/publications/Surveillance92/CONS09.htm. Published August 2011. Accessed August 14, 2012.

190. CBS News and Associated Press. Marijuana use up, alcohol use down among U.S. teens: Report. *CBS News Healthpop.* December 14, 2011. Available at: http://www.cbsnews.

com/8301-504763_162-7343099091704/marijuana-use-up-alcohol-use-down-among-u.s-teens-report/. Accessed August 14, 2012.

191. World Health Organization. WHO expert committee on problems related to alcohol consumption, Geneva, 10–13 October 2006. 2nd report. WHO Report Technical Series no. 944. Geneva: World Health Organization. Available at: http://www.who.int/substance_abuse/expert_committee_alcohol_trs944.pdf. Published 2007. Accessed August 14, 2012.

192. Mosher JF, Johnsson D. Flavored alcoholic beverages: an international marketing campaign that targets youth. *J Public Health Policy*. 2005;26(3):326–342.

193. Mart SM. Alcohol marketing in the 21st century: new methods, old problems. *Subst Use Misuse*. 2011;46(7):889–892.

194. European Centre for Monitoring Alcohol Marketing (EUCAM). Trends in alcohol marketing: Women—the new market. Utrecht, Netherlands: EUCAM. Available at: http://www.eucam.info/eucam/home/trends_in_alcohol_marketing.html. Published February 2008. Accessed August 14, 2012.

195. Crummy M. Chinese continue thirst for international brands. *The Drinks Business*. May 4, 2012. Available at: http://www.thedrinksbusiness.com/2012/05/chinese-alcohol-market-reality-checks/. Accessed August 14, 2012.

Chapter 2 The Public Health Evidence: How Corporate Practices Contribute to Global Epidemics of Chronic Disease and Injuries

1. UN launches global campaign to curb death toll from non-communicable diseases [press release]. United Nations News Center: September 19, 2011. Available at: http://www.un.org/apps/news/story.asp?NewsID=39600&Cr=non-communicable+diseases&Cr1. Accessed August 10, 2012.

2. Cohen D. Will industry influence derail UN summit? *BMJ*. 2011;343:d5328. doi: 10.1136/bmj.d5328.

3. World Health Organization. 2008–2013 Action Plan for the Global Strategy for the Prevention and Control of Noncommunicable Diseases. Geneva: World Health Organization. Available at: http://whqlibdoc.who.int/publications/2009/9789241597418_eng.pdf. Published 2008. Accessed August 10, 2012.

4. Bloom DE, Cafiero ET, Jané-Llopis E, et al. The Global Economic Burden of Noncommunicable Diseases. Geneva: World Economic Forum. Available at: www.weforum.org/EconomicsOfNCD. Published September, 2011. Accessed August 10, 2012.

5. Chan M. Speech of WHO Director General at the NCD Summit, New York. Available at: http://www.seatca.org/index.php?option=com_content&view=article&id=1014:speech-of-who-director-general-at-the-ncd-summit-new-york&catid=3:international-updates&Itemid=66. Published September 19, 2011. Accessed August 10, 2012.

6. Bloom DE, Cafiero ET, Jané-Llopis E, et al. The Global Economic Burden of Noncommunicable Diseases. Geneva: World Economic Forum. Available at: www.weforum.org/EconomicsOfNCD. Published September, 2011. Accessed August 10, 2012.

7. Freid VM, Bernstein AB, Bush MA. Multiple chronic conditions among adults aged 45 and over: trends over the past 10 years. NCHS Data Brief No. 100, Hyattsville, MD: National Center for Health Statistics; 2012.

8. Tackling the burden of chronic diseases in the USA. *Lancet*. 2009;373(9659):185. doi:10.1016/S0140-6736(09)60048-9.

9. Bodenheimer T, Chen E, Bennett HD. Confronting the growing burden of chronic disease: can the U.S. health care workforce do the job? *Health Aff (Millwood)*. 2009;28(1):64–74.

10. Chronic Diseases: The Power to Prevent, the Call to Control: At a Glance, 2009. Centers for Disease Control and Prevention. Available at: http://www.cdc.gov/chronicdisease/resources/publications/AAG/chronic.htm. Updated December 17, 2009. Accessed August 10, 2012.

11. New mindset needed to tackle non-communicable diseases, says UN official. UN News Service. Available at: http://www.un.org/apps/news/story.asp?NewsID=40950&Cr=non_communicable+disease&Cr1=. Published January 16, 2012. Accessed August 10, 2012.

12. World Health Organization. Declaration of Alma-Ata, International Conference on Primary Health Care, Alma-Ata, USSR, September 6–12, 1978. Available at: http://www.who.int/publications/almaata_declaration_en.pdf. Accessed August 10, 2012.

13. U.S. Department of Health and Human Services. *Healthy People 2010: Understanding and Improving Health.* 2nd ed. Washington, DC: U.S. Dept. of Health and Human Services; 2000.

14. Ogden C, Carroll G. Prevalence of overweight, obesity, and extreme obesity among adults: United States, trends 1960–1962 through 2007–2008. Centers for Disease Control and Prevention. Available at: http://www.cdc.gov/NCHS/data/hestat/obesity_adult_07_08/obesity_adult_07_08.pdf. Published June, 2010. Accessed August 10, 2012.

15. Ogden C, Carroll M, Curtin L, Lamb M, Flegal K. Prevalence of high body mass index in U.S. children and adolescents, 2007–2008. *JAMA.* 2010;303(3):242–249.

16. Wang YC, McPherson K, Marsh T, Gortmaker SL, Brown M. Health and economic burden of the projected obesity trends in the U.S.A. and the U.K. *Lancet.* 2011;378(9793): 815–825.

17. *The Weight of the Nation, Part 1: Consequences.* HBO Films and the Institutes of Medicine. 2012. Available at: http://theweightofthenation.hbo.com/. Accessed August 14, 2012.

18. Diabetes: Successes and Opportunities for Population-Based Prevention and Control at a Glance, 2011. Centers for Disease Control and Prevention. Available at:http://www.cdc.gov/chronicdisease/resources/publications/AAG/ddt.htm. Updated August 1, 2011. Accessed August 10, 2012.

19. Olshansky SJ, Passaro DJ, Hershow RC, et al. A potential decline in life expectancy in the United States in the 21st century. *N Engl J Med.* 2005;352(11):1138–1145.

20. Robert Wood Johnson Foundation. Declining childhood obesity rates—where are we seeing the most progress? *Health Policy Snapshot Issue Brief,* September 2012.

21. Pan L, Blanck HM, Sherry B, Dalenius K, Grummer-Strawn LM. Trends in the prevalence of extreme obesity among U.S. preschool-aged children living in low-income families, 1998–2010. *JAMA.* 2012;308(24):2563–2565.

22. Mathers CD, Loncar D. Projections of global mortality and burden of disease from 2002 to 2030. *PLoS Med.* 2006;3(11):e442.

23. Mathers CD, Loncar D. Projections of global mortality and burden of disease from 2002 to 2030. *PLoS Med.* 2006;3(11):e442.

24. Peden M, Scurfield R, Sleet D, Mohan D, Hyder A, Jarawan E, et al., eds. World Report on Road Traffic Injury Prevention. Geneva: World Health Organization. Available at: http://whqlibdoc.who.int/publications/2004/9241562609.pdf. Published 2004. Accessed August 10, 2012.

25. Viner RM, Coffey C, Mathers C, Bloem P, Costello A, Santelli J, et al. 50-year mortality trends in children and young people: a study of 50 low-income, middle-income, and high-income countries. *Lancet.* 2011;377(9772):1162–1174.

26. National Center for Health Statistics. Health, United States, 2010: With Special Feature on Death and Dying. Hyattsville, MD: U.S. Dept. of Health and Human Services; 2011. Available at:http://www.cdc.gov/nchs/data/hus/hus10.pdf. Accessed August 10, 2012.

27. Harper S, Lynch J, Burris S, Davey Smith G. Trends in the black-white life expectancy gap in the United States, 1983–2003. *JAMA.* 2007; 297(11):1224–1232.

28. Williams DR. Race, socioeconomic status, and health. The added effects of racism and discrimination. *Ann NY Acad Sci.* 1999;896:173–188.

29. Shrestha L. Life expectancy in the United States. Washington, D.C.: Congressional Research Service. August 16, 2006. Available at: http://aging.senate.gov/crs/aging1.pdf. Accessed August 10, 2012.

30. Freid VM, Bernstein AB, Bush MA. Multiple chronic conditions among adults aged 45 and over: Trends over the past 10 years. NCHS Data Brief No. 100, Hyattsville, MD: National Center for Health Statistics; 2012.

31. National Resarch Council and Institute of Medicine. U.S. Health in International Perspective:Shorter Lives, Poorer Health. Panel on Understanding Cross-National Health Differences Among High Income Countries. Washington, D.C.: National Academies Press, 2013.

32. Keehan SP, Sisko AM, Truffer CJ, et al. National health spending projections through 2020: economic recovery and reform drive faster spending growth. *Health Aff (Millwood)*. 2011;30(8):1594–1605.

33. Schoen C, Osborn R, How SK, Doty MM, Peugh J. In chronic condition: experiences of patients with complex health care needs, in eight countries, 2008. *Health Aff (Millwood)*. 2009;28(1):w1–w16.

34. Anderson GF, Poullier JP. Health spending, access, and outcomes: trends in industrialized countries. *Health Aff (Millwood)*. 1999;18(3):178–192.

35. Katz D. It does, indeed, take a village: schools, families, and beyond for weight control in children. *Childhood Obesity*. 2010;6(4): 184–192. doi:10.1089/chi.2010.0416.

36. TODAY Study Group, Zeitler P, Hirst K, et al. A clinical trial to maintain glycemic control in youth with type 2 diabetes. *N Engl J Med*. 2012;366(24):2247–2256.

37. Lindbäck SM, Gabbert C, Johnson BL, et al. Pediatric nonalcoholic fatty liver disease: a comprehensive review. *Adv Pediatr*. 2010;57(1):85–140.

38. Stuckler D. Population causes and consequences of leading chronic diseases: a comparative analysis of prevailing explanations. *Milbank Q*. 2008;86(2):273–326.

39. . McMichael AJ, Campbell-Lendrum DH, Corvalán CF, Ebi KL, Githeko A, Scheraga JD, et al., eds. Climate Change and Human Health: Risks and Responses. Geneva: World Health Organization; 2003. Available at: http://www.who.int/globalchange/publications/cchh-book/en/. Accessed August 14, 2012.

40. Pope CA 3rd. The expanding role of air pollution in cardiovascular disease: does air pollution contribute to risk of deep vein thrombosis? *Circulation*. 2009;119(24):3050–3052.

41. Cohen AJ, Anderson HR, Ostro B, Pandey KD, Krzyzanowski M, Kuenzli N, et al., eds. *Comparative Quantification of Health Risks: Global and Regional Burden of Disease Due to Selected Major Risk Factors*, Vol. 2. Geneva: World Health Organization; 2004: 1353–1433.

42. Lim SS, Vos T, Flaxman AD, Danaei G, Shibuya K, Adair-Rohani H, et al. A comparative risk assessment of burden of disease and injury attributable to 67 risk factors and risk factor clusters in 21 regions, 1990–2010: a systematic analysis for the Global Burden of Disease Study 2010. *Lancet*. 2013;380(9859):2224–2260.

43. Pope CA 3rd. The expanding role of air pollution in cardiovascular disease: does air pollution contribute to risk of deep vein thrombosis? *Circulation*. 2009;119(24):3050–3052.

44. Yim SH, Barrett SR. Public health impacts of combustion emissions in the United Kingdom. *Environ Sci Technol*. 2012;46(8):4291–4296.

45. Mitka M. Studies probe U.S. traffic injuries, deaths: focus on factors that reduce, exacerbate toll. *JAMA*. 2009;302(11):1159–11560.

46. Mathers CD, Loncar D. Projections of global mortality and burden of disease from 2002 to 2030. *PLoS Med*. 2006;3(11):e442.

47. UN Road Safety Collaboration. Global Plan for the Decade of Action for Road Safety 2011–2020. New York: United Nations, 2010.

48. Douglas MJ, Watkins SJ, Gorman DR, Higgins M. Are cars the new tobacco? *J Public Health* (Oxon). 2011;33(2):160–169.

49. Norton PD. *Fighting Traffic: The Dawn of the Motor Age in the American City*. Cambridge, MA: MIT Press, 2008.

50. Kohl HW 3rd, Craig CL, Lambert EV, Inoue S, Alkandari JR, Leetongin G, Kahlmeier S; Lancet Physical Activity Series Working Group. The pandemic of physical inactivity: global action for public health. *Lancet*. 2012;380(9838):294–305.

51. Tranter PJ. Speed kills: the complex links between transport, lack of time and urban health. *J Urban Health*. 2010;87(2):155–166.

52. Doyle J. *Taken for a Ride: Detroit's Big Three and the Politics of Pollution*. New York: Four Walls Eight Windows, 2000.

53. Bradsher K. *High and Mighty SUVs: The World's Most Dangerous Vehicles and How They Got That Way.* New York: Public Affairs; 2002:88.

54. Bradsher K. *High and Mighty SUVs: The World's Most Dangerous Vehicles and How They Got That Way.* New York: Public Affairs; 2002.

55. Bradsher K. *High and Mighty SUVs: The World's Most Dangerous Vehicles and How They Got That Way.* New York: Public Affairs; 2002:95.

56. Environmental Protection Agency. *40 CFR 86—Control of Emissions from New and In-Use Highway Vehicles and Engines.* Amended June 14, 2005. Available at: http://law.justia.com/cfr/title40/40-18.0.1.1.1.html. Accessed August 14, 2012.

57. Bradsher K. *High and Mighty SUVs: The World's Most Dangerous Vehicles and How They Got That Way.* New York: Public Affairs; 2002.

58. Ramsey M, Terlep S. We still love SUVs: Trucks drive auto sales growth in U.S. *Wall Street Journal.* December 2, 2011. http://blogs.wsj.com/drivers-seat/2011/12/02/we-still-love-suvs-trucks-drive-auto-sales-growth-in-u-s/. Accessed August 14, 2012.

59. Public Citizen. *Risking America's Health and Safety: George Bush and the Task Force on Regulatory Relief.* Washington, D.C.: Public Citizen, 1988. Available at: http://www.citizen.org/documents/risking-americas-health-and-safety.pdf. Accessed August 14, 2012.

60. Vlasic B. Chrysler rejects regulator's request to recall Jeeps. *New York Times,* June 5, 2013, pp. B1 and B5.

61. Tang R. The Rise of China's Auto Industry and Its Impact on the U.S. Motor Vehicle Industry, 7-5700, R40924. Washington, D.C.: Congressional Research Service; November 16, 2009. Available at: http://www.fas.org/sgp/crs/row/R40924.pdf. Accessed August 14, 2012.

62. China's auto industry caught in dilemma. *Xinhua News.* February 17, 2011. Available at: http://news.xinhuanet.com/english2010/business/2011-07/17/c_13990714.htm. Accessed August 14, 2012.

63. Latin America: The Fastest Growing Latin American Industries for 2013–2015. Global Intelligence Alliance. April 26, 2012. Available at: http://www.globalintelligence.com/insights-analysis/bulletins/the-fastest-growing-latin-american-industries-for-/#ixzz22OM4joRT. Accessed August 14, 2012.

64. Indian automotive industry growing from strength to strength. *Times of India.* December 11, 2010. Available at: http://articles.timesofindia.indiatimes.com/2010-12-11/india-business/28228767_1_exports-of-passenger-cars-indian-automobile-manufacturers-growth-story. Accessed August 14, 2012.

65. Loffredo M, Arruda C, Loffredo L de C. Mortality rate in children caused by traffic accidents according to geographical regions: Brazil, 1997–2005. *Rev Bras Epidemiol.* 2012;15(2):308–314.

66. Confino J. Car manufacturers accused of lower safety standards in Latin America. *Guardian,* July 24, 2013. Available at: http://www.theguardian.com/sustainable-business/blog/car-manufacturers-criticised-safety-latin-america/. Accessed on August 3, 2013.

67. Leland A, Oboroceanu MJ. American War and Military Operations Casualties: Lists and Statistics. Congressional Research Service. Available at: http://www.fas.org/sgp/crs/natsec/RL32492.pdf. Published February 26, 2010. Accessed August 9, 2012.

68. Ringuette A. NRA must drop its campaign of lies against U.N. Global Arms Trade Treaty. Amnesty International press release, December 2012. Available at http://www.amnestyusa.org/news/press-releases/nra-must-drop-its-campaign-of-lies-against-un-global-arms-trade-treaty. Accessed on December 28,2012

69. Hemenway D. *Private Guns, Public Health.* Ann Arbor, MI: University of Michigan Press; 2004.

70. *Frontline.* Hot guns: interview with Jim Waldorf. PBS.org. June 3, 1997. http://www.pbs.org/wgbh/pages/frontline/shows/guns/interviews/waldorf.html. Accessed August 9, 2012.

71. Freedman A. Fire power: behind the cheap guns flooding the U.S. cities is a California family. *Wall Street Journal.* March 9, 1992:1.

72. Hot guns: interview with Jim Waldorf [transcript]. *Frontline.* PBS.org. June 3, 1997. Available at: http://www.pbs.org/wgbh/pages/frontline/shows/guns/interviews/waldorf.html. Accessed August 9, 2012.

73. Freedman A. Fire power: Behind the cheap guns flooding the U.S. cities is a California family. *Wall Street Journal.* March 9, 1992:1.

74. Hot guns: interview with Jim Waldorf [transcript]. *Frontline.* PBS.org. June 3, 1997. Available at: http://www.pbs.org/wgbh/pages/frontline/shows/guns/interviews/waldorf.html. Accessed August 9, 2012.

75. Hot guns: interview with Jim Waldorf [transcript]. *Frontline.* PBS.org. June 3, 1997. Available at: http://www.pbs.org/wgbh/pages/frontline/shows/guns/interviews/waldorf.html. Accessed August 9, 2012.

76. Freedman A. Fire power: behind the cheap guns flooding the U.S. cities is a California family. *Wall Street Journal.* March 9, 1992:1.

77. Levin M. Legal claims get costly for maker of cheap handguns. *Los Angeles Times.* December 27, 1997. http://articles.latimes.com/1997/dec/27/news/mn-2618. Accessed August 9, 2012.

78. Hot guns: interview with BATF agent Daryl McRary [transcript]. *Frontline.* PBS.org. June 3, 1997. Available at: http://www.pbs.org/wgbh/pages/frontline/shows/guns/etc/script.html. Accessed August 9, 2012.

79. Hot guns: interview with Jim Waldorf [transcript]. *Frontline.* PBS.org. June 3, 1997. Available at: http://www.pbs.org/wgbh/pages/frontline/shows/guns/interviews/waldorf.html. Accessed August 9, 2012.

80. Freedman A. Fire power: behind the cheap guns flooding the U.S. cities is a California family. *Wall Street Journal.* March 9, 1992:1.

81. Levin M. Legal claims get costly for maker of cheap handguns. *Los Angeles Times.* December 27, 1997. Available at: http://articles.latimes.com/1997/dec/27/news/mn-2618. Accessed August 9, 2012.

82. Hot guns: interview with Jim Waldorf [transcript]. *Frontline.* PBS.org. June 3, 1997. Available at: http://www.pbs.org/wgbh/pages/frontline/shows/guns/interviews/waldorf.html. Accessed August 9, 2012.

83. ATF Youth Crime Gun Interdiction Initiative. Crime gun trace reports (1999). Washington, DC: Bureau of Alcohol, Tobacco and Firearms. Available at: http://www.atf.gov/publications/download/ycgii/1999/ycgii-report-1999-highlights.pdf. Accessed August 9, 2012.

84. Hot guns: interview with Jim Waldorf [transcript]. *Frontline.* PBS.org. June 3, 1997. Available at: http://www.pbs.org/wgbh/pages/frontline/shows/guns/interviews/waldorf.html. Accessed August 9, 2012.

85. Hot guns: interview with Garen Wintemute [transcript]. *Frontline.* PBS.org. June 3, 1997. Available at: http://www.pbs.org/wgbh/pages/frontline/shows/guns/interviews/wintemute.html. Accessed August 9, 2012.

86. Levin M. Legal claims get costly for maker of cheap handguns. *Los Angeles Times.* December 27, 1997. http://articles.latimes.com/1997/dec/27/news/mn-2618

87. Law Center to Prevent Gun Violence. Regulating Guns in America: An Evaluation and Comparative Analysis of Federal, State, and Selected Local Gun Laws. 2008. Available at: http://smartgunlaws.org/regulating-guns-in-america-an-evaluation-and-comparative-analysis-of-federal-state-and-selected-local-gun-laws/. Accessed on 18 March 2013.

88. Freedman A. Fire power: behind the cheap guns flooding the U.S. cities is a California family. *Wall Street Journal.* March 9, 1992:1.

89. Diaz T. *Making a Killing: The Business of Guns in America.* New York: New Press; 1999.

90. Barrett PM. *Glock: The Rise of America's Gun.* New York: Crown;2012.

91. McIntire M, Luo M. Gun makers saw no role in curbing improper sales. *New York Times,* May 28, 2013, pp. A1 and A12.

92. Business Wire. Research and Markets: U.S. Gun Manufacturing Report: Highly concentrated industry with companies such as Browning, Sturm and S&W and combined annual revenue of $3 billion. *Daily Finance.* September 22, 2010. http://www.dailyfinance.com/

rtn/pr/research-and-markets-us-gun-manufacturing-report-highly-concentrated-industry-with-companies-such-as-browning-sturm-and-sandw-and-combined-annual-revenue-of-3-billion/rfid369766493/. Accessed August 9, 2012.

93. Ibis World Guns & Ammunition Manufacturing in the U.S.: Market Research Report. NAICS 33299a | Apr 2012. Available at http://www.ibisworld.com/industry/default.aspx?indid=662. Accessed August 9, 2012.

94. Jacobs JB. *Can Gun Control Work?* New York: Oxford University Press; 2002.

95. Hemenway D. *Private Guns, Public Health.* Ann Arbor, MI: University of Michigan Press; 2004.

96. Singer N. How Freedom Group became the big shot. *New York Times.* November 27, 2011:BU1.

97. Singer N. How Freedom Group became the big shot. *New York Times,* November 27, 2011: BU1.

98. Gray M. Bushmaster.223: Weapon used in Newtown shooting a lightning rod in gun debate. *Time.* December 19, 2012. Available at http://newsfeed.time.com/2012/12/19/bushmaster-223-weapon-used-in-newtown-shooting-a-lightning-rod-in-gun-debate/#ixzz2GAlfHTMa. Accessed on December 27, 2012.

99. Singer N. How Freedom Group became the big shot. *New York Times,* November 27, 2011: BU1.

100. Singer N. How Freedom Group became the big shot. *New York Times,* November 27, 2011: BU1.

101. Annual Report for the fiscal year ended: December 31, 2011. Freedom Group, Inc. Available at: http://www.freedom-group.com/2011_10-K.pdf. Published March 29, 2012. Accessed August 9, 2012.

102. Landler M, Taylor P. "These tragedies must end," Obama says. *New York Times.* December 17, 2012:A1.

103. Robbins L, Goldstein J. Gunman Who Killed 2 Firefighters Left Chilling Note. *New York Times,* December 26, 2012:A20.

104. Obama B. speech in Newtown, Connecticut, December 16, 2012. http://thelede.blogs.nytimes.com/2012/12/16/sunday-coverage-of-newtown-school-shooting/#full-text-and-video-of-obamas-speech

105. Cerebrus Capital Management. Cerberus Capital Management statement regarding Freedom Group, Inc. December 18, 2012. Available at:http://www.prnewswire.com/news-releases/cerberus-capital-management-statement-regarding-freedom-group-inc-183889361.html. Accessed on December 27, 2012.

106. Nocera J. Guns and their makers. *New York Times,* December 22, 2012:A25.

107. Silton AM. Divesting Gun Ownership: Public Funds Deserves No Credit. December 19, 2012, Revised December 22, 2012. Available at: http://meditationonmoneymanagement.blogspot.com/search?q=Freedom+Group. Accessed on December 27, 2012.

108. Tavernise S, Gebeloff R. Share of homes with guns shows 4-decade decline. *New York Times,* March 10, 2013, pp. A1 and A24.

109. Lazarou J, Pomeranz BH, Corey PN. Incidence of adverse drug reactions in hospitalized patients: a meta-analysis of prospective studies. *JAMA.*1998;279(15):1200–1205.

110. U.S. Food and Drug Administration. FDA's Safe Use Initiative: Collaborating to Reduce Preventable Harm from Medications. Washington DC: U.S. Department of Health and Human Services; November 4, 2009. Available at: http://www.fda.gov/downloads/Drugs/DrugSafety/UCM188961.pdf. Accessed August 14, 2012.

111. Miguel A, Azevedo LF, Araújo M, Pereira AC. Frequency of adverse drug reactions in hospitalized patients: a systematic review and meta-analysis. *Pharmacoepidemiol Drug Saf.* 2012;21(11):1139–1154.

112. Simons J, Stipp D. Will Merck survive Vioxx? *Fortune.* 2004;150(9):90–97.

113. Topol EJ. Failing the public health—rofecoxib, Merck, and the FDA. *N Engl J Med.* 2004;351(17):1707–1709.

114. Berenson A. Merck is said to agree to pay $4.85 billion for Vioxx claims. *New York Times.* November 9, 2007:A1.

115. Hawthorne F. *The Merck Druggernaut: The Inside Story of a Pharmaceutical Giant.* Hoboken, NJ: Wiley and Sons; 2003.

116. Brown D. Promise and peril of Vioxx casts harsher light on new drugs. *Washington Post.* October 3, 2004:A14.

117. Brown D. Maker of Vioxx is accused of deception. *Washington Post,* April 16, 2008. Available at: http://articles.washingtonpost.com/2008-04-16/news/36892398_1_vioxx-bruce-m-psaty-merck. Accessed March 18, 2013.

118. Harris G. Doctor's pain studies were fabricated, hospital says. *New York Times.* March 11, 2009:A22.

119. Nissen SE, Wolski K. Effect of Rosiglitazone on the risk of myocardial infarction and death from cardiovascular causes. *N Engl J Med.* 2007;356:2457–2471.

120. Thomas K, Schmidt MS. Glaxo agrees to pay $3 billion in fraud settlement. *New York Times.* July 3, 2012:A1.

121. Plumridge H. Glaxo pays dearly for past demons. *Wall Street Journal.* July 3, 2012. Available at: http://online.wsj.com/article/SB10001424052702303933404577504794077114750.html?KEYWORDS=%22off-label%22+marketing+drugs. Accessed August 14, 2012.

122. Loftus P. GlaxoSmithKline to Pay $229 Million to Settle U.S. Avandia Suits. *Wall Street Journal,* July 25, 2013, p. B2.

123. Mitka M. FDA: Panel recommends easing restrictions on Rosiglitazone despite concerns about safety. *JAMA* 2013;310(3):246–247.

124. Thomas K, Schmidt MS. Glaxo agrees to pay $3 billion in fraud settlement. *New York Times.* July 3, 2012:A1.

125. Stein R. Painkiller is pulled off market at FDA's request. *Washington Post.* November 20, 2010:A02.

126. Hitti M. FDA updates alert on ADHD drug Cylert. WebMD. October 25, 2005. Available at: http://www.webmd.com/add-adhd/news/20051025/fda-updates-alert-on-adhd-drug-cylert. Accessed August 14, 2012.

127. Petersen M. *Our Daily Meds: How the Pharmaceutical Companies Transformed Themselves into Slick Marketing Machines and Hooked the Nation on Prescription Drugs.* New York: Farrar Straus; 2008:248.

128. Petersen M. *Our Daily Meds: How the Pharmaceutical Companies Transformed Themselves into Slick Marketing Machines and Hooked the Nation on Prescription Drugs.* New York: Farrar Straus; 2008:249.

129. Osterberg L, Blaschke T. Adherence to Medication. *New Engl J Med.* 2005;353:487–497.

130. Sluggish economy forces Americans to cut corners to pay for medications. *Consumer Reports,* September 2012. Available at http://www.consumerreports.org/cro/2012/09/sluggish-economy-forces-americans-to-cut-corners-to-pay-for-medications/index.htm Accessed on December 28,2012.

131. McCarthy R. The price you pay for the drug not taken. *Business Health.* 1998;16:27–33.

132. IMS Institute for Health Care Informatics. The use of medicines in the United States: review of 2011. April 2012. Available at: http://www.imshealth.com/ims/Global/Content/Insights/IMS%20Institute%20for%20Healthcare%20Informatics/IHII_Medicines_in_U.S_Report_2011.pdf. Accessed on December 28, 2012.

133. Keyhani S, Diener-West M, Powe N. Do drug prices reflect development time and government investment? *Med Care.* 2005;43(8):753–762.

134. Moynihan R, Doran E, Henry D. Disease mongering is now part of the global health debate. *PLoS Med.* 2008;5(5):e106.

135. Lacasse JR, Leo J. Questionable advertising of psychotropic medications and disease mongering. *PLoS Med.* 2006;3(7):e321.

136. Tiefer L. Female sexual dysfunction: a case study of disease mongering and activist resistance. *PLoS Med.* 2006;3(4):e178.

137. Moynihan R, Cassels A. *Selling Sickness: How the World's Biggest Pharmaceutical Companies are Turning Us All into Patients.* New York: Nation Books; 2005.

138. Fava M. Prospective studies of adverse events related to antidepressant discontinuation. *J Clin Psychiatry.* 2006;67(Suppl 4):14–21.

139. Angell M. *The Truth About Drug Companies: How they Deceive Us and What to Do About It.* New York: Random House; 2004:182–183.

140. U.S. Congressional Budget Office. Cost Estimate S. 27 Preserve Access to Affordable Generics Act. November 7, 2011. Available at: http://aging.senate.gov/publications/s27.pdf. Accessed August 14, 2012.

141. Wyatt E. For big drug companies, a headache looms. *New York Times.* July 26, 2012:B1.

142. Stohr G. Drugmakers Opened to "Pay for Delay" Suits by High Court. *Bloomberg.* June 17, 2013.Available at: http://www.bloomberg.com/news/2013-06-17/drugmakers-opened-to-pay-for-delay-suits-by-high-court.html. Accessed on July 26, 2013.

143. Kaiser Family Foundation. Prescription drug trends. Available at: http://www.kff.org/rxdrugs/upload/3057-08.pdf. Published May 2010. Accessed August 14, 2012.

144. Truffer CJ, Keehan S, Smith S, Cylus J, Sisko A, Poisal JA, et al. Health spending projections through 2019: the recession's impact continues. *Health Aff (Millwood).* 2010;29(3):522–529.

145. Datamonitor. OTC Pharmaceuticals: Global Industry Guide 2011. March 1, 2012. http://www.datamonitor.com/store/Product/otc_pharmaceuticals_global_industry_guide_2011?productid=65B018C3-A52E-406B-92AF-958011035AA3.

146. Datamonitor. Global Pharmaceuticals, Biotechology and Life Sciences. 0199–2357, 2012.

147. Wilkinson R, Pickett K. *The Spirit Level: Why More Equal Societies Almost Always Do Better.* London: Allen Lane; 2009.

148. Marmot, M. *Status Syndrome: How Your Social Standing Directly Affects Your Health And Life Expectancy.* London: Bloomsbury; 2004.

149. Reardon S. Meeting brings attention but little action on chronic diseases. *Science.* 2011;333:1561.

150. Leeder S. Non-communicable diseases come to the United Nations. *The Conversation.* http://theconversation.edu.au/non-communicable-diseases-come-to-the-united-nations-3480. Published September 22, 2011. Accessed August 14, 2012.

151. Lincoln P, Rundall P, Jeffery B, Kellett G, Lobstein T, Lhotska L, et al. Conflicts of interest and the UN high-level meeting on non-communicable diseases. *Lancet.* 2011;378(9804):e6.

152. ChanM.SpeechofWHODirectorGeneralattheNCDSummit,NewYork.Availableat:http://www.seatca.org/index.php?option=com_content&view=article&id=1014:speech-of-who-director-general-at-the-ncd-summit-new-york&catid=3:international-updates&Itemid=66. Published September 19, 2011. Accessed August 10, 2012.

153. Reardon S. Meeting brings attention but little action on chronic diseases. *Science.* 2011;333:1561.

154. Cohen D. Will industry influence derail UN summit? *BMJ.* 2011;343:d5328.

155. Stuckler D, Basu S, McKee M. Commentary: UN high level meeting on non-communicable diseases: an opportunity for whom? *BMJ.* 2011;343:d5336.

156. Brown D. Battle of commercial interests confound fight against noncommunicable diseases. *Washington Post.* September 20, 2011. Available at: http://www.washingtonpost.com/world/battle-of-commercial-interests-loom-over-fight-against-noncommunicable-diseases/2011/09/20/gIQAy0rZjK_story.html. Accessed August 14, 2012.

157. Fink S, Rabinowitz R. The UN's battle with NCDs. *Foreign Affairs.* September 20, 2011. Available at: http://www.foreignaffairs.com/articles/68280/sheri-fink-and-rebecca-rabinowitz/the-uns-battle-with-ncds?page=show. Accessed August 14, 2012.

158. Reardon S. Meeting brings attention but little action on chronic diseases. *Science.* 2011;333, 1561.

159. Brown D. Battle of commercial interests confound fight against noncommunicable diseases. *Washington Post.* September 20, 2011. Available at: http://www.washingtonpost.com/world/battle-of-commercial-interests-loom-over-fight-against-noncommunicable-diseases/2011/09/20/gIQAy0rZjK_story.html. Accessed August 14, 2012.

160. Fink S, Rabinowitz R. The UN's Battle with NCDs. *Foreign Affairs.* The Council on Foreign Relations. September 20, 2011. Available at: http://www.foreignaffairs.com/articles/68280/sheri-fink-and-rebecca-rabinowitz/the-uns-battle-with-ncds?page=show. Accessed August 14, 2012.

161. Woolf SH. A closer look at the economic argument for disease prevention. *JAMA.* 2009;301(5):536–538.

162. Centers for Medicare and Medicaid Services, Office of the Actuary, National Health Statistics Group. National Health Expenditure Projections 2011–2021. Available at: http://www.cms.gov/Research-Statistics-Data-and-Systems/Statistics-Trends-and-Reports/NationalHealthExpendData/Downloads/Proj2011PDF.pdf. Published June 6, 2012. Accessed August 14, 2012.

163. U.S. Department of Health and Human Services. National Health Expenditure Projections 2011–2021. Washington, D.C.: DHHS; 2011. Available at http://www.cms.gov/Research-Statistics-Data-and-Systems/Statistics-Trends-and-Reports/NationalHealthExpendData/Downloads/Proj2011PDF.pdf. Accessed September 9, 2012.

164. Ford ES, Ajani UA, Croft JB, Critchley JA, Labarthe DR, Kottke TE, et al. Explaining the decrease in U.S. deaths from coronary disease, 1980–2000. *N Engl J Med.* 2007;356:2388–2398.

165. Collins F. Has the revolution arrived? *Nature.* 2010;464:674–675. doi:10.1038/464674a.

166. *US News and World Report.* Health information on bariatric surgery. 2010. Available at: http://health.usnews.com/health-conditions/heart-health/information-on-bariatric-surgery. Accessed on September 9,2012.

167. World Health Organization. WHO Report on the Global Tobacco Epidemic, 2008—The MPOWER Package. Geneva: World Health Organization. Available at: http://www.who.int/tobacco/mpower/2008/en/index.html. Published January 18, 2008. Accessed August 9, 2012.

168. United Nations General Assembly. Political declaration of the high-level meeting of the General Assembly on the prevention and control of non-communicable diseases. New York: September 16, 2011, pp. 5, 11. Available at: http://www.un.org/ga/search/view_doc.asp?symbol=A/66/L.1. Accessed August 14, 2012.

169. Dombrowski SU, Avenell A, Sniehott FF. Behavioural interventions for obese adults with additional risk factors for morbidity: systematic review of effects on behaviour, weight and disease risk factors. *Obes Facts.* 2010;3(6):377–396.

170. Jackson C, Geddes R, Haw S, Frank J. Interventions to prevent substance use and risky sexual behaviour in young people: a systematic review. *Addiction.* 2012;107(4):733–747. doi: 10.1111/j.1360-0443.2011.03751.x.

171. Evans CA Jr., Fielding JE, Brownson RC, England MJ, Fullilove MT, Guerra FA, et al. Motor-vehicle occupant injury: strategies for increasing use of child safety seats, increasing use of safety belts, and reducing alcohol-impaired driving. *MMWR Recomm Rep.* 2001;50(RR-7):1–14.

Chapter 3 Corporations Take Control: A New Political and Economic Order Emerges

1. Jeffries JC Jr. *Justice Lewis Powell, Jr. A Biography.* 2nd ed. New York: Scribner's; 2001.

2. Powell LF, Jr. Confidential Memo: Attack on American Free Enterprise System. August 23, 1971. Available at: http://reclaimdemocracy.org/corporate_accountability/powell_memo_lewis.html. Published April 23, 2004. Accessed August 19, 2012.

3. Powell LF, Jr. Confidential Memo: Attack on American Free Enterprise System. August 23, 1971. Available at: http://reclaimdemocracy.org/corporate_accountability/powell_memo_lewis.html. Published April 23, 2004. Accessed August 19, 2012.

4. Powell LF, Jr. Confidential Memo: Attack on American Free Enterprise System. August 23, 1971. Available at: http://reclaimdemocracy.org/corporate_accountability/powell_memo_lewis.html. Published April 23, 2004. Accessed August 19, 2012.

5. Powell LF, Jr. Confidential Memo: Attack on American Free Enterprise System. August 23, 1971. Available at: http://reclaimdemocracy.org/corporate_accountability/powell_memo_lewis.html. Published April 23, 2004. Accessed August 19, 2012.

6. Schmitt M. The legend of the Powell memo. *American Prospect.* April 27, 2005. Available at: http://prospect.org/article/legend-powell-memo. Accessed August 19, 2012.

7. Green M. The perils of public interest law. *New Republic,* September 20, 1975:20–23.

8. Per capita GDP rankings. No date. Available at: http://www2.econ.iastate.edu/classes/econ355/choi/rank.htm. Accessed on September 12, 2012.

9. Barnet R, Muller R. The global shopping center. In: Green M, Massie R, eds. *The Big Business Reader: On Corporate America.* New York: Pilgrim Press, ; 1980:381–398.

10. Mandel M. Multinationals: are they good for America? *Business Week.* February 28, 2008. Available at: http://www.businessweek.com/magazine/content/08_10/b4074041212646.htm?chan=search. Accessed August 19, 2012

11. Galbraith JK. *American Capitalism: the Concept of Countervailing Power.* Boston, MA: Houghton Mifflin; 1952.

12. Berle AA, Means GC. *The Modern Corporation and Private Property.* New York: Harcourt Brace & World; 1968.

13. Friedman M. *Capitalism and Freedom.* Chicago: University of Chicago Press; 1982.

14. Bakan J. *The Corporation: The Pathological Pursuit of Profit and Power.* New York: Free Press; 2004.

15. Roosevelt FD. President Franklin Roosevelt's radio address unveiling the second half of the New Deal. Campaign address at Madison Square Garden, New York City: We have only just begun to fight [*transcript*]. October 31, 1936. U.S. National Archives and Records Administration. Available at: http://www.ourdocuments.gov/doc.php?doc=69&page=transcript. Accessed August 19, 2012.

16. Reich RB. *Supercapitalism: The Transformation of Business, Democracy and Everyday Life.* New York: Knopf; 2007:81.

17. McChesney R. *The Political Economy of Media: Enduring Issues, Emerging Dilemmas.* New York: Monthly Review Press; 2008.

18. Moyers B. How Wall Street occupied America. *Nation.* November 21, 2011. Available at: http://www.thenation.com/article/164349/how-wall-street-occupied-america. Accessed August 19, 2012.

19. Moyers B. How Wall Street occupied America. *The Nation.* November 21, 2011. Available at: http://www.thenation.com/article/164349/how-wall-street-occupied-america. Accessed August 19, 2012.

20. Moyers B. How Wall Street occupied America. *The Nation.* November 21, 2011. Available at: http://www.thenation.com/article/164349/how-wall-street-occupied-america. Accessed August 19, 2012.

21. Welch J. Growing fast in a slow growth economy. In Welch J, Byrne JA. Jack: *Straight from the Gut.* New York: Business Plus, 2001:447–451.

22. Krippner G. The financialization of the American economy. *Soc Econ Rev.* 2005;3:173–208:174.

23. Khatiwadua S. Did the financial sector profit at the expense of the rest of the economy? Evidence from the United States, DP-206-2010. Geneva: International Institute for Labor Studies, International Labor Organization; 2010. Available at: http://www.ilo.org/public/english/bureau/inst/download/dp206_2010.pdf. Accessed August 19, 2012.

24. Burrough B, Helyar J. *Barbarians at the Gate: The Fall of RJR Nabisco.* New York: Harper and Row; 1990.

25. Burrough B, Helyar J. *Barbarians at the Gate: The Fall of RJR Nabisco.* New York: Harper and Row; 1990.

26. Davis GF. *Managed by the Markets: How Finance Re-shaped America.* New York: Oxford University Press; 2009:21.

27. Cooper PJ. *The War Against Government Regulation. From Jimmy Carter to George W. Bush.* Lawrence: University Press of Kansas; 2009.

28. Gordon M. Will Reagan turn business loose if business wants to stay regulated? *National Journal.* January 3, 1981:10.

29. Vogel D. *Fluctuating Fortunes: The Political Power of Business in America,* 2nd ed. Washington, DC: Beard Books; 2003:246.

30. Clark, TB. OMB to keep regulatory powers in reserve in case agencies lag. *National Journal.* March 14, 1981: 86.

31. Ramsey WA. Rethinking regulation of advertising aimed at children. *Fed Comm Law J.* 2006;58:361–368.

32. Nutritional supplements: your questions answered. *Consumer Reports.* June 14, 2006. Available at: http://www.consumerreports.org/health/free-highlights/manage-your-health/supplements_questions.htm. Accessed August 19, 2012.

33. Harris G. Study finds supplements contain contaminants. *New York Times.* May 25, 2010:A15.

34. Erikson PS. The dangers of alcohol deregulation: The United Kingdom experience. Alexandria, VA: Campaign for a Healthy Alcohol Marketplace; 2010. Available at: http://www.centerforalcoholpolicy.org/wp-content/uploads/2010/11/Dangers_of_Deregulation_UK_Experience.pdf. Accessed August 19, 2012.

35. Erikson PS. The dangers of alcohol deregulation: The United Kingdom experience. Alexandria, VA: Campaign for a Healthy Alcohol Marketplace; 2010. Available at: http://www.centerforalcoholpolicy.org/wp-content/uploads/2010/11/Dangers_of_Deregulation_UK_Experience.pdf. Accessed August 19, 2012.

36. Boseley S. Minimum unit price for alcohol proposal shelved. *Guardian,* July 17, 2013. Available at: http://www.guardian.co.uk/society/2013/jul/17/minimum-unit-price-alcohol-shelved. Accessed on July 29, 2013.

37. Bartlett B. Are taxes in the U.S. high or low? *New York Times,* May 31, 2011. Available at: http://economix.blogs.nytimes.com/2011/05/31/are-taxes-in-the-u-s-high-or-low/ Accessed on September 13, 2012.

38. Hacker P, Pierson J. *Winner-Take-All Politics: How Washington Made the Rich Richer—and Turned Its Back on the Middle Class.* New York: Simon and Schuster; 2010:134.

39. Rattner S. The corporate tax dodge. *New York Times,* May 24, 2013, p. A25.

40. U.S. Government Accountability Office, Comparison of the Reported Tax Liabilities of Foreign- and U.S.-Controlled Corporations, 1998-2005, GAO-08-957. Available at: http://www.gao.gov/new.items/d08957.pdf. Published July, 2008. Accessed August 19, 2012.

41. Keightley MP. An Analysis of Where American Companies Report Profits: Indications of Profit Shifting. Congressional Research Service 7-5700. 2013.

42. Stuckler D, Basu S. *The Body Economic: Why Austerity Kills.* New York: Basic Books, 2013.

43. Saez E, Piketty T. How progressive is the U.S. federal tax system? A historical and international perspective. *J Econ Perspect.* 2007;21(1):3–24.

44. Wilkinson RG, Pickett KE. Income inequality and population health: a review and explanation of the evidence. *Soc Sci Med.* 2006;62(7):1768–1784.

45. Johnson N, Hudgins E, Koulish J. Facing deficits, many states are imposing cuts that hurt vulnerable residents. Center on Budget and Policy Priorities. Available at: http://www.cbpp.org/archiveSite/3-13-08sfp.pdf. Updated November 12, 2008. Accessed August 19, 2012.

46. Keane C, Marx J, Ricci E. The privatization of environmental health services: a national survey of practices and perspectives in local health departments. *Public Health Rep.* 2002;117(1):62–68.

47. Alcohol Justice. Control state politics: Big Alcohol's attempt to dismantle regulation state by state. San Rafael, CA: Alcohol Justice; 2010. Available at: http://http://www.alcoholjustice.org/images/stories/pdfs/controlstate_report_final.pdf. Accessed August 19, 2012.

48. Mattera P. USDA Inc.: How agribusiness has hijacked regulatory policy at the U.S. Department of Agriculture. Washington, D.C: Corporate Research Project of Good Jobs First; 2004. Available at: http://www.nffc.net/Issues/Corporate percent20Control/USDA percent20INC.pdf. Accessed August 19, 2012.

49. Büthe T, Mattli W. *The New Global Rulers: The Privatization of Regulation in the World Economy.* Princeton, NJ: Princeton University Press; 2011.

50. Sclar E. *You Don't Always Get What You Pay For: The Economics of Privatization.* Ithaca, NY: Cornell University Press; 2000.

51. Keane C, Marx J, Ricci E, Barron G. The perceived impact of privatization on local health departments. *Am J Public Health.* 2002 Jul;92(7):1178–1180.

52. Keane, C, Marx J, Ricci, E. Public health privatization: proponents, resisters, and decision makers. *J Public Health Pol.* 2002;23(2):133–152.

53. Himmelstein DU, Woolhandler S. Privatization in a publicly funded health care system: the U.S. experience. *Int J Health Serv.* 2008;38(3):407–419.

54. Gilmore AB, Fooks G, McKee M. A review of the impacts of tobacco industry privatisation: implications for policy. *Glob Public Health.* 2011;6(6):621–642.

55. Mulreany JP, Calikoglu S, Ruiz S, Sapsin JW. Water privatization and public health in Latin America. *Rev Panam Salud Publica.* 2006;19(1):23–32.

56. Tavernise S. FDA says importers must audit food safety. *New York Times,* July 27, 2013, pp. B1 and B2.

57. Martinez S. The U.S. Food Marketing System: Recent Developments, 1997–2006. U.S. Department of Agriculture, Economic Research Service, Economic Research Report No. 42, p. 21. Available at: http://www.ers.usda.gov/publications/err42/err42.pdf. Published May, 2007. Accessed August 20, 2012.

58. Jernigan DJ. The extent of global alcohol marketing and its impact on youth. *Contemp Drug Prob.* 2010;37:57–89.

59. Panoff T. Corporate political strategy: a description of lobbying techniques and an explanation for the shift from personal relationship-based approaches to intricate grassroots coalitions from 1970–2000 [master's thesis]. Ann Arbor, MI: University of Michigan; 2000:12. Available at: http://webuser.bus.umich.edu/classes/ba380/2000/panof/panof.pdf. Accessed August 20, 2012.

60. Birnbaum JH. The road to riches is called K Street: lobbying firms hire more, pay more, charge more to influence government. *Washington Post.* June 22, 2005:A1.

61. Goldstein AO, Bearman NS. State tobacco lobbyists and organizations in the United States: crossed lines. *Am J Public Health.* 1996;86(8):1137–1142.

62. Rush L. Influence: A booming business; record $1.3 billion spent to lobby state government. Center for Public Integrity. Available at: http://www.publicintegrity.org/2007/12/20/5895/influence-booming-business. Published December 20, 2007. Accessed August 20, 2012.

63. Rush L. Influence: A booming business; record $1.3 billion spent to lobby state government. Center for Public Integrity. Available at: http://www.publicintegrity.org/2007/12/20/5895/influence-booming-business. Published December 20, 2007. Accessed August 20, 2012.

64. *Buckley v. Valeo,* 424 U.S. 1 (1976) 424 U.S. 1 Buckley et al. v. Valeo, Secretary of the United States Senate, et al. Appeal from the United States Court of Appeals for the District of Columbia Circuit. No. 75–436.

65. Mullins B. Corporate contributions shift to the left: some companies see Democrats having more sway in Washington after upcoming elections. *Wall Street Journal.* June 19, 2006:A4.

66. Mullins B. Corporate contributions shift to the left: Some companies see Democrats having more sway in Washington after upcoming elections. *Wall Street Journal.* June 19, 2006:A4.

67. Young L. Outside spenders' return on investment. Sunlight Foundation Reporting Group. December 18, 2012. Available at: , http://reporting.sunlightfoundation.com/2012/return_on_investment/. Accessed on December 29, 2012.

68. Yang JL, Hamburger T. For U.S. Chamber of Commerce, election was a money-loser. *Washington Post*, November 07, 2012. Available at: http://articles.washingtonpost.com/2012-11-07/business/35505311_1_republican-candidates-business-organization-thomas-j-donohue. Accessed on December 29, 2012.

69. Nestle M. *Food Politics: How the Food Industry Influences Nutrition and Health*. Berkeley: University of California Press; 2002:100.

70. Pollan M. *The Omnivore's Dilemma*. New York: Penguin Books; 2006:51–52.

71. Cook C. *Diet for a Dead Planet: How the Food Industry Is Killing Us*. New York: New Press; 2006:81.

72. Pollan M. The (agri)cultural contradictions of obesity. *New York Times Magazine*. October 12, 2003:41.

73. Bernays EL. *Biography of an Idea: Memoirs of Public Relations Council Edward L. Bernays*. New York: Simon and Schuster; 1965:, 386.

74. Brandt AM. *The Cigarette Century*. New York: Basic Books; 2007:83–85.

75. Interview with Edward Bernays on his work with Beechnut Packing Company. Available at: http://www.youtube.com/watch?v=KLudEZpMjKU. Accessed on December 29, 2012.

76. Grunig LA, Grunig JE. Public relations in the United States, a generation of maturation. In: Sriramesh K, Verčič D, eds. *The Global Public Relations Handbook: Theory, Research, and Practice*. Mahwah, NJ: Lawrence Erlbaum Associates; 2003:323–355.

77. Michaels D. *Doubt Is Their Product: How Industry's Assault on Science Threatens Your Health*. New York: Oxford University Press; 2008.

78. Vogel D. *Fluctuating Fortunes: The Political Power of Business in America*. Washington, DC: Beard Books; 2003:34.

79. Reich R. Regulation by confrontation or negotiation. *Harv Bus Rev*. 1981;59(3):82–93.

80. Vogel D. *Fluctuating Fortunes: The Political Power of Business in America*. Washington, DC: Beard Books; 2003:198.

81. Gittelsohn J. Foreclosures may delay housing rebound to 2013. Bloomberg.com. Available at: http://www.bloomberg.com/news/2011-12-22/foreclosures-weighing-on-prices-may-stall-u-s-housing-recovery-until-2013.html. Published December 22, 2011. Accessed August 20, 2012.

82. World Bank. Global Economic Prospects: Commodities at the Crossroads. Washington, DC: World Bank; 2009:96. Available at: http://siteresources.worldbank.org/INTGEP2009/Resources/10363_WebPDF-w47.pdf. Accessed August 20, 2012.

83. Ivanic M, Martin W, Zaman H. Estimating the short run poverty impact of the 2010–11 increase in food prices: policy research working paper no. WPS 5633. Washington, DC: World Bank; April 2011.,

84. Schwartz ND. As layoffs rise, stock buybacks consume cash. *New York Times*. November 22, 2011:A1.

85. Armstrong D. Pfizer Announces $10 Billion Share Repurchase Program. *Bloomberg*, June 27, 2013. Available at: http://www.bloomberg.com/news/2013-06-27/pfizer-announces-10-billion-share-repurchase-program.html. Accessed on July 30, 2013.

86. Hungerford TL. Changes in the distribution of income among tax filers between 1996 and 2006: The role of labor income, capital income, and tax policy, 7-5700. Washington, DC: Congressional Research Service, December 29, 2011. Available at: http://www.fas.org/sgp/crs/misc/R42131.pdf. Accessed August 20, 2012.

87. Wilkinson RG, Pickett KE. Income inequality and population health: a review and explanation of the evidence. *Soc Sci Med*. 2006;62(7):1768–1784.

88. Liptak A. Justices offer receptive ear to business interest. *New York Times*. December 18, 2010:A1.

89. Wiist WH. *Citizens United*, public health, and democracy: the Supreme Court ruling, its implications, and proposed action. *Am J Public Health*. 2011;101(7):1172–1179.

90. Plumer B. Supreme Court puts new limits on commerce clause. But will it matter? Wonkblog, washingtonpost.com. Available at: http://www.washingtonpost.com/blogs/ezra-klein/wp/2012/06/28/the-supreme-court-put-limits-on-commerce-clause-but-does-it-matter/. Published June 28, 2012. Accessed August 20, 2012.

91. *National Federation of Independent Business et al. v. Sebelius, Secretary of Health and Human Services, et al.* 567 US (2012), p. 2. Available at: http://www.supremecourt.gov/opinions/11pdf/11-393c3a2.pdf. Accessed August 20, 2012.

92. Plumer B. Supreme Court puts new limits on commerce clause. But will it matter? Wonkblog, washingtonpost.com. Available at: http://www.washingtonpost.com/blogs/ezra-klein/wp/2012/06/28/the-supreme-court-put-limits-on-commerce-clause-but-does-it-matter/. Published June 28, 2012. Accessed August 20, 2012.

93. Drutman L. The political one percent of the one percent. Sunlight Foundation. Available at: http://sunlightfoundation.com/blog/2011/12/13/the-political-one-percent-of-the-one-percent/. Published December 13, 2011. Accessed August 20, 2012.

94. Whoriskey P. Congress looks less like rest of America. *Washington Post.* December 27, 2011:A01.

95. Rutenberg J, Parker A. Romney says remarks on voters help clarify position. *New York Times,* September 19, 2012: A1.

Chapter 4 The Corporate Consumption Complex

1. Eisenhower DD. President Dwight D. Eisenhower's Farewell Address (1961) [*transcript*]. January 17, 1961. U.S. National Archives and Records Administration. Available at: http://www.ourdocuments.gov/doc.php?doc=90&page=transcript. Accessed: August 21, 2012.

2. Rampell C. Big spenders: The consumer economy. Economix Weblog, nytimes.com. Available at: http://economix.blogs.nytimes.com/2010/05/03/big-spenders-the-consumer-economy/. Published May 3, 2010. Accessed August 21, 2012.

3. U.S. Bureau of Labor Statistics. Average annual expenditures and characteristics of all consumer units, Consumer Expenditure Survey, 2006–2010. Available at: http://www.bls.gov/cex/2010/standard/multiyr.pdf. Published September 13, 2011. Accessed August 21, 2012.

4. Eriksen M, Mackay J, Ross H. *The Tobacco Atlas.* 4th ed. Atlanta, GA: American Cancer Society; New York: World Lung Foundation; 2012:44.

5. Bouchery EE, Harwood HJ, Sacks JJ, Simon CJ, Brewer RD. Economic costs of excessive alcohol consumption in the U.S., 2006. *Am J Prev Med.* 2011;41(5):516–524.

6. Christopher C Jr., Johnson E. Monetary matters: emerging consumer markets: the new drivers of global economic growth. *CSCMP's Supply Chain Quarterly.* 2011;Quarter 4. Available at: http://www.supplychainquarterly.com/columns/201104monetarymatters/. Accessed August 21, 2012.

7. Christopher C Jr., Johnson E. Monetary matters: emerging consumer markets: the new drivers of global economic growth. *CSCMP's Supply Chain Quarterly.* 2011; Quarter 4. Available at: http://www.supplychainquarterly.com/columns/201104monetarymatters/. Accessed August 21, 2012.

8. Hedrick-Wong Y, Iacobuzio T, Fonseca C. Consumer spending outlook and value creation in the new global economy. MasterCard. Worldwide Insights. 2011; Quarter 4. Available at: http://insights.mastercard.com/wp-content/uploads/2011/11/consumer_spending_outlook_and_value_creation_in_the_new_global_economy.pdf. Accessed August 21, 2012.

9. Spending power in emerging market economies grows rapidly. *Euromonitor.* Available at: http://blog.euromonitor.com/2010/09/spending-power-in-emerging-market-economies-grows-rapidly.html. Published September 6, 2010. Accessed August 21, 2012.

10. McDonald's Corporation. *2012 Annual Report.* Available at: http://www.aboutmcdonalds.com/content/dam/AboutMcDonalds/Investors/Investor%202013/2012%20Annual%20Report%20Final.pdf. Accessed on July 31, 2013.

11. McDonald's Corp. (MCD) Profitability Analysis. Stock Analysis on Net, EBIT Financial Analyses Center. Available at: http://www.stock-analysis-on.net/NYSE/Company/McDonalds-Corp/Ratios/Profitability#Net-Profit-Margin. Accessed August 21, 2012.

12. Spencer EH, Frank E, McIntosh NF. Potential effects of the next 100 billion hamburgers sold by McDonald's. *Am J Prev Med*. 2005;28(4):379–381.

13. Harris JL, Schwartz MB, Brownell, KD, Sarda V, Ustjanauskas A, Javadizadeh J et al. Fast food f.a.c.t.s. evaluating fast food nutrition and marketing to youth. Yale Rudd Center for Food Policy and Obesity. Available at http://fastfoodmarketing.org/media/FastFoodFACTS_Report.pdf. Published November 2010. Accessed August 21, 2012. p. 118.

14. Morrison M. Is McDonald's losing that lovin' feeling? *Ad Age*, February 20, 2012. Available at: http://adage.com/article/news/mcdonald-s-losing-lovin-feeling/232821/. Accessed on December 31, 2012.

15. Rognlin B. Market research: McDonald's customers aren't lovin' their food quality. *Blisstree*. Available at: http://blisstree.com/eat/mcdonalds-customers-unhappy-food-quality-467/. Published February 22, 2012. Accessed August 21, 2012.

16. Golden arches more familiar than the Cross. *Cleveland Plain Dealer*, August 26, 1995. Cited in Sclosser E. *Fast Food Nation*. Boston: Houghton Mifflin, 2011:277.

17. Jenkins, HW Jr. What Pepsi can learn from McDonald's. *Wall Street Journal*, January 27, 2012. Available at http://online.wsj.com/article/SB10001424052970204661604577186812311784468.html. Accessed on December 31, 2012.

18. Morrison M. Is McDonald's losing that lovin' feeling? *Ad Age*, February 20, 2012. Available at: http://adage.com/article/news/mcdonald-s-losing-lovin-feeling/232821/. Accessed on December 31, 2012.

19. Vega T, Alderman L. Merger is set to create world's Number 1 ad company. *New York Times*, July 29,2013, pp. B1 and B5.

20. Schlosser E. *Fast Food Nation: The Dark Side of the All-American Meal*. Boston: Houghton Mifflin, 2001:41.

21. Schlosser E. *Fast Food Nation: The Dark Side of the All-American Meal*. Boston: Houghton Mifflin, 2001:66.

22. U.S. Federal Trade Commission. *A Review of Food Marketing to Children and Adolescents*, 2012 update. Washington, DC: FTC, 2012. Available at: http://online.wsj.com/public/resources/documents/foodmarketingreport20121221.pdf. Accessed on December 31, 2012.

23. Harris JL, Schwartz MB, Brownell, KD, Sarda V, Ustjanauskas A, Javadizadeh J, et al. Fast food f.a.c.t.s. evaluating fast food nutrition and marketing to youth. Yale Rudd Center for Food Policy and Obesity. Available at http://fastfoodmarketing.org/media/FastFoodFACTS_Report.pdf. Published November 2010. Accessed August 21, 2012.

24. Harris JL, Schwartz MB, Brownell, KD, Sarda V, Ustjanauskas A, Javadizadeh J, et al. Fast food f.a.c.t.s. evaluating fast food nutrition and marketing to youth. Yale Rudd Center for Food Policy and Obesity. Available at: http://fastfoodmarketing.org/media/FastFoodFACTS_Report.pdf, p. 54. Published November 2010. Accessed August 21, 2012.

25. Speers SE, Harris JL, Schwartz MB. Child and adolescent exposure to food and beverage brand appearances during prime-time television programming. *Am J Prev Med*. 2011;41(3):291–296.

26. Robinson TN, Borzekowski DL, Matheson DM, Kraemer HC. Effects of fast food branding on young children's taste preferences. *Arch Pediatr Adolesc Med*. 2007;161(8):792–797.

27. Harris JL, Schwartz MB, Brownell, KD, Sarda V, Ustjanauskas A, Javadizadeh J, et al. Fast food f.a.c.t.s. evaluating fast food nutrition and marketing to youth. Yale Rudd Center for Food Policy and Obesity. Available at http://fastfoodmarketing.org/media/FastFoodFACTS_Report.pdf. Published November 2010. Accessed August 21, 2012.

28. Children, adolescents, and advertising. Committee on Communications, American Academy of Pediatrics. *Pediatrics*. 1995;95(2):295–297.

29. Warner M. Salads or no, cheap burgers revive McDonald's. *New York Times.* April 19, 2006:A1.

30. Harris JL, Schwartz MB, Brownell, KD, Sarda V, Ustjanauskas A, Javadizadeh J, et al. Fast food f.a.c.t.s. evaluating fast food nutrition and marketing to youth. Yale Rudd Center for Food Policy and Obesity. Available at http://fastfoodmarketing.org/media/FastFoodFACTS_Report.pdf. Published November 2010. Accessed August 21, 2012.

31. Currie J, Della Vigna S, Moretti E, Pathania V. The effect of fast food restaurants on obesity and weight gain. *American Econ J.* 2010;2(3):32–63.

32. Huang W. McDonald's China CEO on bringing McMuffins to the masses. *CNN Money.* May 10, 2012. Available at: http://management.fortune.cnn.com/2012/05/10/mcdonalds-china-kenneth-chan/. Accessed on January 26, 2013.

33. Meet Our Experts. McDonald's website. Available at http://www.mcdonalds.com/us/en/food/food_quality/nutrition_choices/kids_nutrition/food_to_feel_goodabout.html. Accessed on December 31, 2012.

34. Barbara Booth, Director of Sensory Science, Quality Systems, U.S. Supply Chain Management. Available at: http://www.mcdonalds.com/us/en/food/food_quality/trends_innovation/barbara_booth.html. Accessed on December 31, 202.

35. Wyant C. McDonald's picks Cargill for trans fat–free oil. *Minneapolis / St. Paul Business Journal,* January 30, 2007. Available at: http://www.bizjournals.com/twincities/stories/2007/01/29/daily20.html. Accessed on January 1, 2013.

36. Statement from McDonald's' Global Advisory Council on Balanced, Active Lifestyles. Undated. Available at: http://www.mcdepk.com/olympicresourcecenter/downloads/0207/gac_statement_3rd_party_quotes.pdf. Accessed on December 31, 2012.

37. Jargon J. Under pressure, McDonald's adds apples to kids' meals. *Wall Street Journal.* July 27, 2011. Available at: http://online.wsj.com/article/SB10001424053111903999904576469982832521802.html. Accessed August 21, 2012.

38. Warner M. Salads or no, cheap burgers revive McDonald's. *New York Times.* April 19, 2006:A1.

39. McDonald's "Breakfast After Midnight" menu makes limited debut. *Huffington Post.* August 8, 2012. Available at: http://www.huffingtonpost.com/2012/08/08/mcdonalds-breakfast-after-midnight_n_1756094.html. Accessed August 21, 2012.

40. Cebrzynski G. "Fourth meal" spurs QSR late-night dining push. *Nation's Restaurant News.* 2006;40(19):6, 123.

41. Mitchell L. Ronald McDonald stands up to playground bullies. *Washington Examiner.* July 9, 2010. Available at: http://washingtonexaminer.com/opinion/opinion-zone/2010/07/ronald-mcdonald-stands-playground-bullies/1548. Accessed August 22, 2012.

42. Kowitt B. Why McDonald's wins in any economy. *Fortune.* September 5, 2011. Available at: http://management.fortune.cnn.com/2011/08/23/why-mcdonalds-wins-in-any-economy/. Accessed August 22, 2012.

43. Mitchell L. Ronald McDonald stands up to playground bullies. *Washington Examiner.* July 9, 2010. Available at: http://washingtonexaminer.com/opinion/opinion-zone/2010/07/ronald-mcdonald-stands-playground-bullies/1548. Accessed August 22, 2012.

44. Dorfman L. *Framing Brief: Reading Between the Lines: Understanding food Industry Responses to Concerns About Nutrition.* Berkeley, CA: Berkeley Media Studies Group; 2007:3. Available at: http://www.bmsg.org/documents/FramingBriefIndustryResponse_000.pdf. Accessed August 22, 2012. Accessed August 22, 2012.

45. Awards and Recognition. McDonald's Corporation. Available at: http://www.about-mcdonalds.com/mcd/our_company/awards_and_recognition.html. Accessed August 22, 2012.

46. Rudawsky, G. McDonald's CEO's $17 million pay tied to performance. *Daily Finance.* Available at: http://www.dailyfinance.com/2010/04/10/mcdonalds-ceos-17-million-pay-tied-to-performance/. Published April 10, 2010. Accessed August 22, 2012.

47. PACs: McDonald's Corp. Summary, 2010. Opensecrets.org, Center for Responsive Politics. Available at: http://www.opensecrets.org/pacs/lookup2.php?strID=C00063164&cycle=2010. Accessed August 22, 2012.

48. McDonald's Corp. Contributions to Federal Candidates, 2012. Opensecrets.org, Center for Responsive Politics. Available at: http://www.opensecrets.org/pacs/pacgot. php?cycle=2012&cmte=C00063164 Accessed on August 1, 2013. Accessed on August 1, 2013

49. Campaign Finance Disclosure Data Search, Individual. Washington, DC: Federal Election Commission. http://query.nictusa.com/cgi-bin/qind/. Accessed December 31, 2012.

50. Lobbying: McDonalds Corp. Opensecrets.org, Center for Responsive Politics. Available at: http://www.opensecrets.org/lobby/clientsum.php?id=D000000373&year=2012. Accessed August 22, 2012.

51. Employment History: Bryant, Chester C., Jr. Opensecrets.org, Center for Responsive Politics. Available at: http://www.opensecrets.org/revolving/rev_summary.php?id=75435. Accessed August 22, 2012.

52. Wilson D, Roberts J. Special report: how Washington went soft on childhood obesity. Reuters. Available at: http://www.reuters.com/article/2012/04/27/us-usa-foodlobby-idUSBRE83Q0ED20120427. Published on April 27, 2012. Accessed on August 21, 2012.

53. Wilson D, Roberts J. Special report: how Washington went soft on childhood obesity Reuters. Available at: http://www.reuters.com/article/2012/04/27/us-usa-foodlobby-idUSBRE83Q0ED20120427. Published on April 27, 2012. Accessed on August 21, 2012.

54. Wilson D, Roberts J. Special report: how Washington went soft on childhood obesity. Reuters. Available at: http://www.reuters.com/article/2012/04/27/us-usa-foodlobby-idUSBRE83Q0ED20120427. Published on April 27, 2012. Accessed on August 21, 2012.

55. Agricultural Technical Advisory Committee for Trade (ATAC). Office of the United States Trade Representative. Available at: http://www.ustr.gov/about-us/intergovernmental-affairs/advisory-committees/agricultural-technical-advisory-committee-tra. Accessed August 22, 2012.

56. Agricultural Technical Advisory Committee for Trade (ATAC). Office of the United States Trade Representative. Available at: http://www.ustr.gov/about-us/intergovernmental-affairs/advisory-committees/agricultural-technical-advisory-committee-tra. Accessed August 22, 2012.

57. National Council of Chain Restaurants and National Restaurant Association—Comment on Proposed Rule: Food Labeling: Nutrition Labeling of Standard Menu Items in Restaurants and Similar Retail Food Establishments. Docket no. FDA 2011-F-0172-0443. July 5, 2011. Available at: http://www.regulations.gov/#!documentDetail;D=FDA-2011-F-0172-0443. Accessed August 22, 2012.

58. Children's Food and Beverage Advertising Initiative. Council of Better Business Bureaus. Available at: http://www.bbb.org/us/childrens-food-and-beverage-advertising-initiative/. Accessed August 22, 2012.

59. McIntire M. Nonprofit acts as a stealth business lobbyist. *New York Times*. April 22, 2012:A1.

60. Rosenwald M. McDonald's targets mothers. *Los Angeles Times*. November 26, 2008. Available at: http://articles.latimes.com/2008/nov/26/business/fi-mcdonalds26. Accessed August 22, 2012.

61. What's wrong with McDonald's? Greenpeace (London); 1986. Available at: http://www.mcspotlight.org/case/factsheet.html. Accessed August 22, 2012.

62. McLibel pair get police payout. BBC News, Wednesday, 5 July, 2000, Available at http://news.bbc.co.uk/2/hi/uk_news/820786.stm. Accessed on March 21, 2013.

63. Pring G, Canan P. *SLAPPs: Getting Sued for Speaking Out*. Philadelphia, PA: Temple University Press; 1996.

64. Andrae C. The big beef over one little name. *Christian Science Monitor*. Available at: http://www.csmonitor.com/1996/1016/101696.home.home.1.html. Published October 16, 1996. Accessed August 22, 2012.

65. State Frivolous-Lawsuit Legislation. National Restaurant Association. Available at: http://www.restaurant.org/advocacy/state/nutrition/bills_lawsuits/index.cfm#overview. Accessed August 22, 2012.

66. Gagnon M, Freudenberg N, Corporate Accountability International. *Slowing Down Fast Food: A Policy Guide for Healthier Kids and Families*. Boston, MA: Corporate Accountability International; 2012. Available at: http://www.stopcorporateabuse.org/sites/default/files/resources/slowing_down_fast_food_corporateaccountabilityinternational.pdf. Accessed August 22, 2012. pp. 26–28.

67. San Francisco McDonald's finds way around toy ban. CBS. November 30, 2011. Available at http://www.cbsnews.com/8301-201_162-57333985/san-francisco-mcdonalds-find-way-around-toy-ban/. Accessed on march 21, 2013

68. Representative Bernie Sanders (S-VT). *Congressional Record*. June 28, 2001. 147;9:12244.

69. About PhRMA. PhRMA. Available at: http://www.phrma.org/about/phrma. Accessed August 22, 2012.

70. About PhRMA. PhRMA. Available at: http://www.phrma.org/about/phrma. Accessed August 22, 2012.

71. Organizations: Pharmaceutical Rsrch & Mfrs of America. Influence Explorer. Available at: http://influenceexplorer.com/organization/pharmaceutical-rsrch-mfrs-ofamerica/b939e8e3b46c4569ae0085b8a3dc38f1. Accessed January 1, 2013.

72. Pharmaceutical Research and Manufacturers of America. Open Secrets. Available at http://www.opensecrets.org/orgs/summary.php?id=D000000504&cycle=2012. Accessed on: January 3, 2013. FRS of America.

73. Organizations: Pharmaceutical Research & Mfrs of America. Influence Explorer. Available at: http://influenceexplorer.com/organization/pharmaceutical-rsrch-mfrs-ofamerica/b939e8e3b46c4569ae0085b8a3dc38f1. Accessed August 22, 2012.

74. Pecquet J. Drug lobby official joins Rep. Bono Mack's office. *The Hill*. Available at: http://thehill.com/blogs/healthwatch/politics-elections/139197-drug-lobby-official-joins-rep-bono-macks-office?tmpl=component&print=1&page=..com/blogs/healthwatch/politics-elections/139197-drug-lobby-official-joins-rep-bono-macks-office?tmpl=component&print=1&page=. Published January 20, 2011. Accessed August 22, 2012.

75. Pharmaceutical Research and Manufacturers of America. Open Secrets. Available at http://www.opensecrets.org/orgs/summary.php?id=D000000504&cycle=A

76. Beckel M. Drug lobby gave $750,000 to pro-Hatch nonprofit in Utah's U.S. Senate race. Center for Public Integrity, November 29, 2012. http://www.publicintegrity.org/2012/11/29/11862/drug-lobby-gave-750000-pro-hatch-nonprofit-utahs-us-senate-race Available at: Accessed on January 3, 2013.

77. California Proposition 79, Prescription Drug Discount Program (2005). Ballotpedia. Available at: http://ballotpedia.org/wiki/index.php/California_Proposition_79,_Prescription_Drug_Discount_Program_%282005%29. Accessed on January 3, 2013.

78. California Proposition 78, Prescription Drug Discounts (2005). Ballotpedia. Available at: http://ballotpedia.org/wiki/index.php/California_Proposition_78,_Prescription_Drug_Discounts_%282005%29. Accessed on January 3, 29013.

79. Hamburger T, McGinley L. Drug lobby wins big with massive spending against Medicare plan. *Wall Street Journal*, November 9, 2000:B1.

80. Hamburger T, McGinley L. Drug lobby wins big with massive spending against Medicare plan. *Wall Street Journal*, November 9, 2000:B1.

81. Congress Watch. Citizens for Better Medicare: the truth behind the drug industry's deception of America's seniors. Public Citizen, 2000. Available at: http://www.citizen.org/documents/Cbm.pdf. Accessed on January 3, 2013.

82. Hamburger T. Drug industry ads aid GOP—"Educational grant" funds seniors' prescription-benefit campaign. *Wall Street Journal*. June 18, 2002:A4.

83. PhRMA appears to have funneled up to $41 million to "stealth PACs" to help elect a drug industry-friendly Congress [press release]. Public Citizen: Sept. 20, 2004. Available

at: http://www.citizen.org/pressroom/pressroomredirect.cfm?ID=1789. Accessed August 22, 2012.

84. Goldstein A, Eilperin J. House backs GOP drug plan for seniors. *Washington Post*, June 29, 2002:A1.

85. Singer M. Under the influence. *60 Minutes*, WCBS. Broadcast April 1, 2007. Available at: http://www.cbsnews.com/stories/2007/03/29/60minutes/main2625305.shtml. Accessed on January 3, 2012.

86. Ridgeway J. Medicare's poison pill. *Mother Jones*. September/October 2008. Available at: http://www.motherjones.com/politics/2008/09/medicares-poison-pill?page=2. Accessed on January 3, 2013.

87. Oliver TR, Lee PR, Lipton H L. A political history of Medicare prescription drug coverage. *Milbank Q.* 2004:82(2):283–354.

88. Connolly, C. Drug makers protect their turf: Medicare bill represents success for pharmaceutical lobby. *Washington Post*, November 21, 2003:A4.

89. Novak R. Blame Karl Rove for Medicare drug blunder. Human Events. Available at: http://www.humanevents.com/2006/01/09/blame-karl-rove-for-medicare-drug-blunder/ Accessed on January 3, 2013.

90. Liberto J. Health care lobbying boom continues. *CNN Money*. Available at: http://money.cnn.com/2011/03/25/news/economy/health_care_lobbying/index.htm. Published March 25, 2011. Accessed August 22, 2012.

91. Committee on Oversight And Government Reform. Medicare Part D: Drug Pricing and Manufacturer Windfalls. U.S. House of Representatives, 2008. Available at: http://assets.sunlightfoundation.com/pdf/blog/Medicare_Windfalls.pdf. Accessed on January 13, 2013.

92. Sarasohn J. Tauzin to head drug trade group. *Washington Post*. December 16, 2004:A35.

93. Pecquet J. Former drug lobby head Tauzin joins Alston & Bird lobby shop. *The Hill Healthwatch.* http://thehill.com/blogs/healthwatch/medical-devices-and-prescription-drug-policy-/140545-former-drug-lobby-head-tauzin-joins-alston-a-bird-lobby-shop. Published January 26, 2011. Accessed August 22, 2012.

94. Bogardus K. The top 10 lobbying victories of 2010. *The Hill*. Available at: http://thehill.com/business-a-lobbying/133691-the-top-10-lobbying-victories-of-2010. Published December 14, 2010. Accessed August 22, 2012.

95. Edsall T. The trouble with that revolving door. *New York Times*, December 18, 2011. Available at: http://campaignstops.blogs.nytimes.com/2011/12/18/the-trouble-with-that-revolving-door/. Accessed on January 27, 2011.

96. O'Donnell J. Willful Misconduct: How Bill Frist and the Drug Lobby Covertly Bagged a Liability Shield. Public Citizen. Washington, D.C., May 2006. Available at: http://www.policyarchive.org/handle/10207/10860. Accessed on January 27, 2011.

97. Appelbaum K. Clean Pharma crusader: Senator Chuck Grassley's enigmatic campaign to combat rising health care costs. Posted January 3, 2012, on Somatosphere. Available at http://somatosphere.net/2012/01/clean-pharma-crusader-senator-chuck-grassleys-enigmatic-campaign-to-combat-rising-health-care-costs.html. Accessed on January 27, 2013.

98. Rep. Thomas denies conflict of interest with pharmaceutical industry lobbyist. *CNN Politics*, June 27, 2000. Available at: http://articles.cnn.com/2000-06-27/politics/thomas.letter_1_pharmaceutical-industry-lobbyist-commitment-or-responsibility?_s=PM:ALLPOLITICS Accessed on January 27, 2013.

99. Bill Thoms. Employment history. Open Secrets. Available at http://www.opensecrets.org/revolving/rev_summary.php?id=70341. Accessed on January 26, 2013.

100. Pecquet J. PhRMA hires Cassidy & Associates to lobby on healthcare regs. Available at: http://thehill.com/blogs/healthwatch/health-reform-implementation/142743-phrma-hires-cassidy-a-associates-to-lobby-on-healthcare-regs. Published February 8, 2011. Accessed August 22, 2012.

101. Neel J. Boehner says old GOP pal aiding schoolyard bully. *NPR Health Weblog.* Available at: http://www.npr.org/blogs/health/2009/08/boehner_says_old_gop_pal_aidin.html. Published August 17, 2009. Accessed August 22, 2012.

102. Pecquet J. Healthcare lobbyists seek to repair relationship with Republicans. *The Hill.* Available at: http://thehill.com/blogs/healthwatch/health-reform-implementation/123735-health-care-lobbyists-seek-to-repair-relationship-with-gop. October 12, 2010. Accessed August 22, 2012.

103. Pecquet J. Healthcare lobbyists seek to repair relationship with Republicans. *The Hill.* Available at: http://thehill.com/blogs/healthwatch/health-reform-implementation/123735-health-care-lobbyists-seek-to-repair-relationship-with-gop. Published October 12, 2010. Accessed August 22, 2012.

104. Pharmaceuticals and Health Products: Top Contributors to Federal Candidates, Parties, and Outside Groups,2008,2010 and 2012. Opensecrets.org, Center for Responsive Politics. Available at: http://www.opensecrets.org/industries/contrib.php?ind=H04&cycle=2008. Accessed on August 1, 2013.

105. Americans value the health benefits of prescription drugs, but say drug makers put profits first, new survey shows [press release]. Kaiser Family Foundation: February 25, 2005. Available at: http://www.kff.org/kaiserpolls/pomr022505nr.cfm. Accessed August 22, 2012.

106. Sillup GP, Trombetta B, Klimberg R. The 2002 PhRMA code and pharmaceutical marketing: did anybody bother to ask the reps? *Health Mark Q.* 2010;27(4):388–404.

107. Weber LJ. *Profits Before People? Ethical Standards and the Marketing of Prescription Drugs.* Bloomington: Indiana University Press; 2006:66–81.

108. Abraham J. The pharmaceutical industry as a political player. *Lancet.* 2002;360:1498–1502.

109. Mathews AW. Drug firms use financial clout to push industry agenda at FDA. *Wall Street Journal.* September 1, 2006. Available at: http://online.wsj.com/article/SB115707824013151485.html. Accessed August 22, 2012.

110. Kao DP. What can we learn from drug marketing efficiency? *BMJ.* 2008;337:a2591.

111. Edwards J. *BMJ*: PDUFA, speedy marketing spread risks of new drugs. *CBS Moneywatch.* Available at: http://www.cbsnews.com/8301-505123_162-42840255/bmj-pdufa-speedy-marketing-spread-risks-of-new-drugs/. Published December 8, 2008. Accessed August 22, 2012.

112. Edwards J. *BMJ*: PDUFA, speedy marketing spread risks of new drugs. *CBS Moneywatch.* Available at: http://www.cbsnews.com/8301-505123_162-42840255/bmj-pdufa-speedy-marketing-spread-risks-of-new-drugs/. Published December 8, 2008. Accessed August 22, 2012.

113. PhRMA takes aim at Thailand for production of generics, hints that it will push for sanctions. *The Hill.* Available at: http://thehill.com/business-a-lobbying/3115-phrma-takes-aim-at-thailand-for-production-of-generics-hints-that-it-will-push-for-sanctions. Published May 23, 2007. Accessed August 22, 2012.

114. Angell M. *The Truth About the Drug Companies: How They Deceive Us and What to Do About It.* New York: Random House; 2004.

115. OECD. *Health at a Glance 2011: OECD Indicators.* OECD Publishing, 2011. Available at: http://dx.doi.org/10.1787/health_glance-2011-en. Accessed on January 4, 2013.

116. Eisenhower DD. President Dwight D. Eisenhower's Farewell Address (1961) [*transcript*]. January 17, 1961. U.S. National Archives and Records Administration. Available at: http://www.ourdocuments.gov/doc.php?doc=90&page=transcript. Accessed: August 6, 2013.

Chapter 5 The Corporate Ideology of Consumption

1. Mackey J. The Whole Foods alternative to ObamaCare. *Wall Street Journal.* August 11, 2009. Available at: http://online.wsj.com/article/SB10001424052970204251404574342170072865070.html. Accessed August 23, 2012.

2. BBC News. Blair calls for lifestyle change. July 26, 2006. Available at: http://news.bbc. co.uk/2/hi/5215548.stm. Accessed August 23, 2012.

3. Dutt. B. Obama now a pro-business leader: Indra Nooyi to NDTV [transcript]. November 10, 2010. Available at: http://www.ndtv.com/article/business/obama-now-a-pro-business-leader-indra-nooyi-to-ndtv-65159. Accessed August 23, 2012.

4. Nooyi IK. A healthy bottom line. Presented at: North Carolina Emerging Issues Forum. February 7, 2011. Available at: http://www.pepsico.com/assets/speeches/Emerging percent20Issues percent20Forum.pdf. Accessed August 23, 2012.

5. Fish JH. Mr. Speaker, the era of big government is over. 1996. RJ Reynolds. Available at: http://legacy.library.ucsf.edu/tid/sob70d00. Accessed August 23, 2012. pp. 9–10.

6. Brito C. Plenary address. Presented at: BSR Conference 2011: Redefining Leadership, November 2, 2011. Available at: http://www.bsr.org/en/bsr-conference/session-summary-view/2011/plenary-carlos-brito. Accessed August 23, 2012.

7. Fonda D. CEO interview: Ford's Alan Mulalley. *Smart Money*. November 3, 2010. Available at: http://www.smartmoney.com/invest/stocks/ceo-interview-fords-alan-mulally/. Accessed August 23, 2012.

8. Allahpundit. McDonald's CEO to food police: The clown's going nowhere. Available at: http://hotair.com/archives/2011/05/20/mcdonalds-ceo-to-food-police-the-clowns-going-nowhere/. Published May 20, 2011. Accessed August 23, 2012.

9. Insights: Interview with Dawn Sweeney, President and CEO, National Restaurant Association. Restaurant Nutrition, Healthy Dining. Available at: http://www.restaurantnu-trition.com/nutrition-insights/Dawn-Sweeney.aspx.Accessed August 23, 2012.

10. Active healthy living: Education. The Coca-Cola Company. Available at: http://www. thecoca-colacompany.com/citizenship/think.html. Accessed August 23, 2012.

11. *Frontline*. Analysis: pros and cons of drug advertising and marketing. PBS.org. Available at: http://www.pbs.org/wgbh/pages/frontline/shows/other/themes/marketing.html. Accessed August 23, 2012.

12. Reagan R. Inaugural Address, January 20, 1981. Available at: http://www.reagan.utexas. edu/archives/speeches/1981/12081a.htm. Accessed August 23, 2012.

13. Berman R. Deep fried hysteria. Center for Consumer Freedom. Available at: http:// www.consumerfreedom.com/2006/09/407-deep-fried-hysteria/.   Accessed   August 23, 2012.

14. Goldstone SF. Remarks of Steven F. Goldstone, Chairman and CEO, RJR Nabisco to the Washington Press Club. RJR Nabisco. April 8, 1998. Available athttp://legacy.library.ucsf. edu/tid/qwn70d00. Accessed August 23, 2012.

15. Frazier K. Will Washington find the cure for cancer? *Wall Street Journal*. July 13, 2011. Available at: http://online.wsj.com/article/SB10001424052702304447804576412084061290852.html. Accessed August 23, 2012.

16. Insights: Interview with Dawn Sweeney, president and CEO, National Restaurant Association. Restaurant Nutrition, Healthy Dining. Available at; http://www.restaurantnu-trition.com/nutrition-insights/Dawn-Sweeney.aspx.Accessed August 23, 2012.

17. Havas S, Dickinson BD, Wilson M. The urgent need to reduce sodium consumption. *JAMA*. 2007;298:1439–1441.

18. Parrish SC. Industry Statement by Steven C. Parrish. Philip Morris. January 2, 1996. Available at http://legacy.library.ucsf.edu/tid/yei61d00. Accessed August 23, 2012.

19. Keynote: Exploring inspiration and leadership with Indra Nooyi. Presented at: BlogHer '11, August 5, 2011. Available at: http://www.blogher.com/liveblog-lunch-keynote-exploring-inspiration-and-leadership-indra-nooyi. Accessed August 23, 2012.

20. Interview: Nissan's Carlos Ghosn seeks revenge for the electric car. *Yale Environment 360*. May 4, 2011. Available at: http://e360.yale.edu/feature/nissans_carlos_ghosn_seeks_revenge_for_the_electric_car/2398/. Accessed August 23, 2012.

21. Paolillo C. Smoke screen: big tobacco's global lobbying: Uruguay vs. Philip Morris. International Consortium of Investigative Journalists. November 15, 2010. Available

at: http://www.icij.org/project/smoke-screen-big-tobaccos-global-lobbying/uruguay-vs-philip-morris. Accessed August 23, 2012, 2012.

22. Corley M. Paul calls White House pressure on BP "un-American," says that "sometimes accidents happen." Available at: http://thinkprogress.org/politics/2010/05/21/98537/paul-bp-unamerican/. Published May 21, 2010. Accessed August 23, 2012.

23. CNN Wire Staff. As movement spreads, NY mayor slams protesters for "trying to destroy" jobs. *CNN*. Available at; http://articles.cnn.com/2011-10-08/politics/politics_occupy-wall-street_1_protest-effort-demonstrators-bloomberg?_s=PM:POLITICS.Published October 08, 2011. Accessed August 23, 2012.

24. Miller SA. Defensive driving. *Washington Times*. August 30, 2007. http://www.washingtontimes.com/blog/fishwrap/2007/aug/30/defensive-driving/. Accessed August 23, 2012.

25. U.S. Chamber's Donohue shrugs off defections. *Business Week*. October 9, 2009. Available at: http://www.businessweek.com/bwdaily/dnflash/content/oct2009/db2009109_253028.htm. Accessed August 23, 2012.

26. Meltzer A. Why capitalism [transcript]? American Enterprise Institute. March 9, 2009. Available at: http://www.aei.org/speech/society-and-culture/free-enterprise/why-capitalism-speech/. Accessed August 23, 2012.

27. Friedman, T. *The Lexus and the Olive Tree*. London: Farrar, Straus & Giroux; 1999:xxi.

28. Taurel S. The worldwide campaign against pharmaceutical innovation [transcript]. American Enterprise Institute. March 18, 2003. Available at: http://aei.org/speech/health/the-worldwide-campaign-against-pharmaceutical-innovation/. Accessed August 23, 2012.

29. Foster SE, Vaughan RD, Foster WH, Califano JA Jr. Estimate of the commercial value of underage drinking and adult abusive and dependent drinking to the alcohol industry. *Arch Pediatr Adolesc Med*. 2006;160(5):473–478.

30. Sen A. *Development as Freedom*. New York: Knopf, 2000.

31. Rothkopf D. *Power, Inc.: The Epic Rivalry Between Big Business and Government and the Reckoning That Lies Ahead*. New York: Farrar, Straus & Giroux; 2012:11.

32. Schor J. The new politics of consumption. *Boston Review*, 1999. Available at: http://bostonreview.net/BR24.3/schor.html. Accessed August 23, 2012.

33. Danner M. Words in a time of war: On rhetoric, truth and power. In: Szántó A, ed., *What Orwell Didn't Know: Propaganda and the New Face of American Politics*. New York: Public Affairs; 2007:16–36; 17.

34. Robbins J. Free market flawed, says survey. *BBC News*. Available at: http://news.bbc.co.uk/2/hi/8347409.stm. Published November 9, 2009. Accessed August 23, 2012.

35. Saad L. Americans decry power of lobbyists, corporations, banks, feds; Independents agree with GOP that federal government has too much power. *Gallup*. April 11, 2011. Available at: http://www.gallup.com/poll/147026/americans-decry-power-lobbyists-corporations-banks-feds.aspx. Accessed August 23, 2012.

36. Saad L. Congress Ranks last in confidence in institutions: Fifty percent "very little"/"no" confidence in Congress reading is record high. *Gallup*. July 22, 2010. Available at: http://www.gallup.com/poll/141512/congress-ranks-last-confidence-institutions.aspx. Accessed August 23, 2012.

37. Mendes E. In U.S., fear of big government at near-record level: Democrats lead increase in concerns about big government. *Gallup*. December 12, 2011. Available at: http://www.gallup.com/poll/151490/fear-big-government-near-record-level.aspx. Accessed August 23, 2012.

38. Big Business. Gallup. Available at: http://www.gallup.com/poll/5248/big-business.aspx. Accessed August 23, 2012.

39. Big Business. Gallup. Available at: http://www.gallup.com/poll/5248/big-business.aspx. Accessed August 23, 2012.

40. Partisan Polarization Surges in Bush, Obama Years Trends in American Values: 1987–2012. Pew Research Center, June 4, 2012. Available at: http://www.people- press.

org/2012/06/04/section-5-values-about-business-wall-street-and-labor/#regulation-divide. Accessed on August 2, 2013.

41. Mixed views of regulation, support for Keystone Pipeline: Auto bailout now backed, stimulus divisive. Pew Research Center. February 23, 2012. Available at: http://www.people-press.org/files/legacy-pdf/2-23-12%20Regulation%20release.pdf. Accessed August 23, 2012.p. 3.

42. Gardner MN, Brandt AM. "The Doctors' Choice Is America's Choice": The physician in US cigarette advertisements, 1930–1953. *Am J Public Health.* 2006;96(2):222–232.

43. Bradsher K. *High and Mighty: SUVs: The World's Most Dangerous Vehicles and How They Got That Way*, New York: Public Affairs; 2002:110–111.

44. Blanding M. Bad Medicine. *Boston Magazine*, February 2005. Available at: http://www.bostonmagazine.com/articles/2006/05/bad-medicine/. Accessed on September 16, 2012.

45. Krimsky S. *Science in the Private Interest: Has the Lure of Profits Corrupted Biomedical Research?* Lanham, MD: Rowman-Littlefield Publishing Co.; 2003.

46. Michaels D. *Doubt Is Their Product: How Industry's Assault on Science Threatens Your Health.* New York: Oxford University Press; 2008.

47. Smoking and health proposal. Brown and Williamson, 1969. Available at: http://legacy.library.ucsf.edu/tid/pmq36b00. Cited by: Michaels D. *Doubt Is Their Product: How Industry's Assault on Science Threatens Your Health.* New York: Oxford University Press; 2008:11.

48. Perera F, Herbstman J. Prenatal environmental exposures, epigenetics, and disease. *Reprod Toxicol.* 2011;31(3):363–373.

49. Brownson RC, Haire-Joshu D, Luke DA. Shaping the context of health: a review of environmental and policy approaches in the prevention of chronic diseases. *Annu Rev Public Health.* 2006;27:341–370.

50. Rauch SA, Lanphear BP. Prevention of disability in children: elevating the role of environment. *Future Child.* 2012;22(1):193–217.

51. The costly war on cancer. *Economist.* May 26, 2011. Available at: http://www.economist.com/node/18743951. Accessed August 23, 2012.

52. Brandt A. *The Cigarette Century.* New York: Perseus; 2007.

53. Klein N. Capitalism vs. the climate. *Nation.* November 9, 2011. Available at: http://www.thenation.com/article/164497/capitalism-vs-climate. Accessed August 23, 2012.

54. Scientific Integrity Program. A climate of corporate control: how corporations have influenced the U.S. dialogue on climate science and policy. Washington, DC: Union of Concerned Scientists; 2012.

55. Borick CP, Lachapelle E, Rabe BG. Climate compared: public opinion on climate change in the United States and Canada. *Issues in Governance Studies.* 2011;39:1–13.

56. Bradsher K. *High and Mighty SUVs: The World's Most Dangerous Vehicles and How They Got That Way.* New York: Public Affairs; 2002:98–99.

57. Cigarette smoking, adults, 1965–2011. Healthy People.gov. Available at: http://healthy-people.gov/2020/topicsobjectives2020/nationalsnapshot.aspx?topicId=41 Accessed on August 7, 2013.

58. LaVallee R, Yi HY. Apparent Per Capita Alcohol Consumption: National, State and Regional Trends, 1977–2009, Surveillance Report no. 92. U.S. Department of Health and Human Services, National Institute on Alcohol Abuse and Alcoholism. Available at: http://pubs.niaaa.nih.gov/publications/Surveillance92/CONS09.htm. Published August 2011. Accessed August 6, 2013.

59. O'Connor. Are Americans Done with Coca-Cola, Pepsi, and Dr Pepper? *The Daily Beast*, July 31, 2013. Available at: http://www.thedailybeast.com/articles/2013/07/31/are-americans-done-with-coca-cola-pepsi-and-dr-pepper.html.Accessed on August 7,2013.

60. Dutzik D, Baxandall P. A New Direction: Our Changing Relationship with Driving and the Implications for America's Future. U.S. PIRG Education Fund and Frontier Group. Washington, D.C., 2013. Available at: http://uspirg.org/sites/pirg/files/reports/A%20New%20Direction%20vUS.pdf Accessed on August 7, 2013.

61. Beauchamp DE. Public health as social justice. *Inquiry.* 1976;12:3–14.
62. Wallack L, Lawrence R. Talking about public health: developing America's "second language." *Am J Public Health.* 2005;95(4):567–570.
63. Mills CW. *The Sociological Imagination.* 2nd ed. New York: Oxford University Press, 2000. p. 186.
64. Brown P, Zavestoski S, McCormick S, Mayer B, Morello-Frosch R, Gasior Altman R. Embodied health movements: new approaches to social movements in health. *Sociol Health Illn.* 2004;26(1):50–80.
65. Hersey JC, Niederdeppe J, Ng SW, Mowery P, Farrelly M, Messeri P. How state counter-industry campaigns help prime perceptions of tobacco industry practices to promote reductions in youth smoking. *Tob Control.* 2005 Dec;14(6):377–383.
66. Associated Press. Super Bowl ads cost an average of $3.5M. ESPN.com. Available at: http://espn.go.com/nfl/playoffs/2011/story/_/id/7544243/super-bowl-2012-commercials-cost-average-35m. Accessed August 23, 2012.
67. Venutolo A. The 2012 Super Bowl commercials: watch them here. *Star-Ledger* (Newark, NJ). February 5, 2012. Available at: http://www.nj.com/super-bowl/index.ssf/2012/02/super_bowl_commercials_2012_watch_them_here.html. Accessed August 23, 2012.
68. Barber BR. *Consumed: How Markets Corrupt Children, Infantilize Adults and Swallow Citizens Whole.* New York: Norton; 2007:3.
69. Bullard, RD. *The Quest for Environmental Justice:Human Rights and the Politics of Pollution.* San Francisco: Sierra Club Books, 2005.
70. Gottlieb R, Joshi A. *Food Justice* Cambridge, MA: MIT Press, 2010.
71. Rasmussen Polls. 47% say media bias bigger problem than campaign contributions, 42% disagree. August 21, 2012. Available at: http://www.rasmussenreports.com/public_content/politics/general_politics/august_2012/47_say_media_bias_bigger_problem_than_campaign_contributions_42_disagree. Accessed on September 16, 2012.
72. Colón RL. An unlikely alliance: religious institutions as a necessary partner in promoting sustainable consumption. In: Sustainable Consumption and Production: Framework for Action. 2nd Conference of the Sustainable Consumption Research 2008, Brussels, Belgium, pp. 51–67. Available at: http://www.score-network.org/files//24119_CF2_session_5.pdf
73. Burkeman O. "What would Jesus drive?" gas-guzzling Americans are asked. *Guardian,* November 13, 2002. Available at: http://www.guardian.co.uk/world/2002/nov/14/usa.oliverburkeman. Accessed on January 5, 2013.
74. McKibben B. *Eaarth: Making Life on a Tough New Planet.* New York: Times Books; 2010.
75. The unsustainable cost of health care. Social Security Advisory Board. September 2009, p. i. Available at: http://www.ssab.gov/documents/TheUnsustainableCostofHealthCare_graphics.pdf. Accessed August 23, 2012.

Chapter 6 The Health Impact of Corporate Managed Globalization

1. Gossner CM, Schlundt J, Ben Embarek P, Hird S, Lo-Fo-Wong D, Beltran JJ, et al. The melamine incident: implications for international food and feed safety. *Environ Health Perspect.* 2009;117(12):1803–1808.
2. Hawkes C. Uneven dietary development: linking the policies and processes of globalization with the nutrition transition, obesity and diet-related chronic diseases. *Global Health.* 2006;28;2:4.
3. Clark SE, Hawkes C, Murphy SM, Hansen-Kuhn KA, Wallinga D. Exporting obesity: US farm and trade policy and the transformation of the Mexican consumer food environment. *Int J Occup Environ Health.* 2012;18(1):53–65.
4. Chase K. NAFTA: The politics in the United States. In: Chase K. *Trading Blocs: States, Firms, and Regions in the World Economy.* Ann Arbor, : University of Michigan Press; 2005:181–221.
5. Berlind M. Testimony of Mark Berlind, Executive Vice-President, Global Corporate Affairs, Kraft Foods, Inc., to the United States Senate Committee on Finance. Hearing on

U.S-Central America-Dominican Republic Free Trade Agreement, April 13, 2005, p. 2. Available at: http://www.finance.senate.gov/imo/media/doc/mbtest041205.pdf. Accessed August 28, 2012.

6. Remarks by President Clinton, President Bush, President Carter, President Ford, and Vice President Gore in signing of NAFTA side agreements. September 14, 1993. National Archives and Records Administration. Available at: http://clinton6.nara.gov/1993/09/1993-09-14-remarks-by-clinton-and-former-presidents-on-nafta.html. Accessed August 28, 2012.

7. Clark SE, Hawkes C, Murphy SM, Hansen-Kuhn KA, Wallinga D. Exporting obesity: US farm and trade policy and the transformation of the Mexican consumer food environment. *Int J Occup Environ Health*. 2012;18(1):53–65.

8. Hawkes C. Uneven dietary development: linking the policies and processes of globalization with the nutrition transition, obesity and diet-related chronic diseases. *Global Health*. 2006;2(4). doi:10.1186/1744-8603-2-4.

9. United States Economic Research Service. Mexico Trade, Policy and FDI. United States Department of Agriculture. Last updated September 12, 2012. Available at: http://www.ers.usda.gov/topics/international-markets-trade/countries-regions/nafta-canada-mexico/mexico-trade-policy-fdi.aspx#Mexicofdi. Accessed on September 18, 2012.

10. United States Economic Research Service. Mexico Trade &, FDI. United States Department of Agriculture. Last updated May 15, 2013., Available at: http://www.ers.usda.gov/topics/international-markets-trade/countries-regions/nafta,   -canada-mexico/mexico-trade-fdi.aspx#.Uf_MCKx15EM. Accessed on August 5, 2013

11. Cervantes-Godoy D, Sparling D, Avendano B, Calvin L. North American retailers and their impact on food chains. Presented at: North American Agrifood Market Integration Consortium; June 15, 2007; Cancun, Mexico. Available at: http://naamic.tamu.edu/cancun2/sparling.pdf. Accessed August 28, 2012.

12. Cervantes-Godoy D, Sparling D, Avendano B, Calvin L. North American Retailers and their impact on food chains. Presented at: North American Agrifood Market Integration Consortium; June 15, 2007; Cancun, Mexico. Available at: http://naamic.tamu.edu/cancun2/sparling.pdf. Accessed August 28, 2012.

13. Barstow D, Von Bertrab AX. The bribery aisle: how Wal-Mart got its way in Mexico. *New York Times*, December 18, 2012:, A1.

14. Clifford S. Bribery case at Wal-Mart may widen. *New York Times*. May 18, 2012:B1.

15. Wohl. J. Wal-Mart CEO's Pay Jumps 14.1 Percent To $20.7 Million. *Huffington Post*, April 22, 2013. Available at: http://www.huffingtonpost.com/2013/04/22/walmart-ceo-pay-2012_n_3134515.html. Accessed on August 7, 2013.

16. Iacovone L, Javorcik B, Keller W, Tybout J. Supplier responses to Wal-Mart's invasion in Mexico. NBER Working Paper No. 17204. July 2011. National Bureau of Economic Research. Available at: http://www.nber.org/papers/w17204. Accessed August 28, 2012.

17. McDonald's. McDonald's Mexico Corporativo: *Quienes Somos*. Available at: http://www.McDonald's.com.mx/#/NPC%253AInstitutional%25231List1. Accessed August 28, 2012.

18. Hawkes C. Uneven dietary development: linking the policies and processes of globalization with the nutrition transition, obesity and diet-related chronic diseases. *Global Health*. 2006;2(4). doi:10.1186/1744-8603-2-4.

19. Arroyo P, Loria A, Mendez O. Changes in the household calorie supply during the 1994 economic crisis in Mexico and its implications for the obesity epidemic. *Nutrition Reviews*. 2004;62:S163–S168.

20. Hawkes C. Uneven dietary development: linking the policies and processes of globalization with the nutrition transition, obesity and diet-related chronic diseases. *Global Health*. 2006;2(4). doi:10.1186/1744-8603-2-4.

21. Hawkes C. Uneven dietary development: linking the policies and processes of globalization with the nutrition transition, obesity and diet-related chronic diseases. *Global Health*. 2006;2(4). doi:10.1186/1744-8603-2-4.

22. Barquera S, Campirano F, Bonvecchio A, Hernández-Barrera L, Rivera JA, Popkin BM. Caloric beverage consumption patterns in Mexican children. *Nutr J.* 2010;9(47). doi:10.1186/1475-2891-9-47.

23. Clark SE, Hawkes C, Murphy SM, Hansen-Kuhn KA, Wallinga D. Exporting obesity: US farm and trade policy and the transformation of the Mexican consumer food environment. *Int J Occup Environ Health.* 2012;18(1):53–65.

24. Rivera JA, Barquera S, Gonzalez-Cossyo T, Olaiz G, Sepulveda J. Nutrition transition in Mexico and in other Latin American countries. *Nutrition Reviews.* 2004;62:S149–S157.

25. Bonvecchio A, Safdie M, Monterrubio EA, Gust T, Villalpando S, Rivera JA. Overweight and obesity trends in Mexican children 2 to 18 years of age from 1988 to 2006. *Salud Publica Mex.* 2009;51(Suppl 4):S586–S594.

26. Rivera JA, Barquera S, Gonzalez-Cossyo T, Olaiz G, Sepulveda J. Nutrition transition in Mexico and in other Latin American countries. *Nutr Rev.* 2004;62:S149–S157.

27. Rivera JA, Barquera S, Campirano F, Campos I, Safdie M, Tovar V. Epidemiological and nutritional transition in Mexico: rapid increase of non-communicable chronic diseases and obesity. *Public Health Nutr.* 2002;5(1A):113–122. doi:10.1079/PHN2001282.

28. Baillie K. Health implications of transition from a planned to a free-market economy—an overview. *Obes Rev.* 2008;9(Suppl 1):146–150.

29. Misra A, Singhal N, Khurana L. Obesity, the metabolic syndrome, and type 2 diabetes in developing countries: role of dietary fats and oils. *J Am Coll Nutr.* 2010;29 (Suppl 3):289S–301S.

30. Igumbor EU, Sanders D, Puoane TR, Tsolekile1 L, Schwarz C, Purdy C, et al. "Big Food, " the consumer food environment, health, and the policy response in South Africa. *PLoS Med.* 2012;9(7):e1001253. doi:10.1371/journal.pmed.1001253.

31. Wallach LM. Accountable governance in the era of globalization: The WTO, NAFTA, and international harmonization of standards. *U Kan L Rev.* 2002;50:823–865; 828.

32. Wallach LM. Accountable governance in the era of globalization: The WTO, NAFTA, and international harmonization of standards. *U Kan L Rev.* 2002;50:823–865.

33. Wallach LM. Accountable governance in the era of globalization: The WTO, NAFTA, and international harmonization of standards. *U Kan L Rev.* 2002;50:823–865; 828.

34. Wallach LM. Accountable governance in the era of globalization: The WTO, NAFTA, and international harmonization of standards. *U Kan L Rev.* 2002;50:823–865.

35. Wallach LM. Accountable governance in the era of globalization: The WTO, NAFTA, and international harmonization of standards. *U Kan L Rev.* 2002;50:823–865.

36. De Jonquieres G. Network guerillas. *Financial Times.* April 30, 1998:12.

37. Fast Track—Presidential trade negotiating authority. *Public Citizen.* Available at: http://www.citizen.org/trade/fasttrack/. Accessed August 28, 2012.

38. Pecquet J. White House still looking to get fast-track trade authority through Congress. *The Hill,* July 30, 2013. Available at: http://thehill.com/blogs/global-affairs/global-economy/314315-white-house-still-looking-to-get-fast-track-trade-authority-through-congress-by-years-end#ixzz2b7OY0iRF. Accessed on August 5, 2013.

39. Wallach LM. Accountable governance in the era of globalization: The WTO, NAFTA, and international harmonization of standards. *U Kan L Rev.* 2002;50:823–865.p. 836.

40. Wallach LM. Accountable governance in the era of globalization: The WTO, NAFTA, and international harmonization of standards. *U Kan L Rev.* 2002;50:823–865.

41. Stiglitz J. *Globalization and Its Discontents.* New York, : Norton; 2002:67.

42. Hertz N. *The Silent Takeover.* New York, : Free Press; 2001:26.

43. Schrecker T. The power of money: global financial markets, national politics, and social determinants of health. In: Williams OD, Kay A, eds. *Global Health Governance: Crisis, Institutions and Political Economy.* Houndmills, UK: Palgrave Macmillan; 2009:160–181.

44. Norris F. Globalization, measured by investment, takes a step backward. *New York Times,* March 2, 2013, p. B3.

45. Hawkes C. The role of foreign direct investment in the nutrition transition. *Public Health Nutr*. 2005;8(4):357–365.

46. Labonté R, Mohindra KS, Lencucha R. Framing international trade and chronic disease. *Global Health*. 2011;7:21. doi: 10.1186/1744-8603-7-21.

47. Gilmore AB, McKee M. Exploring the impact of foreign direct investment on tobacco consumption in the former Soviet Union. *Tob Control*. 2005;14(1):13–21.

48. Labonté R, Mohindra K, Schrecker T. The growing impact of globalization for health and public health practice. *Annu Rev Public Health*. 2011;32:263–283.

49. Wahl P. Food Speculation: the main factor of the price bubble in 2008, Briefing Paper. Berlin, Germany: World Economy, Ecology and Development; 2009. Available at: http://www2. weed-online.org/uploads/weed_food_speculation.pdf. Accessed August 28, 2012.

50. Euromonitor International. Tobacco multinationals assess opportunities in China. *Market Research World*. Available at: http://www.marketresearchworld.net/index. php?option=com_content&task=view&id=214&Itemid=77. Accessed August 28, 2012.

51. World Bank, Human Development Unit, East Asia and Pacific Region. Toward a healthy and harmonious life in China: Stemming the rising tide of non-communicable diseases. Washington, DC: World Bank; 2011. Available at: http://www.worldbank.org/content/ dam/Worldbank/document/NCD_report_en.pdf. Accessed August 28, 2012.p. 4.

52. American Cancer Society. *The Tobacco Atlas*. 4th ed. Atlanta, GA: American Cancer Society, 2012. Available at: http://tobaccoatlas.org/uploads/Images/PDFs/Tobacco_ Atlas_2ndPrint.pdf. Accessed on September 18, 2012.

53. The big smoke. Graphic Detail weblog, *The Economist*. March 21, 2012. Available at:http:// www.economist.com/blogs/graphicdetail/2012/03/daily-chart-14. Accessed on August 28, 2012.

54. Proctor R. *Golden Holocaust*. Berkeley, : University of California Press; 2011:546.

55. Mäkelä P, Osterberg E. Weakening of one more alcohol control pillar: a review of the effects of the alcohol tax cuts in Finland in 2004. *Addiction*. 2009;104(4):554–563.

56. Labonte R, Sanger M. Glossary of the World Trade Organisation and public health: Part 1. *J Epidemiol Community Health*. 2006;60(8):655–661.

57. Relinger R. NAFTA and U.S. corn subsidies: explaining the displacement of Mexico's corn farmers. *Prospect: Journal of International Affairs at UCSD*. April, 2010. Available at:http:// prospectjournal.ucsd.edu/index.php/2010/04/nafta-and-u-s-corn-subsidies-explaining- the-displacement-of-mexicos-corn-farmers/. Accessed August 28, 2012.

58. Chang HJ. *Kicking Away the Ladder: Development Strategy in Historical Perspective*. London: Anthem Press; 2002.

59. Kushwaha S, Sachan R, Maheshwari S, Kushwaha N, Rai AK. An overview on: Trade-related aspects of intellectual property rights. *J Appl Pharm Sci*. 2001;1(03):01–05.

60. Labonte R, Sanger M. Glossary on the World Trade Organisation and public health: Part 2. *J Epidemiol Community Health*. 2006;60(9):738–744.

61. Ip S, Chung M, Raman G, Chew P, Magula N, DeVine D, et al. Breastfeeding and maternal and infant health outcomes in developed countries. *Evid Rep Technol Assess*. 2007;(153):1–186.

62. Montague P. Corporate rights vs. human need. Environmental Research Foundation, Rachel's Newsletter, No. 677. Available at: http://www.rachel.org/?q=en/node/4964. Published November 17, 1999.Accessed August 28, 2012.

63. Shiva V. Stolen harvest: the hijacking of the food supply. In: Fort M, Mercer MA, Gish O, eds. *Sickness and Wealth: The Corporate Assault on Global Health*. Cambridge, MA: South End Press; 2004:107–117.

64. Shiva V. Stolen harvest: The hijacking of the food supply. In: Fort M, Mercer MA, Gish O, eds. *Sickness and Wealth: The Corporate Assault on Global Health*. Cambridge, MA: South End Press; 2004:107–117; 114.

65. Rai S. India–U.S. fight on Basmati rice is mostly settled. *New York Times*. August 25, 2001:C1.

66. Mulle ED, Ruppanner V. Exploring the global food supply chain markets, companies, systems. Geneva, Switzerland: 3D → Trade—Human Rights—Equitable Economy, 2010. 4 Available at: http://www.3dthree.org/pdf_3D/3D_ExploringtheGlobalFoodSupplyChain.pdf. Accessed August 28, 2012.

67. Parthasarathi S. Food Security in Knowledge-Based Economy: Role of Trans-national Seed Corporations in *Sustainable Food Security in the Era of Local and Global Environmental Change*, M. Behnassi et al., eds. New York: Springer; 2013:245–267.

68. Angell M. *The Truth About the Drug Companies: How They Deceive Us and What to Do About It*. New York, : Random House; 2004.

69. DOHA World Trade Organization Ministerial Declaration WT/MIN(01)/DEC/120, November 2001, p. 4. Available at http://www.wto.org/english/thewto_e/minist_e/min01_e/mindecl_e.htm. Accessed on September 18, 2012.

70. TRIPS and Health: Frequently asked questions; compulsory licensing of pharmaceuticals and TRIPS. World Health Organization. Available at: http://www.wto.org/english/tratop_e/trips_e/public_health_faq_e.htm. Published September, 2006. Accessed August 28, 2012.

71. Beall R, Kuhn R. Trends in compulsory licensing of pharmaceuticals since the Doha Declaration: a database analysis. *PLoS Med.* 2012;9(1):e1001154.

72. Maskus KE. Reforming U.S. patent policy: getting the incentives right. Council on Foreign Relations, Council Special Report No. 19. November, 2006. Available at: http://www.ipeg.com/_UPLOAD percent20BLOG/MaskusForeignRelations.pdf. Accessed August 28, 2012.

73. Maskus KE. Reforming U.S. patent policy: getting the incentives right. Council on Foreign Relations, Council Special Report No. 19. November, 2006. Available at: http://www.ipeg.com/_UPLOAD percent20BLOG/MaskusForeignRelations.pdf. Accessed August 28, 2012.

74. Beall R, Kuhn R. Trends in compulsory licensing of pharmaceuticals since the Doha Declaration: a database analysis. *PLoS Med.* 2012;9(1):e1001154.

75. Smith RD, Correa C, Oh C. Trade, TRIPS, and pharmaceuticals. *Lancet.* 2009;373 (9664):684–691.

76. Garrett L. *Betrayal of Trust: The Collapse of Global Public Health*. New York, : Hyperion; 2001.

77. Bussard S. The price for private funding of the World Health Organization. *Le Temps* (Geneva). May 20, 2011. Available at: http://www.worldcrunch.com/price-private-funding-world-health-organization/world-affairs/the-price-for-private-funding-of-the-world-health-organization/c1s3121/#.UPWBqKx0SSp.Accessed on January 15, 2013.

78. Stuckler D, Basu S, McKee M. Global health philanthropy and institutional relationships: how should conflicts of interest be addressed? *PLoS Med.* 2011;8(4):e1001020.

79. Collin J. Global health, equity and the WHO Framework Convention on Tobacco Control. *Global Health Promotion.* 2010;17(Supp 73–75);1757–9759. doi: 10.1177/1757975909358363.

80. World Health Organization, Commission on Social Determinants of Health. Closing the gap in a generation: health equity through action on the social determinants of health. Geneva, Switzerland: World Health Organization; 2008, p. 142. Available at: http://whqlibdoc.who.int/publications/2008/9789241563703_eng.pdf. Accessed August 28, 2012.

81. World Health Organization, Commission on Social Determinants of Health. Closing the gap in a generation: health equity through action on the social determinants of health. Geneva, Switzerland: World Health Organization; 2008. Available at: http://whqlibdoc.who.int/publications/2008/9789241563703_eng.pdf. Accessed August 28, 2012.

82. Proctor R. *Golden Holocaust*. Berkeley, CA: University of California Press; 2011:547.

83. World Health Organization. WHO Framework Convention on Tobacco Control: Guidelines for implementation of the WHO FCTC. Geneva, Switzerland: World Health Organization; 2011, p. 51. Available at: http://whqlibdoc.who.int/publications/2011/9789241501316_eng.pdf. Accessed August 28, 2012.

84. World Health Organization. WHO Framework Convention on Tobacco Control: Guidelines for implementation of the WHO FCTC. Geneva, Switzerland: World Health Organization; 2011. Available at: http://whqlibdoc.who.int/publications/2011/9789241501316_eng. pdf. Accessed August 28, 2012.

85. About Us: What is the Framework Convention Alliance? Framework Convention Alliance. Available at: http://www.fctc.org/index.php?option=com_content&view=article&id=2&I temid=277. Accessed August 28, 2012.

86. Mamudu HM, Glantz SA. Civil society and the negotiation of the Framework Convention on Tobacco Control. *Glob Public Health*. 2009;4(2):150–168; 156.

87. Collin J. Global health, equity and the WHO Framework Convention on Tobacco Control. *Global Health Promotion*. 2010;17(Suppl 1):73–75. doi: 10.1177/1757975909358363.

88. Collin J. Global health, equity and the WHO Framework Convention on Tobacco Control. *Global Health Promotion*. 2010;17(Suppl 1):73–75. doi: 10.1177/1757975909358363.

89. Collin J. Global health, equity and the WHO Framework Convention on Tobacco Control. *Global Health Promotion*. 2010;17(Suppl 1):73–75. doi: 10.1177/1757975909358363.

90. Carter SM. Mongoven, Biscoe & Duchin: destroying tobacco control activism from the inside. *Tob Control*. 2002;11(2):112–118.

91. Brandt A. *The Cigarette Century*. New York, : Basic Books; 2007:477.

92. Chan M. The changed face of the tobacco industry. Presented at 15th World Conference on Tobacco or Health; March 20, 2012; Singapore. Available at:http://www.who.int/dg/ speeches/2012/tobacco_20120320/en/index.html. Accessed August 28, 2012.

93. World Health Organization. Small Arms and Global Health. Geneva, Switzerland: World Health Organization; 2001,. Available at http://whqlibdoc.who.int/hq/2001/WHO_ NMH_VIP_01.1.pdf. Accessed August 29, 2012.

94. World Health Organization. Small Arms and Global Health. Geneva, Switzerland: World Health Organization; 2001, p. 1. Available at http://whqlibdoc.who.int/hq/2001/WHO_ NMH_VIP_01.1.pdf. Accessed August 29, 2012.

95. Hemenway D. *Private Guns, Public Health*. Ann Arbor, : University of Michigan Press; 2004.

96. Krug EG, Dahlberg LL, Mercy JA, Zwi AB, Lozano R, eds. World report on violence and health. Geneva, Switzerland; World Health Organization; 2002, p. 254. Available at: http:// whqlibdoc.who.int/publications/2002/9241545615_eng.pdf. Accessed August 28, 2012.

97. Zavala DE et al. Implementing a hospital based injury surveillance system in Africa. Lessons learned. *Medicine, Conflict and Survival*. 2008;24(4):260–272. doi:10.1080/ 13623690802373884.

98. Valenti M, Ormhaug CM, Mtonga RE, Loretz J. Armed violence: a health problem, a public health approach. *J Public Health Pol*. 2007;28(4):389–400.

99. Nichols M. United Nations fails to agree landmark arms-trade treaty. Reuters. Available at: http:// www.reuters.com/article/2012/07/27/us-arms-treaty-idUSBRE86Q1MW20120727. Published July 27, 2012.Accessed August 28, 2012.

100. SAAMI testifies at U.N. arms trade treaty negotiations [press release]. National Shooting Sports Foundation: July 12, 2012. Available at: http://nssf.org/NewsRoom/releases/show. cfm?PR=071212_SAAMI_UN.cfm&path=2012. Accessed August 28, 2012.

101. About Us. International Action Network on Small Arms. Available at: http://www.iansa. org/aboutus. Accessed August 28, 2012.

102. Drajem M. Two U.S. agencies object to Obama proposal to ease gun exports. *Bloomberg Business Week*. May 3, 2012. Available at: http://www.businessweek.com/news/2012-05- 02/homeland-security-objects-to-obama-s-plan-for-eased-gun-exports. Accessed August 28, 2012.

103. Horowitz S. Obama plan would ease weapons export rules. *Washington Post*. May 2, 2012:A03.

104. Urqhhart C. Arms trade treaty failure is disappointing, says William Hague. *Guardian*. July 28, 2012. Available at: http://www.guardian.co.uk/world/2012/jul/28/arms-trade-treaty- william-hague. Accessed on August 26, and August 28, 2012.

105. The Arms Trade Treaty Has Been Approved! *Control Arms*. Available at: http://controlarms.org/en/att/Accessed on August 5, 2013.
106. Swinburn B, Sacks G, Lobstein T, Rigby N, Baur LA, Brownell KD, et al. The "Sydney Principles" for reducing the commercial promotion of foods and beverages to children. *Public Health Nutr.* 2008;11(9):881–886;. 881.
107. Kumanyika SK. A question of competing rights, priorities, and principles: a postscript to the Robert Wood Johnson Foundation symposium on the ethics of childhood obesity policy. *Prev Chronic Dis.* 2011;8(5):A97. Available at: http://www.cdc.gov/pcd/issues/2011/sep/10_0289.htm. Accessed August 28, 2012.
108. Urgently needed: a framework convention for obesity control. Editorial. *Lancet.* 2011;378(9793):741.
109. Galvão J. Access to antiretroviral drugs in Brazil. *Lancet.* 2002;360:1862–1865.
110. Brazil Ministry of Health. National AIDS drug policy. Brasília: Coordenação Nacional de DST e AIDS, Ministério da Saúde, 2002.
111. Galvão J. Access to antiretroviral drugs in Brazil. *Lancet.* 2002;360:1862–1865.
112. Cohen J. AIDS drugs: Brazil, Thailand override Big Pharma patents. *Science.* 2007;316:816. doi: 10.1126/science.316.5826.816.
113. Cohen J. AIDS drugs: Brazil, Thailand override Big Pharma patents. *Science.* 2007;316:816. doi: 10.1126/science.316.5826.816.
114. Cohen J. AIDS drugs: Brazil, Thailand override Big Pharma patents. *Science.* 2007;316:816. doi: 10.1126/science.316.5826.816.
115. Indian government allows legal generic cancer drug under TRIPS. *Genglob Magazine.* March 13, 2012. Available at: http://www.genglob.com/genglobmag/2012/03/indian-government-allow-legal-generic-cancer-drug-under-trips/. Accessed August 28, 2012.
116. Ahmed R. India Appeals Body Rejects Bayer's Plea on Nexavar. *Wall Street Journal.* March 4, 2013. Available at: http://online.wsj.com/article/SB10001424127887324178904578340013954624212.html. Accessed on August 7, 2013.
117. World Health Organization. The world medicines situation. Geneva, Switzerland: World Health Organization; 2004. Available at: http://www.searo.who.int/LinkFiles/Reports_World_Medicines_Situation.pdf. Accessed August 28, 2012.
118. Koivusalo M, Mackintosh M. Commercial influence and global nongovernmental public action in health and pharmaceutical policies. *Int J Health Serv.* 2011;41(3):539–563; 545.
119. About the Treatment Action Campaign. Treatment Action Campaign. Available at: http://www.tac.org.za/community/about. Accessed August 28, 2012.
120. Das P. Zackie Achmat—head of the Treatment Action Campaign. *Lancet Infectious Diseases.* 2004;4(7):467–470; 468.
121. Heywood M. South Africa's Treatment Action Campaign (TAC): An example of a successful human rights campaign for health. Treatment Action Campaign. Available at: http://www.tac.org.za/community/node/2064. Published March 26, 2008.Accessed August 28, 2012.
122. Loff B, Heywood M. Patents on drugs: manufacturing scarcity or advancing health. *J, Law Med Ethics.* 2002;30:621–631.
123. Heywood M. South Africa's Treatment Action Campaign (TAC): An example of a successful human rights campaign for health. Treatment Action Campaign. Available at: http://www.tac.org.za/community/node/2064. Published March 26, 2008. Accessed August 28, 2012.
124. Fisher WW, Rigamonti CP. The South Africa AIDS controversy. A case study in patent law and policy. *The Law and Business of Patents.* Harvard Law School; 2005. Available at: http://cyber.law.harvard.edu/people/tfisher/South   percent20Africa.pdf.   Accessed   August 28, 2012.
125. Fisher WW, Rigamonti CP. The South Africa AIDS controversy. A case study in patent law and policy. *The Law and Business of Patents.* Harvard Law School; 2005. Available at: http://cyber.law.harvard.edu/people/tfisher/South   percent20Africa.pdf.   Accessed   August 28, 2012.

126. Weissman R. AIDS drugs for Africa: grassroots pressure overcomes U.S.-industry "full court press" to block South Africa's affordable medicine program. *Multinational Monitor.* 1999;20(9). Available at: http://www.multinationalmonitor.org/mm1999/091999/weissman.html. Accessed August 28, 2012.

127. Heywood M. South Africa's Treatment Action Campaign (TAC): An example of a successful human rights campaign for health. Treatment Action Campaign. Available at: http://www.tac.org.za/community/node/2064. Published March 26, 2008. Accessed August 28, 2012.

128. Heywood M. South Africa's Treatment Action Campaign (TAC): An example of a successful human rights campaign for health. Treatment Action Campaign. Available at: http://www.tac.org.za/community/node/2064. Published March 26, 2008. Accessed August 28, 2012.

129. Heywood M. South Africa's Treatment Action Campaign (TAC): An example of a successful human rights campaign for health. Treatment Action Campaign. Available at: http://www.tac.org.za/community/node/2064. Published March 26, 2008. Accessed August 28, 2012.

130. Oseid BJ. Breast-feeding and infant health. *Clin Obstet Gynecol.* 1975;18(2):149–173.

131. Bader MB. Breast-feeding: the role of multinational corporations in Latin America. *Int J Health Serv.* 1976;6(4):609–626.

132. Carter SM. Mongoven, Biscoe & Duchin: destroying tobacco control activism from the inside. *Tob Control.* 2002;11(2):112–118.

133. Thirty-Fourth World Health Assembly, International Code of Marketing of Breast Milk Substitutes, Res. WHA34.22, Annex WHO Doc. A341VRlI5, (Fifteenth Plenary, Meeting, May 21, 1981).

134. Walker M. International breastfeeding initiatives and their relevance to the current state of breastfeeding in the United States. *J Midwifery Women's Health.* 2007;52(6):549–555.

135. History: Challenging corporate abuse for over 35 years. Corporate Accountability International. Available at: http://www.stopcorporateabuse.org/history. Accessed August 28, 2012.

136. International Baby Food Action Network, International Code Documentation Centre. *Breaking the Rules, Stretching the Rules 2010.* Penang, Malaysia: International Baby Food Action Network; 2010.

137. Baby Milk Action. *Breaking the Rules—Stretching the Rules 2010.* Available at: http://info.babymilkaction.org/update/update43page9. Accessed on September 16, 2012.

Chapter 7 Optimism Past, Present, and Future: The Building Blocks for a Movement

1. Bunker JP, Frazier HS, Mosteller F. Improving health: measuring effects of medical care. *Milbank Q.* 1994;72:225–258.

2. Sinclair U. *The Jungle.* New York: Doubleday, Page and Co.; 1906:328.

3. Hilts P. *Protecting America's Health: The FDA, Business, and One Hundred Years of Regulation.* New York: Knopf; 2003.

4. Hilts P. *Protecting America's Health: The FDA, Business, and One Hundred Years of Regulation.* New York: Knopf; 2003:52.

5. Hilts P. *Protecting America's Health: The FDA, Business, and One Hundred Years of Regulation.* New York: Knopf; 2003:51.

6. Hilts P. *Protecting America's Health: The FDA, Business, and One Hundred Years of Regulation.* New York: Knopf; 2003:51.

7. Adams SH. The great American fraud. *Colliers.* 1905;36(2):14–15. Cited by: Young JH. *The Medical Messiahs: A Social History of Health Quackery in Twentieth-Century America.* Princeton, NJ: Princeton University Press; 1967:31.

8. Hilts P. *Protecting America's Health: The FDA, Business, and One Hundred Years of Regulation.* New York: Knopf; 2003:44.

9. Law MT, Libecap GD. The determinants of Progressive Era reform: The Pure Food and Drugs Act of 1906. NBER Working Paper No.10984. December 2004. National Bureau of

Economic Research. Available at: http://www.nber.org/papers/w10984. Accessed October 1, 2012.

10. CDC. Achievements in public health, 1900–1999: safer and healthier foods. *MMWR*. 1999;48(40):905–913.

11. Hilts P. *Protecting America's Health: The FDA, Business, and One Hundred Years of Regulation*. New York: Knopf; 2003.

12. No author. Microbe Killer defeated. *Medical and Surgical Reporter*. 1893(68):790–791.

13. Law MT, Libecap GD. The determinants of Progressive Era reform: The Pure Food and Drugs Act of 1906. NBER Working Paper No.10984. December 2004. National Bureau of Economic Research. Available at: http://www.nber.org/papers/w10984. Accessed October 1, 2012.

14. Hilts P. *Protecting America's Health: The FDA, Business, and One Hundred Years of Regulation*. New York: Knopf; 2003:39–40.

15. CDC. Achievements in public health, 1900–1999: safer and healthier foods. *MMWR*. 1999;48(40):905–913.

16. Hilts P. *Protecting America's Health: The FDA, Business, and One Hundred Years of Regulation*. New York: Knopf; 2003.

17. Hilts P. *Protecting America's Health: The FDA, Business, and One Hundred Years of Regulation*. New York: Knopf; 2003:xii.

18. Hilts P. *Protecting America's Health: The FDA, Business, and One Hundred Years of Regulation*. New York: Knopf; 2003:55.

19. Reeve AB. The death roll of industry. *Charities and the Commons*. 1907;17(14):791. Cited by: Rosner D, Markowitz G. Introduction: Workers' health and safety: Some historical notes. In: Rosner D, Markowitz G, eds. *Dying for Work*, 2nd ed. Bloomington: Indiana University Press; 1989:ix–xviii; xi.

20. Rosner D, Markowitz G. Introduction: Workers' health and safety: Some historical notes. In: Rosner D, Markowitz G, eds. *Dying for Work*, 2nd ed. Bloomington: Indiana University Press; 1989:ix–xviii; ix–xix.

21. Centers for Disease Control and Prevention. Achievements in public health, 1900–1999: improvements in workplace safety—United States, 1900–1999. *MMWR*. 1999;48(22):461–469.

22. National Safety Council. *Accident Facts, 1998 edition*. Itasca, IL: National Safety Council, 1998.

23. Centers for Disease Control and Prevention. Achievements in public health, 1900–1999: improvements in workplace safety—United States, 1900–1999. *MMWR*. 1999;48(22):461–469.

24. Centers for Disease Control and Prevention. Achievements in public health, 1900–1999: improvements in workplace safety—United States, 1900–1999. *MMWR*. 1999;48(22):461–469.

25. Centers for Disease Control and Prevention. Achievements in public health, 1900–1999: improvements in workplace safety—United States, 1900–1999. *MMWR*. 1999;48(22):461–469.

26. Clopper EN. Child labor and public health. *J Am Public Health Assoc*. 1911;1(5):322–328.

27. Clopper EN. Child labor and public health. *J Am Public Health Assoc*. 1911;1(5):322–328.

28. Sanderson AR. Child-labor legislation and the labor force participation of children. *Journal of Economic History*. 1974;34(1):297–299.

29. Keating-Owen Child Labor Act of 1916. September 1, 1916. U.S. National Archives and Records Administration. Available at: http://www.ourdocuments.gov/doc.php?doc=59. Accessed October 1, 2012.

30. Postol P. Public health and working children in twentieth-century America: An historical overview. *J Public Health Pol*. 1993;14 (3):348–354.

31. Landrigan PJ, McCammon JB. Child labor still with us after all these years. *Public Health Rep*. 1997;112(6):466–473.

32. International Programme on the Elimination of Child Labour (IPEC). *Children in Hazardous Work: What We Know, What We Need to Do.* Geneva, Switzerland: International Labor Organization; 2011:xiii.

33. Levy, AR. Interview with Nancy Romer [transcript]. *Connect the Dots.* Progressive Radio Network. May 23, 2012. Available at: http://prn.fm/2012/05/23/connect-dots-052312/#axzz1xhoXB9vP. Accessed October 1, 2012.

34. Reynolds L. In anticipation of the Brooklyn Food Conference: an interview with Nancy Romer. *Nourishing the Planet.* Available at: http://blogs.worldwatch.org/nourishingthe-planet/in-anticipation-of-the-brooklyn-food-conference-an-interview-with-nancy-romer/. Published May 11, 2012. Accessed October 1, 2012.

35. Reynolds L. In anticipation of the Brooklyn Food Conference: an interview with Nancy Romer. *Nourishing the Planet.* Available at: http://blogs.worldwatch.org/nourishingthe-planet/in-anticipation-of-the-brooklyn-food-conference-an-interview-with-nancy-romer/. Published May 11, 2012.Accessed October 1, 2012.

36. Nestle M. Advocacy groups join for N.Y. candidates forum. *San Francisco Chronicle.* August 4, 2013. Available at: http://www.sfchronicle.com/food/foodmatters/article/Advocacy-groups-join-for-N-Y-candidates-forum-4704079.php. Accessed on August 8, 2013.

37. Beckford B. School districts soon will be able to opt out of a common ammonia-treated ground-beef filler critics have dubbed "pink slime." Brooklyn Food Coalition. Available at: http://brooklynfoodcoalition.ning.com/group/schoollunchreform/forum/topics/school-districts-soon-will-be-able-to-opt-out-of-a-common-ammonia. Published March 15, 2012. Accessed October 1, 2012.

38. Romer N. Where do we go from here? Presented at: Brooklyn Food Conference. Brooklyn, NY: May 12, 2012.

39. Romer N. Where do we go from here? Presented at: Brooklyn Food Conference. Brooklyn, NY: May 12, 2012

40. Gustafson K. *Change Comes to Dinner: How Vertical Farmers, Urban Growers, and Other Innovators Are Revolutionizing How America Eats.* New York: St. Martin Griffins, 2012: 256.

41. Graham C. St. Ides and hip-hop: would today's rappers endorse malt liquor? October 24, 2011. Available at: http://blogs.houstonpress.com/rocks/2011/10/st_ides_and_hip-hop_would_toda.php. Accessed October 2, 2012.

42. Emeno A. Coalition protests sale of malt liquor in "40s": black leaders called the 40-ounce bottles "Liquid Crack." They want brewers to fund anti–alcohol abuse messages. *Philadelphia Inquirer,* July 10, 2000. Available at http://articles.philly.com/2000-07-10/news/25609390_1_malt-liquor-40-ounce-bottles-state-owned-liquor-stores.Accessed October 2, 2012.

43. Herd D. Community mobilization and the framing of alcohol-related problems. *Int J Environ Res Public Health.* 2010;7(3):1226–1247:1236.

44. Popova S, Giesbrecht N, Bekmuradov D, Patra J. Hours and days of sale and density of alcohol outlets: impacts on alcohol consumption and damage: a systematic review. *Alcohol.* 2009;44(5):500–516.

45. Alaniz ML, Wilkes C. Pro-drinking messages and message environments for young adults: The case of alcohol industry advertising in African American, Latino, and Native American communities. *J Public Health Pol.* 1998;19(4):447–472.

46. Alaniz ML, Wilkes C. Pro-drinking messages and message environments for young adults: the case of alcohol industry advertising in African American, Latino, and Native American communities. *J Public Health Pol.* 1998;19(4):447–472.

47. Center on Alcohol Marketing and Youth. *Exposure of African-American youth to alcohol advertising, 2003 to 2004.* Baltimore, MD: Center on Alcohol Marketing and Youth; 2006.

48. Douglass F. *Narrative of the Life of Frederick Douglass, An American Slave,* 6th ed. London: H.G. Collins; 1851:70.

49. Herd DA. Contesting culture: alcohol related identity movements in contemporary African-American communities. *Contemp Drug Probs.* 1993;20(4):739–758.

50. Herd DA. Voices from the field: the social construction of alcohol problems in inner-city communities. *Contemp Drug Problems*. 2011;38(1):7–39.

51. Alaniz ML, Wilkes C. Pro-drinking messages and message environments for young adults: the case of alcohol industry advertising in African American, Latino, and Native American communities. *J Public Health Pol*. 1998;19(4):447–472.

52. Black Expo ties to beer, tobacco hit. *Chicago Tribune*. July 14, 1991. Available at: http://articles.chicagotribune.com/1991-07-14/news/9103190532_1_tobacco-and-alcohol-billboards-addictive-black-people. Accessed October 1, 2012.

53. McClory R. Blacks and Catholics are joint ventures at Chicago parish—St. Sabina Church led by a priest, Michael Pfleger. *National Catholic Reporter*. March 13, 1998.

54. Spielman F. Billboard blitz in Chicago. *Chicago-Sun Times*. September 11, 1997.

55. Meyerson C. Billboard protest gets quick response. *Chicago Tribune*. August 29, 2000. Available at: http://articles.chicagotribune.com/2000-08-29/news/0008300061_1_alcohol-billboards-billboard-s-owner-tobacco-and-alcohol. Accessed: October 1, 2012.

56. National Association of African Americans for Positive Imagery. Defeat of PowerMaster malt liquor. Available at http://www.naaapi.org/documents/powermaster.asp

57. Eichenwald K. U.S. rescinds approval of a malt liquor. *New York Times*. July 4, 1991:D3.

58. National Association of African Americans for Positive Imagery. Defeat of PowerMaster malt liquor. Available at http://www.naaapi.org/documents/powermaster.asp. Accessed on October 6, 2012.

59. Cawley J. Brewer to drop controversial malt liquor. *Chicago Tribune*. July 4, 1991. Available at: http://articles.chicagotribune.com/1991-07-04/news/9103160613_1_powermaster-heileman-officials-rev-george-clements. Accessed October 2, 2012.

60. Herd D. Community mobilization and the framing of alcohol-related problems. *Int J Environ Res Public Health*. 2010;7(3):1226–1247.

61. Lopez-Garza M. *State of South Los Angeles 1990–2010: A Community Coalition Perspective*. Los Angeles, CA: Community Coalition; 2001.

62. Brown J. Speech on National Association of African Americans for Positive Imagery at World Health Organization, Global Tobacco Convention hearings, Geneva, Switzerland, October 12–13, 2000. Text at: http://www.who.int/tobacco/framework/public_hearings/national_association_of_african_americans_for_positive_imagery.pdf. Accessed October 6, 2012.

63. The History of the California Environmental Protection Agency: Air Resources Board. California Environmental Protection Agency. Available at: http://www.calepa.ca.gov/about/history01/arb.htm. Updated October 20, 2008.Accessed October 2, 2012.

64. Hayes SP. *Explorations in Environmental History*. Pittsburgh, PA: University of Pittsburgh Press; 1998:221–279.

65. Fimrite P. The high price of polluted air: illnesses costing almost $200 million per year. *San Francisco Chronicle*. March 2, 2010:C1.

66. [65] California Air Resources Board. Scientists present findings on black carbon and climate change. Press release. May 24, 2012. Available at http://www.arb.ca.gov/newsrel/newsrelease.php?id=306. Accessed on April 28,2013.

67. Costello A, Abbas M, Allen A, Ball S, et al. Managing the health effects of climate change: *Lancet* and University College London Institute for Global Health Commission. *Lancet*. 2009;373(9676):1693–1733.

68. Global Warming Solutions Act, Assembly Bill 32. Environmental Protection Agency, September 27, 2006. Available at: http://www.leginfo.ca.gov/pub/05-06/bill/asm/ab_0001-0050/ab_32_bill_20060927_chaptered.pdf. Accessed October 2, 2012.

69. Blake M. California ready to cut greenhouse gases. Next, doing it. *Christian Science Monitor*. March 13, 2012. Available at: http://www.csmonitor.com/layout/set/print/content/view/print/479229. Accessed October 2, 2012.

70. Barnes R, Eilperin J. High court faults EPA inaction on emissions. *Washington Post*. April 3, 2007:A01.

71. California's Clean Cars law. Environmental Defense Fund. Available at: http://www.edf. org/transportation/policy/california-clean-cars-law. Accessed October 2, 2012.

72. Eilperin J. U.S., auto industry agree on long-range fuel efficiency rules. *Washington Post.* July 28, 2011:A17

73. Eilperin J. U.S., auto industry agree on long-range fuel efficiency rules. *Washington Post.* July 28,2011:A17.

74. Blake M. California ready to cut greenhouse gases. Next, doing it. *Christian Science Monitor.* March 13, 2012. Available at: http://www.csmonitor.com/layout/set/print/content/view/ print/479229. Accessed October 2, 2012.

75. Blake M. California ready to cut greenhouse gases. Next, doing it. *Christian Science Monitor.* March 13, 2012. Available at: http://www.csmonitor.com/layout/set/print/content/view/ print/479229. Accessed October 2, 2012.

76. Sweeney JL, Kahn ME. A flawed cost/benefit study of a greener California. *Los Angeles Times.* March 24, 2010. Available at: http://articles.latimes.com/2010/mar/24/opinion/ la-oe-sweeney24-2010mar24. Accessed October 2, 2012.

77. Carlson A. AB32 lawsuit: Assessing the environmental justice arguments against cap and trade. *Legal Planet.* Available at: http://legalplanet.wordpress.com/2011/03/22/ab-32-law-suit-assessing-the-environmental-justice-arguments-against-cap-and-trade/. Published March 22, 2012. Accessed October 2, 2012.

78. The History of the California Environmental Protection Agency: Air Resources Board. California Environmental Protection Agency. Available at http://www.calepa.ca.gov/ about/history01/arb.htm.Updated October 20, 2008. Accessed October 2, 2012.

79. Rogers P. California's clean car rules help remake U.S. auto industry: interview with Mary Nichols. *Yale Environment 360.* February 8, 2012. Available at: http://e360.yale.edu/feature/californias_ clean_car_rules_help_remake_us_auto_industry/2492/. Accessed October 2, 2012.

80. Wood DB. Can California change U.S. cars forever? New zero-emission rules take aim. *Christian Science Monitor.* January 27, 2012. Available at: http://www.csmonitor.com/ USA/2012/0127/Can-California-change-US-cars-forever-New-zero-emissions-rules-take-aim. Accessed October 2, 2012.

81. Kahn M. Don't make fun of California's carbon reduction efforts. *Christian Science Monitor.* November 2, 2011. Available at: http://www.csmonitor.com/Business/Green-Economics/2011/1102/Don-t-make-fun-of-California-s-carbon-reduction-efforts. Accessed October 2, 2012.

82. Cruising 55 panel discussion [podcast]. The Commonwealth Club of California. February 13, 2012. Available at: http://www.commonwealthclub.org/events/2012-02-13/cruis-ing-55. Accessed October 2, 2012.

83. Dal Bó E. Regulatory capture: a review. *Oxf Rev Econ Policy.* 2006;22(2):203–225.

84. Wallack L, Winett L, Nettekoven L. The million mom march: engaging the public on gun policy. *J Public Health Pol.* 2003;24(3/4);355–379.

85. Wallack L, Winett L, Nettekoven L. The million mom march: Engaging the public on gun policy. *J Public Health Pol.* 2003;24(3/4);355–379.

86. Wallack L, Winett L, Nettekoven L. The million mom march: Engaging the public on gun policy. *J Public Health Pol.* 2003;24(3/4);355–379; 364.

87. Brown PH, Abel DG. *Outgunned: Up Against the NRA.* New York: Free Press; 2003:240.

88. Fortune releases annual survey of most powerful lobbying organizations [press release]. Time Warner: November 15, 1999. Available at: http://www.timewarner.com/news-room/press-releases/1999/11/FORTUNE_Releases_Annual_Survey_Most_Powerful_ Lobbying_11-15-1999.php. Accessed October 2, 2012.

89. Dickinson A. Mothers against guns. *Time.* May 15, 2000. Available at: http://www.time. com/time/magazine/article/0,9171,996903,00.html. Accessed October 2, 2012.

90. Brown PH, Abel DG. *Outgunned: Up Against the NRA.* New York: Free Press; 2003.

91. Dickinson A. Mothers against guns. *Time.* May 15, 2000. Available at: http://www.time. com/time/magazine/article/0,9171,996903,00.html. Accessed October 2, 2012.

92. Wallack L, Winett L, Nettekoven L. The million mom march: engaging the public on gun policy. *J Public Health Pol.* 2003;24(3/4);355–379; 367

93. Ponte W. Million mom march: speaking up for safer gun laws. *Mothering.* 2000;102. Available at: http://mothering.com/parenting/million-mom-march-speaking-up-for-safer-gun-laws. Accessed October 2, 2012.

94. Dickinson A. Mothers against guns. *Time.* May 15, 2000. Available at: http://www.time.com/time/magazine/article/0,9171,996903,00.html. Accessed October 2, 2012.

95. Wallack L, Winett L, Nettekoven L. The million mom march: engaging the public on gun policy. *J Public Health Pol.* 2003;24(3/4);355–379; 364.

96. Brown PH, Abel DG. *Outgunned: Up Against the NRA.* New York: Free Press; 2003:242.

97. Brown PH, Abel DG. *Outgunned: Up Against the NRA.* New York: Free Press; 2003:245.

98. Goss KG, Heaney MT. Organizing women as women: hybridity and grassroots collective action in the 21st century. *Perspectives on Politics.* 2010;8(1):2752.

99. Ponte W. Million mom march: speaking up for safer gun laws. *Mothering.* 2000;102. Available at: http://mothering.com/parenting/million-mom-march-speaking-up-for-safer-gun-laws. Accessed October 2, 2012.

100. Wallack L, Winett L, Nettekoven L. The million mom march: engaging the public on gun policy. *J Public Health Pol.* 2003;24(3/4);355–379; 359.

101. Goss KG. *Disarmed: The Missing Movement for Gun Control in America.* Princeton, NJ: Princeton University Press; 2009:184.

102. Wallack L, Winett L, Nettekoven L. The million mom march: engaging the public on gun policy. *J Public Health Pol.* 2003;24(3/4);355–379.

103. Thomas SB, Leite B, Duncan T. Breaking the cycle of violence among youth living in metropolitan Atlanta: a case history of kids alive and loved. *Health Educ Behav.* 1998;25(2):160–174.

104. Schwartz J. Conflicting rulings on guns open way to Supreme Court review. *New York Times.* June 17, 2009:A14.

105. Wallack L, Winett L, Nettekoven L. The million mom march: engaging the public on gun policy. *J Public Health Pol.* 2003;24(3/4);355–379.

106. Million Mom Chapters. Brady campaign to end gun violence. Available at http://www.bradycampaign.org/chapters/.Accessed October 2, 2012.

107. Goss KG. *Disarmed: The Missing Movement for Gun Control in America.* Princeton, NJ: Princeton University Press; 2009:377.

108. Wallack L, Winett L, Nettekoven L. The million mom march: engaging the public on gun policy. *J Public Health Pol.* 2003;24(3/4);355–379.

109. Weise E. Gun-control advocates blast NRA statement. *USA Today,* December 21, 2012. Available at: http://www.usatoday.com/story/news/nation/2012/12/21/nra-gun-control-newton-shooting/1784457/. Accessed on January 17, 2013.

110. MacGillis A. This Is How the NRA Ends. *New Republic,* May 28, 2013. Available at: http://www.newrepublic.com/node/113292/print. Accessed on August 8, 2013.

111. Johnson T. The media myth of NRA electoral dominance should end with 2012. *Media Matters,* December 21, 2012. Available at: http://mediamatters.org/blog/2012/12/21/the-media-myth-of-nra-electoral-dominance-shoul/191944. Accessed on January 16, 2013.

112. MacGillis A. This Is How the NRA Ends. *New Republic,* May 28, 2013. Available at: http://www.newrepublic.com/node/113292/print. Accessed on August 8, 2013.

113. Violence Prevention Policy Center. Blood money: how the gun industry bankrolls the NRA. Washington, D.C., 2011.

114. Kaiser Public Opinion Spotlight: Views on prescription drugs and the pharmaceutical industry. Kaiser Family Foundation. Available at: http://www.kff.org/spotlight/rxdrugs/upload/rx_drugs.pdf. Updated April, 2008. Accessed October 2, 2012.

115. Public perception of U.S. pharmaceutical industry at all-time low. *Pharmaceutical Business Review.* October 18, 2005. Available at: http://www.commercialalert.org/news/

archive/2005/10/public-perception-of-us-pharmaceutical-industry-at-all-time-low. Accessed October 2, 2012.

116. Sillup GP, Porth SJ. Pharm Exec's seventh annual media audit. PharmExec.com. March 1, 2011. Available at: http://www.pharmexec.com/pharmexec/Noteworthy/Pharm-Execs-Seventh-Annual-Media-Audit/ArticleStandard/Article/detail/711575. Accessed October 2, 2012.

117. Gagnon MA, Lexchin J. The cost of pushing pills: a new estimate of pharmaceutical promotion expenditures in the United States. *PLoS Med*.5(1):e1. doi:10.1371/journal.pmed.0050001.

118. Grande D. Prescriber profiling: time to call it quits. *Ann Intern Med*. 2007;146:751–752.

119. Rodwin MA. Drug advertising, continuing medical education, and physician prescribing: a historical review and reform proposal. *J Law Med Ethics*. 2010;38(4):807–815.

120. Spurling GK, Mansfield PR, Montgomery BD, Lexchin J, Doust J, Othman N, et al. Information from pharmaceutical companies and the quality, quantity, and cost of physicians' prescribing: a systematic review. *PLoS Med*. 2010;7(10):e1000352. doi:10.1371/journal.pmed.1000352.

121. About Us. No Free Lunch. Available at: http://www.nofreelunch.org/aboutus.htm. Accessed October 2, 2012.

122. Patients. No Free Lunch. Available at: http://www.nofreelunch.org/patients.htm. Accessed October 2, 2012.

123. Campbell EG, Gruen RL, Mountford J, Miller LG, Cleary PD, Blumenthal D. A national survey of physician–industry relationships. *N Engl J Med*. 2007;356(17):1742–1750.

124. Evans DV, Hartung DM, Andeen G, Mahler J, Haxby DG, Kraemer DF, et al. One practice's experiment in refusing detail rep visits. *J Fam Pract*. 2011;60(8):E1–E6.

125. Evans DV, Hartung DM, Andeen G, Mahler J, Haxby DG, Kraemer DF, et al. One practice's experiment in refusing detail rep visits. *J Fam Pract*. 2011;60(8):E1–E6.

126. Ehringhaus SH, Weissman JS, Sears JL, Goold SD, Feibelmann S, Campbell EG. Responses of medical schools to institutional conflicts of interest. *JAMA*. 2008;299(6):665–671.

127. Bekelman JE, Li Y, Gross CP. Scope and impact of financial conflicts of interest in biomedical research: a systematic review. *JAMA*. 2003;289(4):454–465.

128. AMSA Pharm Free Scorecard 2011–12. American Medical Student Association. Available at: http://www.amsascorecard.org/executive-summary. Updated March 7, 2012. Accessed October 2, 2012.

129. McCarthy M. U.S. campaign tackles drug company influence over doctors. *Lancet*. 2007;730(369):9563.

130. Harris G. Senators seek public listing of payments to doctors. *New York Times*. Sept. 7, 2007:A20.

131. The Unbranded Doctor. The National Physicians Alliance. Available at: http://npalliance.org/action/the-unbranded-doctor/. Accessed October 2, 2012.

132. Rx Democracy. The National Physicians Alliance. Available at: http://salsa.democracyinaction.org/o/1021/p/dia/action/public/?action_KEY=4627. Accessed October 2, 2012.

133. Ornstein C, Weber T, Nguyen D. Docs on Pharma payroll have blemished records, limited credentials *Pro Publica*. October 18, 2010. Available at: http://www.propublica.org/article/dollars-to-doctors-physician-disciplinary-records. Accessed October 2, 2012.

134. Ornstein C, Weber T, Nguyen D. Docs on Pharma payroll have blemished records, limited credentials. *Pro Publica*. October 18, 2010. Available at: http://www.propublica.org/article/dollars-to-doctors-physician-disciplinary-records. Accessed October 2, 2012.

135. Sorrell WH. Supreme Court strikes down Vermont prescription privacy law [press release]. Office of the Attorney General, Vermont: June 23, 2011. Available at: http://www.atg.state.vt.us/news/supreme-court-strikes-down-vermont-prescription-privacy-law.php. Accessed October 2, 2012.

136. Mello MM, Messing NA. Restrictions on the use of prescribing data for drug promotion. *N Engl J Med*. 2011;365(13):1248–1254.

137. Fact Sheet: Physician payments sunshine provisions in health care reform. Pew Prescription Project. Available at: http://www.pewhealth.org/uploadedFiles/PHG/Supporting_Items/ IB_FS_PPP_Sunshine-fact-sheet.pdf. Updated March 23, 2010. Accessed October 2, 2012.

138. Schneider ME. Implementing health reform: The Physician Payments Sunshine Act. *Internal Medicine News.*December 15, 2011. Available at: http://www.internalmedicinenews.com/ index.php?id=514&tx_ttnews%5btt_news%5d=93972&cHash=489de78db9. Accessed October 2, 2012.

139. Corporate Accountability International: Global action challenging unhealthy corporate practices. *Corporations and Health Watch.* September 1, 2007. Available at:http:// corporationsandhealth.org/2007/09/01/corporate-accountability-international-global- action-challenging-unhealthy-corporate-practices/. Accessed October 2, 2012.

140. Kellett G. Big Tobacco: stop interfering in public health [press statement]. Corporate Accountability International: May 31, 2012. Available at: http://www.stopcorporatea- buse.org/press-statement/big-tobacco-stop-interfering-public-health. Accessed October 2, 2012.

141. *Alternative Annual Report: Philip Morris International Exposed.* Boston, MA: Corporate Accountability International; 2011:1.

142. Kattalia K. Philip Morris CEO tells cancer nurse: Quitting isn't hard for smokers. *NY Daily News.* May 14, 2011. Available at: http://articles.nydailynews.com/2011-05-14/enter- tainment/29558015_1_smokers-philip-morris-ceo-tobacco-products. Accessed October 2, 2012.

143. WHO, UN poised to allow corporations' input in global public health decisions [press release]. Corporate Accountability International: June 16, 2011. Available at: http://www. stopcorporateabuse.org/press-release/who-un-poised-allow-corporations-input-global- public-health-decisions. Accessed October 2, 2012.

144. *Corporate Accountability International 2009 Annual Report.* Boston, MA: Corporate Accountability International; 2009:9. Available at: http://www.stopcorporateabuse.org/ sites/default/files/resources/2009-annual-report.pdf. Accessed October 3, 2012.

145. Corporate Accountability International. Press Release: Report finds Big Tobacco continuing to obstruct health treaty. March 22, 2012. Available at: http://www. stopcorporateabuse.org/press-release/mayor-bloomberg-honors-corporate-accountability- international-fundaci%C3%B3n-fes-global. Accessed October 6, 2012.

Chapter 8 Wanted: A Movement for a Healthier, More Sustainable Future

1. Schor J. The New Politics of Consumption. *Boston Review,* 1999. Available at: http://bos- tonreview.net/BR24.3/schor.html

2. Market Wire. Online word-of-mouth turned controversial *trans* fat lawsuit against Kraft into major food industry PR crisis, August 16, 2004. Available at: http://findarticles.com/p/ articles/mi_pwwi/is_200408/ai_n8556894/.

3. Sen A. *Development as Freedom,* Oxford, UK: Oxford University Press; 1999.

4. Freudenberg N, McDonough J, Tsui E. Can a food justice movement improve nutrition and health? A case study of the emerging food movement in New York City. *J Urban Health.* 2011 Aug;88(4):623–636.

5. Wiist WH. *Citizens United,* public health, and democracy: the Supreme Court ruling, its implications, and proposed action. *Am J Public Health.* 2011;101(7):1172–1179.

6. Goodwin J, Jasper JM, eds. *The Social Movements Reader: Cases and Concepts, 2nd ed.* Hoboken NJ: Wiley-Blackwell; 2009.

7. Freudenberg N, McDonough J, Tsui E. Can a food justice movement improve nutrition and health? A case study of the emerging food movement in New York City. *J Urban Health.* 2011 Aug;88(4):623–636.

8. O'Riordan B. Australian smokers will be extinct by 2030, researchers say. *Guardian,* 29 July 2005. Available at: http://www.guardian.co.uk/world/2005/jul/30/australia.smoking

9. Chapman S. Global perspective on tobacco control. Part II. The future of tobacco control: making smoking history? *Int J Tuberc Lung Dis.* 2008 Jan;12(1):8–12.

10. New Mexico Department of Health. Data and confidence limits for alcohol-related chronic disease death rates by county, New Mexico 2007–2009, and United States, 2005–2007. Last updated December 2010. Available at: http://ibis.health.state.nm.us/indicator/view_numbers/AlcoholRelatedDthChronic.Cnty.html

11. OECD. Road motor vehicles and road fatalities. *OECD Handbook,* 2006. http://www.oecd.org/dataoecd/44/48/36340933.pdf

12. Welsh JA, Sharma A, Abramson JL, Vaccarino V, Gillespie C, Vos MB. Caloric sweetener consumption and dyslipidemia among US adults. *JAMA.* 2010;303(15):1490–1497.

13. Wackernagel M, Galli A. An overview on ecological footprint and sustainable development: a chat with Mathis Wackernagel. *International Journal of Ecodynamics,* 2007;2(1):1–9.

14. MacDonald JM, Stokes RJ, Cohen DA, Kofner A, Ridgeway GK. The effect of light rail transit on body mass index and physical activity. *Am J Prev Med.* 2010 Aug;39(2):105–112.

15. Friel S, Bowen K, Campbell-Lendrum D, Frumkin H, McMichael AJ, Rasanathan K. Climate change, non-communicable diseases, and development: the relationships and common policy opportunities. *Annu Rev Public Health.* 2011;32:133–147;

16. O'Rourke D. Citizen consumer. *Boston Review.* November/December 2011. Available at: http://www.bostonreview.net/BR36.6/ndf_dara_orourke_ethical_consumption.php

17. O'Rourke D. Citizen Consumer. *Boston Review.* November/December 2011. Available at: http://www.bostonreview.net/BR36.6/ndf_dara_orourke_ethical_consumption.php

18. Council on Economic Priorities. *Shopping for a Better World: The Quick and Easy Guide to All Your Socially Responsible Shopping.* San Francisco: Sierra Club Books; 1994.

19. Littler J. What's wrong with ethical consumption? *Ethical Consumption: A Critical Introduction,* ed. T. Lewis & E. Potter. London: Routledge; 2011:27–39.

20. Schor J. The new politics of consumption. *Boston Review,* 1999. Available at: http://bostonreview.net/BR24.3/schor.html.

21. Cohen MJ, Comrov A, Hoffner B. The new politics of consumption: promoting sustainability in the marketplace. *Sustainability: Science, Practice & Policy* 2005;1(1):58–76.

22. Oxfam. The food transformation. Harnessing consumer power to create a fair food future. 2012. Available at: http://www.oxfam.org/sites/www.oxfam.org/files/food-transformation-grow-report-july2012.pdf.

23. Pibel D. Communities in transition yes! February 1, 2008. Available at: http://www.yesmagazine.org/issues/climate-solutions/communities-in-transition. Accessed on October 20, 2012.

24. Social Investment Forum Foundation. 2010 Report on Socially Responsible Investing Trends in the United States. 2010. Available at: http://ussif.org/resources/research/documents/2010TrendsES.pdf.

25. Sullivan P. With impact investing, a focus on more than returns. *New York Times,* April 23, 20101. Available at: http://www.nytimes.com/2010/04/24/your-money/24wealth.html?pagewanted=all.

26. Happy returns: The birth of a virtuous new asset class. *The Economist,* Sept. 10, 2011. Available at: http://www.economist.com/node/21528678.

27. Pons E, Long M-A, Pomares R. Promoting sustainable food systems through impact investing. The Springcreek Foundation, 2011. Available at: http://www.thespringcreekfoundation.org/images/download/tsf_Promoting_Sustainable_Food_Systems.pdf.

28. Hernandez M, Syme SL, Brush R. *A Market for Health: Shifting the Paradigm for Investing in Health.* San Francisco, The California Endowment, 2012.

29. Wood D, Thornley B, Grace K. Impact at scale policy innovation for institutional investment with social and environmental benefit. Insight at Pacific Community ventures and the Initiative for Responsible Investment at Harvard University, 2012. Available at: http://www.pacificcommunityventures.org/uploads/reports-and-publications/Impact_at_Scale_ExecutiveSummary_FINAL.2.10.12.pdf.

30. Kim EH, Lyon T. When does institutional investor activism increase shareholder value? The carbon disclosure project, *Berkeley Electronic Journal of Economic Analysis & Policy.* 2011;11:(1). Available at: http://www.bepress.com/bejeap/vol11/iss1/art50.

31. Barber BM. Pension fund activism: the double-edged sword. In *The Future of Public Employee Retirement Systems,* Anderson G, Mitchell O, eds. New York: Oxford University Press; 2009:271–293.

32. Lifsher M. Teachers pension fund votes to sell holdings in firearms, ammo clips. *Los Angeles Times,* January 9, 2013. Available at http://www.latimes.com/business/money/la-fi-mo-pension-votes-firearms-divestment-20130109,0,4942689.story. Accessed on January 20, 2013.

33. Jarley P, Maranto CL., Union corporate campaigns: an assessment. *Indus. & Lab. Rel. Rev.* 1990;43(5):505–524.

34. Herder RA. Strategies of narrative disclosure in the rhetoric of anti-corporate campaigns (2012). *Communication Dissertations.* Paper 32. http://digitalarchive.gsu.edu/communication_diss/32.

35. Dorfman L, Cheyne A, Friedman LC, Wadud A, Gottlieb M. Soda and tobacco industry corporate social responsibility campaigns: how do they compare? *PLoS Med* 2012;9(6):e1001241. doi:10.1371/journal.pmed.1001241.

36. Ford CEO: global warming is real. *Detroit News,* April 24, 2007. Available at: http://www.hybridcars.com/news2/ford-mulally-global-warming-042407.html.

37. Strom S. Has "organic" been oversized? *New York Times,* July 8, 2012:BU1.

38. Liu P. Sustainable consumerism begins with China. *Solutions Journal* 2012;3(3). Available at: http://www.thesolutionsjournal.com/node/1122.

39. Qingfen D, Ying D. Domestic consumption takes the driver's seat. *China Daily,* March 22, 2012:2.

40. Black R. China "won't follow US" on carbon emissions. October 25, 2011. Available at: http://www.bbc.co.uk/news/science-environment-15444858

41. Liu P. Sustainable consumerism begins with China. *Solutions Journal* 2012;3(3). Available at: http://www.thesolutionsjournal.com/node/1122.

42. Monteiro CA, Cannon G. The impact of transnational "big food" companies on the south: a view from Brazil. *PLoS Med* 2012;9(7):e1001252.

43. Bajaj V. India weighs providing free drugs at state-run hospitals. *New York Times,* July 5, 2012. Available at: http://www.nytimes.com/2012/07/06/business/india-may-provide-free-drugs-at-state-run-hospitals.html?_r=2&pagewanted=1&partner=rssnyt&emc=rss.

44. Muro M, Rothwell J, Saha D, Battelle Technology Partnership Practice. Sizing the clean economy: a national and regional green jobs assessment. Washington, DC: Brookings Institution, 2011. Available at: http://www.surdna.org/what-we-fund/sustainable-environments/sustainable-environments-whats-new/365-sizing-the-clean-economy-a-national-and-regional-green-jobs-assessment-a-new-study-from-the-brookings-institution-.html. Accessed on October 20,2012.

45. Schor J. The new politics of consumption. *Boston Review,* 1999. Available at: http://bostonreview.net/BR24.3/schor.html.

46. Story L. Anywhere the eye can see, it's likely to see an ad. *New York Times,* January 15, 2007. Available at: http://www.nytimes.com/2007/01/15/business/media/15everywhere.html?pagewanted=all.

47. Pomeranz JL. Television food marketing to children revisited: the Federal Trade Commission has the constitutional and statutory authority to regulate. *J Law Med Ethics.* 2010 Spring;38(1):98–116.

48. Graff S, Kunkel D, Mermin SE. Government can regulate food advertising to children because cognitive research shows that it is inherently misleading. *Health Aff (Millwood).* 2012 Feb;31(2):392–398.

49. Schor JB. *Born to Buy: The Commercialized Child and the New Consumer Culture.* New York: Scribner; 2004:11.

50. Schor JB. *Born to Buy: The Commercialized Child and the New Consumer Culture.* New York: Scribner; 2004:11.

51. Cairns G, Angus K, Hastings G, Caraher M. Systematic reviews of the evidence on the nature, extent and effects of food marketing to children. A retrospective summary. *Appetite.* May 2, 2012.

52. Grier SA, Kumanyika S. Targeted marketing and public health. *Annu Rev Public Health.* 2010;31:349–369.

53. Pechmann C, Shih C-F. Smoking scenes in movies and antismoking advertisements before movies: effects on youth. *J Marketing.* 1999;63(3). http://www.marketingpower.com/ResourceLibrary/JournalofMarketing/Pages/1999/63/3/2026300.aspx (accessed July 21, 2011).

54. Flay BR. Mass media and smoking cessation: a critical review. *Am J Public Health* 1987;7(2): 153–160.

55. Farrelly MC, Nonnemaker J, Davis KC, Hussin A. The influence of the national Truth Campaign on smoking initiation. *Am J Prev Med.* 2009 May;36(5):379–384.

56. Gagnon M, Freudenberg N, and Corporate Accountability International. *Slowing Down Fast Food: A Policy Guide for Healthier Kids and Families.* Boston, MA: Corporate Accountability International, 2012. Available at: www.StopCorporateAbuse.org

57. Haas A, Sherman J. Eliminating alcohol advertising on Philadelphia's public property: a case study. Baltimore, MD: Center on Alcohol Marketing and Youth; 2005. Available at: http://www.camy.org/action/case_studies/Case_Philadelphia.pdf. Accessed on January 20, 2013.

58. Rocheleau M. MBTA to bar alcohol ads on all property, including trains, buses. www.Boston.com, January 24, 2012. Available at: http://articles.boston.com/2012-01-24/yourtown/30660001_1_alcohol-ads-transit-agency-ad-revenue#.Tx_7I30u99U.email. Accessed on October 6, 2012.

59. Lee J. Nourishing change. Partnership enlists dozens of hospitals to put healthier food on their menus and kick junk food out of the cafeteria. *Mod Healthc.* 2012;42(41):6–7; 1.

60. Wiist WH. *Citizens United,* public health, and democracy: the Supreme Court ruling, its implications, and proposed action. *Am J Public Health.* 2011;101(7):1172–1179.

61. Poinski M. Public financing of election campaigns makes another try. Marylandreporter.com, February 16, 2011. http://marylandreporter.com/2011/02/16/public-financing-of-election-campaigns-makes-another-try/#ixzz20ydtjrhU

62. Cicilline D. Stopping the lobbyist revolving door. RIFutures.org. March 6, 2012. Available at: http://www.rifuture.org/stopping-the-revolving-door.html

63. H.R. 4030: Stop the Revolving Door in Washington Act. Govtrack.us. 2012. Available at: http://www.govtrack.us/congress/bills/112/hr4030

64. US Environmental Protection Agency. Emergency Planning and Community Right-to-Know Act Overview. Last updated January 2011. Available at: http://www.epa.gov/oem/content/lawsregs/epcraover.htm

65. Harmon A, Pollack A. Battle brewing over labeling of genetically modified food. *New York Times,* May 25, 2012, p. A1.

66. Sutton CD. The Coalition Against Uptown Cigarettes: Marketing practices and community mobilization (unpublished report). Philadelphia: Coalition Against Uptown Cigarettes; 1993:11.

67. Community Environmental Legal Defense Fund, Linzey T. A citizen's guide to corporate charter revocation under state law. Community Environmental Legal Defense Fund, no date. Available at: http://webcache.googleusercontent.com/search?q=cache:P2GZyP0T1CUJ:www.sierraclub.org/committees/cac/corporatepower/Manual%2520for%2520Revoking%2520Corporate%2520Charters.rtf+%22a+citizen%27s+guide+to+charter+revocation%22&cd=1&hl=en&ct=clnk&gl=us&client=firefox-a.

68. FAQs on corporate death penalty legislation. Reclaimdemocracy.org, 2011. Available at: http://reclaimdemocracy.org/corporate_accountability/death_penalty.php.

69. Letter from Ralph Nader, John Richard, and Charlie Cray to Attorney General Eric Holder, February 20, 2009. Available at: http://www.corporatepolicy.org/issues/lettertoAGHolder. htm.

70. Parmet WE, Daynard RA. The new public health litigation. *Annu Rev Public Health*. 2000;21: 437–454.

71. Rutkow L, Teret SP. Role of state attorneys general in health policy. *JAMA*. 2010;304(12): 1377–1378.

72. Parmet WE, Daynard RA. The new public health litigation. *Annu Rev Public Health*. 2000;21: 437–454.

73. U.S. General Accounting Office. Environmental Protection: Assessing the Impacts of EPA's Regulations Through Retrospective Studies, GAO/RCED-99-250, September 1999.

74. Cooper PJ. *The War Against Regulation from Jimmy Carter to George W. Bush*. Lawrence, KS: University Press of Kansas; 2009.

75. Letter from National Consumers League and seven other organizations to Harold Rogers, Chairman, Committee on Appropriations, United States House of Representatives, May 27, 2011. Available at: http://npalliance.org/wp-content/uploads/ChairmanRogersFDAbudget May25.pdf.

76. Chan S. Financial crisis was avoidable, inquiry finds. *New York Times*, January 26, 2011:A1.

77. Cooper MN. "Too big to fail?": the role of antitrust law in government-funded consolidation in the banking industry. Hearing Before the Subcommittee on Courts and Competition Policy of the Committee on the Judiciary House of Representatives. 111th Congress, First Session. March 17, 2009. Available at: http://judiciary.house.gov/hearings/ printers/111th/111-33_48102.PDF. Accessed on January 20, 2013.

78. Breuer L. Prison for executives, deferrals for corporations. *Corporate Crime Reporter 2012*, October 23, 2012. Available at: http://www.corporatecrimereporter.com/news/200/ breuerprisondpas10232012/. Accessed on January 20, 2013.

79. Uhlmann on BP, manslaughter, and the case against deferred prosecution. *Corporate Crime Reporter.* 2011;25(8). Available at: http://www.corporatecrimereporter.com/uhlmann021611.htm. Accessed on January 20,2013.

80. Black F. A moral economy. *Nation*. March 20, 2006:16–19.

81. Tobacco Control Legal Consortium. *The Verdict Is In: Findings From* United States v. Philip Morris, *Suppression of Information* (2006).

82. Hastings G. *The Marketing Matrix. How the corporation gets its power—and how we can reclaim it*. London: Routledge; 2013:58.

83. Gangarosa RE, Vandall FJ, Willis BM. Suits by public hospitals to recover expenditures for the treatment of disease, injury and disability caused by tobacco and alcohol. *Fordham Urb Law J.* 1994;22(1):81–139.

84. Sugarman SD. Performance-based regulation: enterprise responsibility for reducing death, injury, and disease caused by consumer products. *J Health Polit Policy Law.* 2009;34(6):1035–1077.

85. Caraher M, Cowburn G. Taxing food: implications for public health nutrition. *Public Health Nutr.* 2005 Dec;8(8):1242–1249.

86. Skov SJ; Royal Australasian College of Physicians Alcohol Advisory Group. Alcohol taxation policy in Australia: public health imperatives for action. *Med J Aust.* 2009 Apr 20;190(8):437–439.

87. Lewin A, Lindstrom L, Nestle M. Food industry promises to address childhood obesity: preliminary evaluation. *J Public Health Policy.* 2006;27(4):327–348.

88. Brownell KD. Thinking forward: the quicksand of appeasing the food industry. *PLoS Med.* 2012 Jul;9(7):e1001254.

89. Vendrame A, Pinsky I. [Inefficacy of self-regulation of alcohol advertisements: a systematic review of the literature]. *Rev Bras Psiquiatr.* 2011 Jun;33(2):196–202.

90. Grande D. Limiting the influence of pharmaceutical industry gifts on physicians: self-regulation or government intervention? *J Gen Intern Med.* 2010 Jan;25(1):79–83.

91. Chinn D. Critical health literacy: a review and critical analysis. *Soc Sci Med.* 2011 Jul;73(1):60–67.

92. Goldberg JP, Sliwa SA. Communicating actionable nutrition messages: challenges and opportunities. *Proc Nutr Soc.* 2011 Feb;70(1):26–37.

93. Hasler CM. Health claims in the United States: an aid to the public or a source of confusion? *J Nutr.* 2008 Jun;138(6):1216S–1220S.

94. Kuo M. NRA stymies firearms research, scientists say. *New York Times,* January 25, 2011:A1.

95. Washburn J. *University, Inc.: The Corporate Corruption of Higher Education.* New York: Basic Books, 2006.

96. Angell M. Industry-sponsored clinical research: a broken system. *JAMA.* 2008;300(9): 1069–1071.

97. Srinivasan UT, Carey SP, Hallstein E, Higgins PA, Kerr AC, Koteen LE, et al. The debt of nations and the distribution of ecological impacts from human activities. *Proc Natl Acad Sci USA.* 2008 Feb 5;105(5):1768–1773.

Afterword

1. Picchi A. GM discloses CEO pay details after gender-bias question. *CBS MoneyWatch,* February 11, 2014.

2. Spector M, Matthews CM. U.S. Charges GM with Wire Fraud, Concealing Facts on Ignition Switch. *Wall Street Journal,* September 17, 2015.

3. Office of Inspector General. Inadequate Data and Analysis Undermine NHTSA's Efforts to Identify and Investigate Vehicle Safety Concerns. Washington, D.C. National Highway Traffic Safety Administration. Report Number: ST-2015–063, June 18, 2015.

4. Boston W. Volkswagen Emissions Investigations Should Widen to Entire Auto Industry, Officials Say. *Wall Street Journal,* September 22, 2015.

5. Hakim D. U.S. Chamber travels the world, fighting curbs on smoking. *New York Times,* July 1, 2015, pp. A1 and B8.

6. AlKhater SA. Paediatric non-alcoholic fatty liver disease: an overview. Obes. Rev. 2015;16(5):393–405.

7. World Health Organization. Tuberculosis WHO Global Tuberculosis Report 2014. Geneva, WHO. Available at: http://www.who.int/tb/publications/factsheet_global.pdf

8. Boseley S. Drug-resistant tuberculosis poses global threat, warn doctors. *The Guardian,* 22 October 2014.

9. Frick M. Tuberculosis Research and Development: 2014 Report on Tuberculosis Research Funding Trends, 2005–2013. New York: Treatment Action Group, 2015.

10. Sum of Us. Bad Medicine: How the pharmaceutical industry is contributing to the global rise of antibiotic-resistant superbugs. New York, 2015.

11. Roland D. Multibillion-Dollar Investment Needed to Fight Drug-Resistant "Superbugs." *Wall Street Journal,* May 13, 2015.

12. Beaglehole R, Bonita R, Ezzati M, Alleyne G, Dain K, Kishore SP, Horton R. NCD Countdown 2025: accountability for the 25 × 25 NCD mortality reduction target. *The Lancet* 2014; 384 (9938): 105–107.

13. Rehm J, Mathers C, Popova S, Thavorncharoensap M, Teerawattananon Y, Patra J. Global burden of disease and injury and economic cost attributable to alcohol use and alcohol-use disorders. *Lancet.* 2009 ;373(9682):2223–33.

14. Mathers CD, Loncar D. Projections of global mortality and burden of disease from 2002 to 2030. *PLoS Med* 2006; 3(11): e442.

15. Balakrishnan A. Soft drink sales hit a decade of decline. CNBC. 26 Mar 2015 http://www.cnbc.com/2015/03/26/soft-drink-sales-hit-a-decade-of-decline.html

16. Follman M, Lurie J, Lee J, West J. The true cost of gun violence in America. *Mother Jones* May/June 2015. Available at: http://www.motherjones.com/politics/2015/04/true-cost-of-gun-violence-in-america

17. Klein N. *The Shock Doctrine The Rise of Disaster Capitalism*. New York: Metropolitan Books, 2008.

18. Woolf SH, Aron L, eds., *U.S. Health in International Perspective Shorter Lives, Poorer Health*. Washington, D.C.: National Research Council and Institute of Medicine of The National Academies, 2013.

19. Hide No Harm Act. Introduced in 113th Congress, Available at: http://www.foreffectivegov.org/files/regs/hide-no-harm-act-2014.pdf

20. Ruane, KA. Fairness Doctrine: History and Constitutional Issues. Journal of Current Issues in Media & Telecommunications, 2012; 4(3).

21. Opinion of Stevens, J. Supreme Court of the United States Citizens United, Appellant v. Federal Election Commission (No. 08–205), 2010.

22. Banks CP. Reversals of precedent and judicial policy-making: how judicial conceptions of stare decisis in the U.S. Supreme Court influence social change. Akron L. Rev. 32(1999):233.

23. Hoover K. Public opinion of big business improves, but small business still rules. *The Business Journals*, Aug 5, 2014. Available at: http://www.bizjournals.com/bizjournals/washington-bureau/2014/08/public-opinion-of-big-business-improves-but-small.html

24. Scheiber N, Sussman D. Inequality Troubles Americans Across Party Lines, Times/CBS Poll Finds. *New York Times*, June 4, 2015, p. A1.

25. Penders B, Nelis AP. Credibility engineering in the food industry: Linking science, regulation, and marketing in a corporate context. *Science in context*, 2011;24(04),487–515.

26. Thorup M. *Pro Bono?* London: Zero Books, 2015.

27. National Council of Farmer Cooperatives. About Coops, 2015. Available at: http://www.ncfc.org/about-ncfc/about-co-ops

Index